DRUG DISCOVERY APPROACHES FOR THE TREATMENT OF NEURODEGENERATIVE DISORDERS

DRUG DISCOVERY APPROACHES FOR THE TREATMENT OF NEURODEGENERATIVE DISORDERS

ALZHEIMER'S DISEASE

Edited by

ADEBOYE ADEJARE
Philadelphia College of Pharmacy, University of the Sciences, Philadelphia, PA, United States

ELSEVIER

AMSTERDAM • BOSTON • HEIDELBERG • LONDON
NEW YORK • OXFORD • PARIS • SAN DIEGO
SAN FRANCISCO • SINGAPORE • SYDNEY • TOKYO
Academic Press is an imprint of Elsevier

Academic Press is an imprint of Elsevier
125 London Wall, London EC2Y 5AS, United Kingdom
525 B Street, Suite 1800, San Diego, CA 92101-4495, United States
50 Hampshire Street, 5th Floor, Cambridge, MA 02139, United States
The Boulevard, Langford Lane, Kidlington, Oxford OX5 1GB, United Kingdom

Library of Congress Cataloging-in-Publication Data
A catalog record for this book is available from the Library of Congress

British Library Cataloguing-in-Publication Data
A catalogue record for this book is available from the British Library

ISBN: 978-0-12-802810-0

For information on all Academic Press publications
visit our website at https://www.elsevier.com/

Publisher: Mica Haley
Acquisition Editor: Kristine Jones
Editorial Project Manager: Molly McLaughlin
Production Project Manager: Chris Wortley
Designer: Mark Rogers

Typeset by TNQ Books and Journals

Dedication

I would like to dedicate this book to my teachers and students. I am extremely fortunate to have had a great set of mentors in research from undergraduate (Dr. Harold M. Goff, The University of Iowa) to MS (Dr. David F. Weimer, The University of Iowa) to Ph.D. (Dr. Duane D. Miller, The Ohio State University) and finally postdoctoral studies (Dr. Kenneth L. Kirk, National Institutes of Health). I have also been blessed by a great set of students and postdoctoral associates. Many of them are authors of several of the chapters in the book.

Finally, I would like to dedicate the book to my greatest teacher, I. Abiola Adejare, none other than my father. Though you have moved on to "ibi agba re" (where elders go), the seeds that you sowed continue to bear great fruits.

Contents

4. Current Medications for the Treatment of Alzheimer's Disease: Acetylcholinesterase Inhibitors and NMDA Receptor Antagonist

L.A. FINN

5. Physicochemical Properties for Potential Alzheimer's Disease Drugs

Z. ATES-ALAGOZ AND A. ADEJARE

6. Receptor Targets in Alzheimer's Disease Drug Discovery

J. WALLACH, T. COLESTOCK AND A. ADEJARE

7. Amyloid β Hypothesis in the Development of Therapeutic Agents for Alzheimer's Disease

A.O. ADENIJI, P.W. ADAMS AND V.V. MODY

8. Tau Proteins

S. MONDRAGÓN-RODRÍGUEZ, G. PERRY AND F. PEÑA-ORTEGA

9. Cholesterol and Fat Metabolism in Alzheimer's Disease

C. TAGHIBIGLOU AND S. KHALAJ

List of Contributors

P.W. Adams South University School of Pharmacy, Savannah, GA, United States

A. Adejare University of the Sciences in Philadelphia, Philadelphia, PA, United States

A.O. Adeniji South University School of Pharmacy, Savannah, GA, United States

M. Alamri University of the Sciences in Philadelphia, Philadelphia, PA, United States

Z. Ates-Alagoz University of the Sciences in Philadelphia, Philadelphia, PA, United States; Ankara University, Tandogan, Ankara, Turkey

J.E. Barrett Drexel University College of Medicine, Philadelphia, PA, United States

S.W. Caito Albert Einstein College of Medicine, Bronx, NY, United States

J.B. Camacho Universidad del Valle de México, Querétaro, México

E. Carlson University of Kansas, Lawrence, KS, United States

T. Colestock University of the Sciences in Philadelphia, Philadelphia, PA, United States

E. Corum Georgetown Living Home Health, Georgetown, TX, United States

L.A. Finn University of the Sciences, Philadelphia, PA, United States

M. Glenn Widener University, Chester, PA, United States

D.D. Hu Memorial Hermann Memorial City Medical Center, Houston, TX, United States

C. Hu Georgetown Living Certified Alzheimer's Community, Georgetown, TX, United States

S. Khalaj University of Saskatchewan, Saskatoon, SK, Canada

L. Mace University of the Sciences, Philadelphia, PA, United States

P. McGonigle Drexel University College of Medicine, Philadelphia, PA, United States

V.V. Mody Philadelphia College of Osteopathic Medicine, Suwanee, GA, United States

S.T. Moelter University of the Sciences, Philadelphia, PA, United States

S. Mondragón-Rodríguez CONACyT National Council for Science and Technology, México, México; National Autonomous University of México, Querétaro, México

J.L. Newell-Caito University of the Sciences in Philadelphia, Philadelphia, PA, United States

F. Peña-Ortega National Autonomous University of México, Querétaro, México

G. Perry University of Texas at San Antonio, San Antonio, TX, United States

M. Sheerin University of the Sciences, Philadelphia, PA, United States

C. Taghibiglou University of Saskatchewan, Saskatoon, SK, Canada

K.R. Valasani University of Kansas, Lawrence, KS, United States

J.R. Vangavaragu University of Kansas, Lawrence, KS, United States

J. Wallach University of the Sciences in Philadelphia, Philadelphia, PA, United States

T.A. Yacoubian University of Alabama at Birmingham, Birmingham, AL, United States

S.S.D. Yan University of Kansas, Lawrence, KS, United States

Foreword

Despite vastly increased understanding of the pathogenic cascades that underlie numerous neurodegenerative disorders, the last two decades have seen few inroads in terms of development of successful therapies. For the most, those therapies that have been approved are symptomatic in nature and do not significantly alter disease course. It is important that we learn from both our failures and our successes so that we may more efficiently develop therapies that meet our medical needs. Indeed, given the economic, societal, and personal toll of common and less common neurodegenerative diseases, we cannot collectively afford to fail. This book provides an overview, using Alzheimer's disease for illustration and a review of successes and failures to date, to help point out the paradigms necessary for successful therapeutic discovery and their translation into therapies that benefit patients. Diagnostic paradigms, epidemiology studies, current therapeutics targets (eg, amyloid, tau, APOE, energy metabolism, various receptors, cholesterol, and fat metabolism), and strategies for drug discovery are described. The value and also limits of preclinical models are also elaborated. The book also provides insights into the physicochemical properties that are necessary for such drugs, the role of in vivo models in evaluating potential efficacy, and a compendium of current agents in clinical trials. In addition, nonpharmacological treatment approaches and the national plan and resources available for anyone embarking on research in this area are discussed.

The editor, Adeboye Adejare, is an outstanding medicinal chemist and a professor at the Philadelphia College of Pharmacy, University of the Sciences, in Philadelphia. He has over 40 publications and four issued patents. He has served on many grant review committees that focus on CNS drug discovery including the National Institutes of Health, National Science Foundation, and Alzheimer's Association panels. He has also served as a consultant to the Food and Drug Administration, the Educational Testing Service (College Board, Princeton, New Jersey), as well as to many companies. He is editor of the Pharmaceutical Chemistry section of the 22nd edition of *Remington: The Science and Practice of Pharmacy*. The authors are experts in their various areas and several have industrial and/or clinical experiences.

The book is designed for college graduates involved in the drug discovery process, whether in academia, research institutes, or the pharmaceutical industry, and for chemists who are involved in drug design and those involved in clinical trials. Also laboratories and start-up companies that do not have access to extensive resources may find the book useful.

Todd E. Golde, M.D., Ph.D.
Director, Center for Translational Research in Neurodegenerative Diseases
Professor, Department of Neuroscience, College of Medicine, University of Florida

Preface

The incidence of neurodegenerative disorders (NDs) keeps increasing. This increase is in part due to the fact that we are living longer, thanks to advances in the treatments of microbial infections, cardiovascular disorders, cancer, and other diseases. A good illustration of the dilemma presented by NDs is with Alzheimer's disease (AD). Prevalence has a high correlation with age. The Alzheimer Association estimates that there are about 5.4 million people living with AD and that given the current trajectory in longevity, as many as 13.8 million people may be battling the disease by 2050 (www.alz.org). The last US Food and Drug Administration-approved new chemical entity for AD was in 2003. So, while the need is increasing, treatment options have been very limited and stagnant for over a decade. Many clinical trials have failed to yield promising results. The costs to society using social or financial measures are staggering and increasing. A similar scenario holds for other NDs such as Parkinson's disease, amyotrophic lateral sclerosis, and Huntington's disease though the numbers of people affected and therefore societal burden are lower. This situation calls for a fresh look at drug discovery for NDs, hence this book.

From reading literature and serving on many NDs drug discovery grant review panels, it became clear to me that while many of those efforts may be good science and certainly worthwhile, they may not necessarily lead to the main goals of the investigators, which in many instances are drugs for AD. This observation is further supported by the many clinical trials that failed to reach desired end points. A goal of this book is to provide a comprehensive look at drug discovery in this space. The approach to drug discovery for NDs is necessarily very different from those for microbial infections, cardiovascular disorders, cancer, and others. We have to deal with blood–brain barrier permeability issues in addition to complexity of the neuron and the chronic nature of the disease. The book provides information that investigators may find very useful, from where to go for research funding to which drugs are in clinical trials, what are their mechanisms of action, and by which company.

The editor is extremely grateful to the outstanding scientists who opted to write chapters in their various areas of expertise despite their very busy schedules. Broadly, the book can be divided into five parts. Part I has four chapters and deals with an introduction to NDs, AD diagnosis, national plan and resources to address AD, and current medications. Chapter 3 on national plan and resources to address AD is fairly unique to this book. Part II consists of Chapter 5, which deals with physicochemical properties desired for an AD medication especially if it is to be administered orally, which is the preferred route in most cases. These guidelines are for potential small molecule therapies, regardless of mechanisms of action. Part III deals with drug targets, from various pharmacological receptors to the amyloid hypothesis, tau proteins, cholesterol and fat metabolism as well as energy metabolism. These were covered in Chapters 6 to 10. Part IV deals with in vivo models that can be utilized in drug discovery, from simple ones such as *Caenorhabditis elegans* (Chapter 11) to rodents (Chapter 12), as well as advantages and limitations presented by each model. The last part deals with relevant topics that are not necessarily covered in many drug discovery books but which are very relevant in these efforts. Chapter 13 deals with drugs at different phases of clinical trials including mechanisms of action and sponsoring companies. The final chapter deals with nonpharmacological treatment approaches, which range from cognitive training to diet and environmental modification. These approaches can attenuate AD and therefore be part of a comprehensive plan where they exert synergistic effects with drugs.

The book is designed for scientists involved in drug discovery, from chemists to pharmacologists and clinicians; be they in academia, research institutes, or the pharmaceutical industry. Others such as physicians, patients, and their families may find it useful, for example, in deciding in which clinical trials to participate. The book has been written in such a manner that anyone with a college education especially in the sciences can read and understand the many topics. It can also be used as a textbook for upper-level undergraduate and graduate courses on drug discovery in the area of neuroscience addressed.

Adeboye Adejare, Ph.D.
Professor, Philadelphia College of Pharmacy
University of the Sciences
Philadelphia, PA, USA
July 2016

Acknowledgments

The good news is that we are living longer! This development is in part because of progress in addressing several health care challenges such as microbial infections, cardiovascular disorders, and even cancer. The not-so-good news is that diseases associated with aging such as neurodegenerative disorders are increasing. Examples of these neurodegenerative disorders are Alzheimer's and Parkinson's diseases. Given the limited availability of medications, the unmet needs, and the very high failure rate in clinical trials, it appeared to me that a comprehensive look at addressing drug discovery for neurodegenerative disorders in the form of a book was clearly needed. The paradigm for drug discovery for neurodegeneration is certainly very different from those for antiinfectives, cancer, and many other diseases. Around 2012, I began discussions with Elsevier, Inc. about such a book. In the meantime, I was fortunate to be able to attend two relevant National Institutes of Health meetings, namely, Alzheimer's Disease Research Summit 2012: Path to Treatment and Prevention (May 14–15, 2012) and Alzheimer's Disease-Related Dementias: Research Challenges and Opportunities (ADRD) (May 1–2, 2013). This period was when the idea of this book began to take hold. I then set out to teach a graduate-level special topics course on "Drug Discovery for Neurodegenerative Disorders" in 2013. By the end of the course, the outline for the book began to emerge.

I would like to thank all authors in the book. I set out to identify the broad areas for drug discovery for neurodegenerative disorders using Alzheimer's disease as an illustration since it is the most prevalent and has major increasing need. I contacted several experts in the various areas and in different countries since the matter is global in nature. I am thankful and grateful that they responded in a positive manner, resulting in an outstanding piece of work.

I am also thankful to the reviewers for providing excellent feedback to the authors. The reviewers include Laura Finn, Michael Dybek, Mohammed Alamri, Drs. Adegoke Adeniji, Hadiyah-Nicole Green, Joy L. Britten-Webb, Jason Wallach, and Zeynep Ates-Alagoz. The gentle persistence of Kristine Jones, Senior Acquisitions Manager, and help of Molly McLaughlin, Editorial Project Manager, both of Elsevier, Inc., are also gratefully acknowledged. I am also grateful to Dr. Todd E. Golde for the Foreword.

I would also like to acknowledge the support for my career in academia and for this book granted by my family, starting from my lovely wife Adekemi to our children Adeboye Jr. (AJ), Adekunle, Aderonke, and Adeola. I would also like to thank many people who have been helpful in one way or another, with special thanks going to my mother, Ayoola Adejare.

CHAPTER

1

Neurodegenerative Disorders: Why Do We Need New Therapies?

T.A. Yacoubian

OUTLINE

INTRODUCTION

Neurodegeneration covers a wide spectrum of neurological disorders. These disorders can manifest with many different symptoms, including cognitive impairment, speech difficulties, and motor dysfunction. The underlying pathological hallmark shared by neurodegenerative disorders is the loss of neuronal populations in the brain and/or spinal cord. The particular areas of the brain and spinal cord in which neuronal loss occurs dictate the clinical features of a given neurodegenerative disorder. Neurodegenerative disorders include common and uncommon diseases including Alzheimer's disease (AD), Parkinson's disease (PD), amyotrophic lateral sclerosis (ALS), Huntington's disease (HD), dementia with Lewy bodies (DLB), progressive supranuclear palsy (PSP), multiple system atrophy (MSA), corticobasal

Drug Discovery Approaches for the Treatment of Neurodegenerative Disorders
http://dx.doi.org/10.1016/B978-0-12-802810-0.00001-5

degeneration (CBD), frontotemporal dementia (FTD), spinocerebellar ataxia (SCA) disorders, and spinal muscular atrophy, among others. This chapter is not meant to be an all-inclusive review of this large and diverse group of disorders but to serve as an introduction to neurodegeneration in general. In this chapter, we will focus on AD, along with PD, HD, and ALS, as examples of the more common neurodegenerative disorders to discuss some of the similarities and differences among this broad class of neurological disorders.

As a whole, neurodegenerative disorders are common. AD is the most common neurodegenerative disorder. AD is the sixth-leading cause of death in the United States (Murphy et al., 2013). Approximately 5 million Americans over the age of 65 had AD in 2010, which translates to about 11% of Americans over age 65 as having AD (Alzheimer's Association, 2014; Hebert et al., 2013). With the expected aging of the US population, it is estimated that 13.8 million older Americans will have AD in 2050 (Hebert et al., 2013). The second most common neurodegenerative disorder is PD, with an estimated prevalence of PD in the United States of about 630,000 cases in 2010 (Kowal et al., 2013). As with AD, the prevalence of PD is age related, with a dramatic increase in prevalence after age 65. While the prevalence is estimated at 0.3% in the general US population, the prevalence rate is 1–2% over age 65 and 4–5% over age 85 (Dorsey et al., 2007; Hirtz et al., 2007; Kowal et al., 2013; Noyes et al., 2006; Weintraub et al., 2008). As with AD, the prevalence of PD is dramatically increasing, with an expected doubling of PD prevalence by the year 2040 (Dorsey et al., 2007; Kowal et al., 2013).

With the anticipated rise in AD and PD cases in the next several decades, the expected societal burden and financial costs of these two disorders are sky-rocketing. In the case of AD and related dementias, the estimated total health care costs were $214 billion in 2014, with about 70% paid by Medicare and Medicaid (Alzheimer's Association, 2014). Additionally, it is estimated that 17.7 billion hours of unpaid care was provided by caregivers for patients with AD and other dementias in 2013, valued at about $220.2 billion (Alzheimer's Association, 2014). Given the expected increase in AD prevalence, the predicted health care costs for AD will reach $1.2 trillion in 2050 (Alzheimer's Association, 2014). The anticipated costs for PD are less, because of the lower prevalence, but are still considerable. Estimated medical costs secondary to PD were about $8 billion in the United States in 2010, and costs caused by reduced employment and other indirect costs were estimated at $6.3 billion in 2010 (Kowal et al., 2013). By 2050, the projected medical costs secondary to PD will reach $18.5 billion (Kowal et al., 2013). While other neurodegenerative disorders are less common, they still cause considerable disability and loss of life.

CLINICAL FEATURES OF COMMON NEURODEGENERATIVE DISORDERS

While all neurodegenerative diseases are marked by neuronal loss and atrophy, these disorders vary greatly in the clinical manifestations of the disorder. Some disorders, such as AD or FTD, are marked by significant cognitive decline, while other disorders, such as PD and ALS, are initially marked by motor impairment. Some disorders, such as HD, can have motor, psychiatric, and cognitive impairment as predominant features early on. The common neurodegenerative disorders can usually be distinguished by a thorough neurological evaluation, yet the rarer disorders, such as PSP and MSA, can often be difficult to distinguish from their more common relatives early on in the disease course. While each neurodegenerative disorder has its distinguishing features, these diseases can look somewhat similar at the end stage with patients becoming bed bound, mute, incontinent, and unable to care for self.

Alzheimer's disease, the most common neurodegenerative disorder, is marked by memory impairment. Patients initially present with memory dysfunction. Episodic memory is typically affected, with more recent events being more difficult to remember and a tendency of more distant memories preserved initially. Patients also have early impairment in semantic memory, memory involving knowledge of facts about the world, but procedural memory is not affected. Other cognitive dimensions involved in AD include language, visuospatial function, praxis, and executive function. AD patients have language difficulties that manifest early in the disease as reduced verbal fluency and naming. Anosognosia, or lack of awareness of cognitive decline, is common in AD. Patients often have neuropsychiatric disturbances, including depression, delusions, hallucinations, behavioral disturbances such as agitation, and personality changes. However, these features can be seen in other neurodegenerative dementias, such as FTD and DLB, and the constellation of other neurological features is used for distinguishing these disorders.

PD has been classically defined as a motor disorder. The cardinal motor features of PD include resting tremor, bradykinesia, rigidity, and gait imbalance. However, the nonmotor features of PD have been increasingly recognized in the last decade. Nonmotor features of PD include cognitive impairment, psychiatric symptoms, autonomic dysfunction, and sleep disturbances. Autonomic dysfunction includes constipation, gastrointestinal motility issues, urinary symptoms, orthostatic hypotension, and sexual dysfunction. Common psychiatric features include depression and anxiety. In later stages of PD, patients develop cognitive decline and potentially full-blown dementia. In contrast to AD, memory impairment is not typically seen in PD, but cognitive impairment in PD is marked by deficits in attention and executive function, hallucinations, and psychosis. Sleep disturbances include sleep apnea, daytime sleepiness, and rapid eye movement sleep behavior disorder (RBD). Certain nonmotor features, such as RBD, loss of sense of smell, and constipation, are likely the initial features of PD that may predate the motor features by 10 or more years.

ALS presents with weakness and atrophy in a focal group of muscles and then spreads to contiguous muscles before spreading to other parts of the body. Typically, the weakness first develops in one limb, although in some patients the weakness can begin in bulbar muscles, affecting speech and swallowing. Patients also note fasciculations or muscle twitches. Traditionally, cognitive and behavioral impairments have not been viewed as a feature of ALS, yet patients can have deficits in executive function, anomia, impaired verbal fluency, apathy, and personality changes (Phukan et al., 2007; Ringholz et al., 2005; Witgert et al., 2010). If not the presenting feature of their disease, patients eventually develop severe dysarthria and dysphagia, which impedes their caloric intake and thus worsens their weakness. Patients with ALS decline relatively rapidly and eventually develop respiratory failure.

HD presents clinically with a triad of psychiatric illness, cognitive impairment, and motor dysfunction. When HD manifests during adulthood, patients can present with either motor symptoms or behavioral symptoms initially. Psychiatric symptoms include depression, anxiety, and less likely mania and psychosis. Rates of suicide are very high in patients with HD. Behavioral disturbances are common. HD patients may have aggressive behaviors toward others. Patients also develop cognitive impairment, with decline in attention, motivation, insight, problem solving, and executive function. They often lack insight into their own illness. The motor dysfunction is typically marked by choreiform movements, which are excessive, involuntary movements involving the limbs, face, tongue, and trunk. Patients develop incoordination, bradykinesia, impaired eye movements, dysarthria, dysphagia, and gait difficulty. The clinical presentation in childhood is quite different. Juvenile HD is marked by akinesia and rigidity along with cerebellar ataxia and seizures. Diagnosis of the disorder is made by genetic testing for the CAG repeat expansion in the *huntingtin* (*htt*) gene.

For many of these disorders, including AD, PD, and ALS, the diagnosis is made based on clinical criteria. There is no specific imaging or laboratory test that can confirm the diagnosis, leading to some diagnostic uncertainty for some patients with evidence of neurodegeneration. This lack of diagnostic uncertainty not only affects individual patients with questions regarding treatment options and prognosis, but affects the field of neurodegeneration as a whole, particularly in the development of new therapies. The lack of clear biomarkers for many of these disorders complicates the design and interpretation of clinical trials. For example, the lack of a therapeutic effect of a new drug in a clinical trial could be affected if a fair number of patients are misdiagnosed and included in the trial. It is also difficult to measure disease progression objectively without distinct biomarkers. For certain disorders, the diagnosis can be confirmed irrefutably. This is true of those diseases caused by genetic mutations, such as HD and SCAs. However, the current cost of genetic testing can be a significant barrier for diagnosis for many patients, as many insurance policies will not cover genetic testing.

PATHOLOGICAL FEATURES OF COMMON NEURODEGENERATIVE DISORDERS

Common pathological features shared among the neurodegenerative disorders are neuronal cell loss, gliosis, atrophy, and pathological protein inclusions. These disorders differ in the details of the neuropathology—which neuronal populations are lost, what proteins are found in inclusions, and the subcellular localization of these inclusions.

In AD, the key pathological features include neuron loss, amyloid plaques, and neurofibrillary tangles. Atrophy is predominant in temporal and parietal cortex because of neuronal loss. Neuron loss is predominant in layers 3 and 5 of the neocortex, CA1 region of the hippocampus, and layers 2 and 5 in the entorhinal cortex. Plaques are composed of abnormal neurites and glial processes surrounding a central core composed of β-amyloid. β-Amyloid can also be found in the cerebral blood vessels. Plaques are mostly found in cerebral cortex and hippocampus. Neurofibrillary tangles are composed of excessively phosphorylated tau protein that form paired helical filaments that are deposited in soma and processes of neurons. In the earliest stages, neurofibrillary tangles develop in the transentorhinal cortex and then spread to the entorhinal cortex and hippocampus prior to neocortical regions (Braak and Braak, 1991, 1995). These tangles are not specific to AD, but are found in other neurodegenerative disorders, including PSP and dementia pugilistica.

PD was classically described as caused by loss of dopaminergic neurons within the substantia nigra with associated Lewy bodies, cytoplasmic aggregates made up predominantly of alpha-synuclein (Spillantini et al., 1997). The motor features of this disorder are caused by the loss of these nigral neurons, but many other brain areas are also involved in PD. Braak and colleagues have shown that the likely first regions involved in PD include the olfactory bulb and dorsal motor nucleus of vagus, which may explain the common symptoms of constipation and hyposmia, which predate the motor findings by many years (Braak et al., 2003). In stage II, alpha-synuclein pathology is found in pontine structures, such as the locus coeruleus and raphe nuclei, but it is not until stage III when nigral involvement is predominant (Braak et al., 2003). In more advanced disease, cortical involvement is seen (Braak et al., 2003).

ALS is marked by the loss of lower motor neurons in the anterior horn of the spinal cord and cranial motor nuclei. In addition, there is degeneration and loss of upper motor neurons in the motor cortex, particularly involving Betz cells. With the loss of these upper motor neurons, there is gliosis of the lateral corticospinal tracts. Affected muscles show grouped atrophy caused by denervation of muscle fibers. Ubiquitin-positive, proteinaceous inclusions are seen but are of variable composition compared to AD and PD, in which β-amyloid and tau or alpha-synuclein, respectively, are the predominant components. In certain familial forms of ALS, proteins that are the product of the related gene mutation can be found within the inclusions, including superoxide dismutase 1 (SOD1), TAR DNA-binding protein 43 (TDP-43), and fused in sarcoma (FUS), among others (Al-Chalabi et al., 2012).

HD is marked by predominant atrophy of the striatum and cortex. The caudate is particularly affected with significant loss of medium spiny neurons and less loss of glial cells. Inclusions found in the disorder are composed predominantly of the huntingtin protein and tend to be localized to the nucleus.

Neurodegenerative disorders are often classified into groups based on the predominant protein that is found aggregated in the brains. Tauopathies are disorders in which neurofibrillary tangles are found and other tau-based aggregates. These include PSP, FTD, and CBD, among other disorders, and the clinical phenotype and thus clinical and neuropathological diagnosis are related to the specific brain areas affected in each disorder. Synucleinopathies are those disorders in which alpha-synuclein aggregates are found in the brain, and include PD, DLB, and MSA, among others. In PD and DLB, the alpha-synuclein aggregates are found in neurons, while in MSA the aggregates are predominantly in glial cells. Other newer classifications being recognized include disorders marked by deposition of TDP-43 or other RNA-binding proteins.

CURRENT TREATMENT OPTIONS

None of the current therapies for any of the neurodegenerative disorders slow or stop neurodegeneration, and patients with these disorders progressively get worse. Current treatment options are aimed at treating the symptoms of the disease. For several of the neurodegenerative disorders, these therapies can make a big difference in the quality of life of patients. Therapies for PD are perhaps the most effective at improving the symptoms and keeping patients more active. Most of the therapies in PD are targeted toward treating the motor symptoms, including tremor, slowness, stiffness, and gait difficulties. As these motor symptoms are secondary to the loss of dopaminergic neurons in the substantia nigra, treatments aimed at promoting dopaminergic function are effective at treating these symptoms. Most PD medications act on dopamine neurochemistry (Fig. 1.1). The most effective medication for PD is levodopa, which is a precursor for dopamine. Dopamine receptor agonists can act on

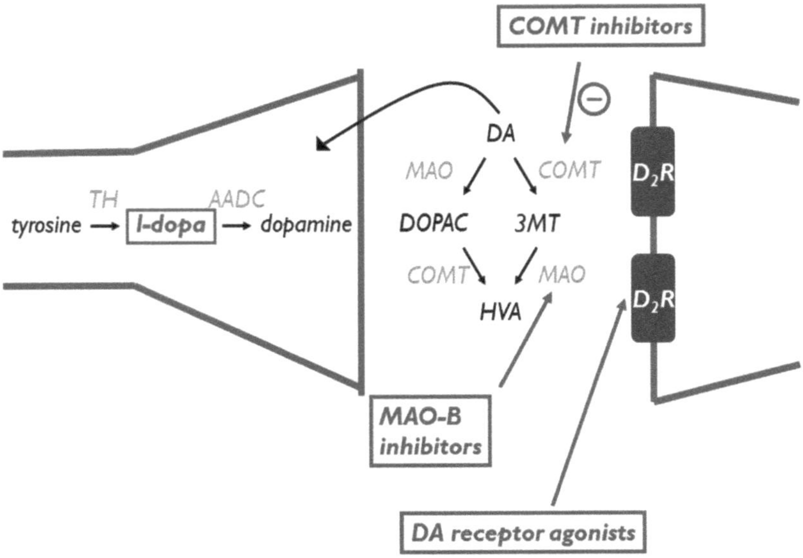

FIGURE 1.1 **Dopamine-based medications for use in Parkinson's disease.** *3-MT*, 3-methoxytyramine; *AADC*, aromatic amino acid decarboxylase; *COMT*, catechol-*o*-methyltransferase; D_2R, D2 dopamine receptor; *DA*, dopamine; *DOPAC*, 3,4-dihydroxyphenylacetic acid; *HVA*, homovanillic acid; *MAO*, monoamine oxidase; *TH*, tyrosine hydroxylase.

postsynaptic receptors to activate dopamine signaling in the basal ganglia. Other dopamine-based drugs include inhibitors of monoamine oxidase or catechol-*o*-methyltransferase, two enzymes that metabolize dopamine in the synaptic cleft into inactive metabolites. Beyond pharmaceutical agents, surgical interventions, particularly deep brain stimulation, are other effective therapies for treating the motor symptoms of PD.

While these PD medications are effective at controlling tremor, stiffness, and slowness, there are many limitations to these drugs. None of these medications fail to slow the continued degeneration of neurons in the brain, and these medications treat only the motor symptoms. PD also causes a range of nonmotor symptoms, including autonomic dysfunction, depression, anxiety, sleep disorders, and cognitive impairment, but the dopamine-based medications fail to treat these symptoms. Available therapies, particularly levodopa, can eventually lead to motor complications, including dyskinesias and motor fluctuations, which are difficult to treat.

In the case of most other neurodegenerative disorders, the therapeutic options are much more limited. In AD, acetylcholinesterase inhibitors and memantine have been approved to treat the cognitive disorder, yet these therapies have a small but significant impact on cognitive dysfunction in AD (Reisberg et al., 2003; Rogers et al., 1998; Tariot et al., 2004). In ALS, riluzole has been shown to extend the lifespan of treated patients by a few months (Miller et al., 2009). No other therapy tested in clinical trials has been shown to impact disease progression. In HD, treatments are also symptomatic. The choreiform movements can be controlled with dopamine inhibitors, such as tetrabenazine or dopamine receptor antagonists. No treatments are effective at treating the cognitive deficits. Psychiatric disorders can be treated with psychiatric medications, such as antidepressants for depression and dopamine receptor antagonists for psychosis.

Because of the lack of effective therapies, the prognosis is poor for most of these disorders. ALS perhaps has the grimmest prognosis. Median survival of patients with ALS ranges from 2 to 5 years. Patients succumb to respiratory failure. Median survival in AD is about 8 years, and the common cause of death is pneumonia. Median survival in HD is more variable, ranging usually between 10 and 20 years from symptom onset. An inverse correlation exists between CAG repeat size and progression of the disorder. With longer repeats, the disorder starts at an earlier age and progresses more rapidly. Patient often die from aspiration, but suicide is a common cause of death. The effect of PD on survival is less clear—mortality rates for patients with PD are estimated to be increased at least twofold compared to persons without PD (Louis et al., 1997; Morens et al., 1996; Morgante et al., 2000). While survival rates in PD are not clear-cut, this disorder has been shown in longitudinal studies to cause significant disability over time. A longitudinal study of 136 newly diagnosed PD patients in Australia revealed that nearly 75% had died by 20 years, and among those who were still living at 20 years, 83% had dementia and 48% were living in a nursing home, with only one patient still living independently (Hely et al., 2008).

To ultimately change the poor prognoses of these disorders, better therapies need to be developed to target the underlying causes of neuronal loss. To achieve this, we need a better understanding of the underlying mechanisms of neurodegeneration.

COMMON MECHANISMS IMPLICATED IN NEURODEGENERATION

HD is a purely genetic disorder caused by the CAG repeat expansion in the *huntingtin* gene. ALS, AD, and PD are more commonly sporadic in nature, but specific gene mutations can cause autosomal dominant or autosomal recessive forms of these disorders, often starting earlier in life than sporadic forms of these illnesses. In addition, genetic factors are recognized to play a role in the risk of these disorders.

While the cause of each neurodegenerative disorder differs, these clinically disparate disorders do share commonalities in molecular mechanisms involved in neurodegeneration once the disease process has been initiated. For many neurodegeneration disorders, mechanisms leading to cell death include mitochondrial dysfunction, oxidative stress, loss of growth factors, proteasomal dysfunction, autophagic/lysosomal dysfunction, excitotoxicity, protein aggregation, prion-like spread, and neuroinflammation. No one mechanism appears to be primary in neurodegeneration, and these pathogenic mechanisms likely act synergistically through complex interactions to promote neurodegeneration.

Mitochondrial Dysfunction

The role of mitochondrial dysfunction and oxidative stress has been implicated in neurodegeneration for a long time. Oxidative stress results from an overabundance of reactive free radicals secondary to either an overproduction of reactive species and/or a failure of cell buffering mechanisms that normally limit their accumulation. Excess reactive species can react with cellular macromolecules and thereby disrupt their normal functions. Alterations in mitochondrial function and evidence of oxidative damage to proteins, lipids, and nucleic acids have been found in human AD (Hensley et al., 1995; Markesbery and Lovell, 1998;

Wang et al., 2014) and PD (Alam et al., 1997; Dexter et al., 1994; Schapira et al., 1989; Schapira et al., 2014). In HD, mutant huntingtin causes mitochondrial dysfunction with impaired calcium homeostasis, mitochondrial membrane potential, and complex II and III activity, and alterations in mitophagy (Gu et al., 1996; Panov et al., 2002; Schapira et al., 2014; Song et al., 2011). Epidemiological studies have shown that pesticides that inhibit mitochondrial function can increase the risk of PD, AD, and ALS (Baltazar et al., 2014). Complex I inhibitors can induce Parkinsonism in animal models (Betarbet et al., 2000; Langston et al., 1983; Langston et al., 1984), and the mitochondrial inhibitor 3-nitropropionic acid can cause a Huntington-like phenotype in animals (Brouillet et al., 1999).

There is also evidence of impairment of endogenous protective mechanisms. The antioxidant protein glutathione is reduced in postmortem PD nigra (Perry and Yong, 1986; Sian et al., 1994; Sofic et al., 1992), while activity of antioxidants, such as SOD, catalase, and glutathione peroxidase are reduced in AD brain (Marcus et al., 1998; Omar et al., 1999; Wang et al., 2014). Several genes linked to familial forms of ALS and PD play a role in protection against oxidative stress, including phosphatase and tensin homolog-induced putative kinase (PINK1), DJ-1, and SOD1 (Clark et al., 2006; Kim et al., 2005; Lee, Hyun, Jenner and Halliwell, 2001; Park et al., 2006; Yokota et al., 2003).

Protein Aggregation and Clearance

Protein aggregation and misfolding have emerged as important mechanisms in many neurodegenerative disorders. While the proteins involved in these disorders are different, each is associated with characteristic aggregates of misfolded protein, and these abnormal aggregates appear to acquire toxic properties. The mechanism by which overabundance or aggregation of the pathogenic protein, whether alpha-synuclein, huntingtin, SOD, TDP-43, or tau, causes neuronal injury is not well understood. Hypotheses include toxic effects of aggregates on proteasomal or autophagic function, effects on gene transcription, interactions of pathogenic proteins with cell signaling and cell death cascades, and aggregate-mediated activation of inflammatory mechanisms.

Protein misfolding observed in neurodegeneration can be placed in the broader context of proteostasis, the homeostatic balance of the proteins within cells, which is maintained by cellular mechanisms regulating protein synthesis, folding, trafficking, and degradation (Balch et al., 2008; Lim and Yue, 2015; Morimoto, 2008; Prahlad and Morimoto, 2009). The capacity of cells to clear misfolded proteins is limited and cell-type specific, with neurons being particularly vulnerable to the build-up of aggregated proteins (Balch et al., 2008; Lim and Yue, 2015; Morimoto, 2008; Prahlad and Morimoto, 2009). Clearance requires the coordinated activity of chaperones, proteasomal degradation, and autophagy–lysosomal mechanisms, and these mechanisms may become overwhelmed if a large number of aberrant proteins are present. Evidence for disrupted protein clearance in many neurodegenerative disorders is growing. Autophagic failure has been noted in animal models or postmortem brains for AD, PD, and HD (Anglade et al., 1997; Kegel et al., 2000; Martinez-Vicente, 2015; Nixon et al., 2005). Disease-associated mutations or accumulation of alpha-synuclein, mutant htt, and Aβ peptide is associated with disruption of autophagy and lysosomal function (Cuervo et al., 2004; Heng et al., 2010; Lee et al., 2010; Martinez-Vicente, 2015; Martinez-Vicente et al., 2010; Pickford et al., 2008; Winslow et al., 2010). In addition, failure of protein quality control mechanisms can itself initiate neurodegeneration. For example, proteasomal inhibitors cause Parkinsonism and loss of nigral neurons in animals (McNaught et al., 2004). Conditional knockout of key genes required for proteasome function can cause Parkinsonism or motor neuron disease (Bedford et al., 2008; Tashiro et al., 2012), and similarly conditional knockout of autophagy genes can cause neurodegeneration in mice (Hara et al., 2006; Komatsu et al., 2006). Genes linked to PD, such as PINK1, parkin, ATP13A2, and glucocerebrosidase, play roles in mitophagy and lysosomal function (Martinez-Vicente, 2015). Aging, the key risk factor for neurodegeneration, has been associated with reduced proteasomal function (Tonoki et al., 2009) and autophagy (Yamaguchi and Otsu, 2012), which may explain the increasing prevalence of neurodegenerative disorders with age.

Prion-Like Spread

A new concept in neurodegeneration is the potential for key aggregation-prone proteins observed in neurodegenerative disorders to spread from one neuron to another (Brundin et al., 2010; Costanzo and Zurzolo, 2013; Lim and Yue, 2015; Polymenidou and Cleveland, 2012). In PD, HD, and AD, brain regions affected are synaptically connected regions, suggesting that some "signal" may be spread from earlier involved regions to new regions. In all three disorders, the progression of disease follows a predictable and stereotyped pattern. This was first described in PD and AD by Braak and colleagues (Braak and Braak, 1991, 1995; Braak et al., 2003). Detection of alpha-synuclein, tau, and SOD in cerebrospinal fluid suggest that these proteins can be released by cells and thus become available for uptake by neighboring neurons or glia (Arai et al., 1995; Borghi et al., 2000; El-Agnaf et al., 2003; Zetterstrom et al., 2011). Animal studies in which rodents were injected with aggregated tau or alpha-synuclein have demonstrated the spread of the aggregating protein from one brain region to another in vivo (de Calignon et al., 2012; Liu et al., 2012; Luk et al., 2012). Injection of brain lysates from patients with PD or MSA into rodents caused alpha-synuclein aggregation and neurodegeneration (Recasens et al., 2014; Watts et al., 2013). Cell-to-cell spread has been demonstrated in cell culture and/or in vivo for alpha-synuclein (Desplats et al., 2009; Hansen et al., 2011), tau (Kfoury et al., 2012; Sanders et al., 2014), and htt (Costanzo et al., 2013). Evidence for prion-like spread of SOD1, TDP-43, and FUS is also accumulating for ALS (S. Lee and Kim, 2015). How these pathogenic proteins are transferred is not well understood, but potential cellular pathways involved, including exosomes, tunneling nanotubes, synaptic release, recycling endosomal pathways, fluid-phase or receptor-mediated endocytosis, and direct translocation across plasma membrane, are among those mechanisms invoked (Costanzo and Zurzolo, 2013).

Inflammation

The role of inflammation has been long ignored in neurodegenerative disorders, but neuroinflammation has been increasingly recognized as a primary mechanism involved in neurodegeneration. Epidemiological studies have suggested that certain nonsteroidal anti-inflammatory drugs and statin drugs may reduce the risk of PD and AD (Bower et al., 2006; Chen et al., 2003, 2005; Hernan et al., 2006; Jick et al., 2000; Launer, 2003; Ton et al., 2006; Wahner et al., 2008; Wolozin et al., 2000, 2007). Genes associated with immune function, including *Triggering receptor expressed on myeloid cells 2* and *CD33*, are associated with risk of AD (Guerreiro et al., 2013; Hollingworth et al., 2011; Naj et al., 2011). Microglial activation is observed in postmortem AD, ALS, HD, and PD brains, as well as in animal models (Chao et al., 2014; Crotti and Glass, 2015; Heneka et al., 2015; Henkel et al., 2009). Proinflammatory cytokines and chemokines are elevated in human AD, ALS, HD, and PD and animal models (Chao et al., 2014; Crotti and Glass, 2015; Heneka et al., 2015; Henkel et al., 2009). A potential role of peripheral immune cells is suggested by the evidence of T cells in human PD brain in human ALS spinal cord (Brochard et al., 2009; Engelhardt et al., 1993).

A central issue is how the inflammatory process is related to neurodegeneration. Until recently, inflammation was viewed primarily as a secondary consequence of cell death, with microglia playing a role in removing cellular debris. Recent work, however, has pointed to a much earlier and active role of inflammation and has suggested that inflammation may promote the progression of neural injury. Expression of mutant proteins associated with neurodegenerative disorders, such as mutant htt, Leucine-rich repeat kinase 2, or SOD1, is associated with activation of microglia and astrocytes and impairment of normal astrocytic function, such as glutamate uptake (Almer et al., 1999; Crotti et al., 2014; Gillardon et al., 2012; Hall et al., 1998; Lievens et al., 2001; Shin et al., 2005). Expression of mutant proteins in inflammatory cells is at least partially responsible for neurodegeneration. For example, expression of mutant htt in only microglia or astrocytes can cause increased brain inflammation and neurological symptoms (Bradford et al., 2009; Hsiao et al., 2013), while reduction of mutant SOD1 expression in microglia slowed disease progression and death in SOD1 transgenic mice (Beers et al., 2006; Boillee et al., 2006). Protein aggregates could serve as a trigger for the inflammatory response in neurodegeneration. For example, aggregated or nitrated alpha-synuclein can directly trigger microglial and humoral responses (Benner et al., 2008; Reynolds, et al., 2008a,b; Theodore et al., 2008; Zhang et al., 2005). Aβ aggregates can also bind and activate microglia (Bamberger et al., 2003; El Khoury et al., 2003; Paresce et al., 1996). Excessive activation of microglia and astrocytes in response to mutant and/or aggregated proteins can lead to the death of more neurons, resulting in a vicious feed-forward cycle in which the release of more proteins from dying cells can induce further microglia and astrocytic activation (Crotti and Glass, 2015).

GOALS FOR NEW DRUG THERAPIES FOR NEURODEGENERATION

Ultimately, better understanding of the mechanisms underlying neurodegeneration should lead to better therapeutic options. As noted earlier, current therapies at best treat the symptoms of the disease but fail to slow disease progression. The goal of therapeutic development for neurodegenerative disorders is to develop drugs that slow down or stop the neurodegenerative process. So-called neuroprotective, or disease-modifying, therapies would not only treat the symptoms but slow the continued loss of neurons in disease. While such disease-modifying therapies may not be curative and restore those cells already lost by the time of diagnosis, such therapies would thus dramatically change the grim prognosis for most of these disorders. Patients afflicted with these disorders would develop disability at a much slower pace and median survival would also improve. The earlier the therapies are started, the slower that neurons are lost and thus the slower that clinical features present. Advances in presymptomatic diagnosis of many neurodegenerative disorders suggest that detection of the disease process before the onset of visible symptoms will become practical in the near future. Indeed, for those neurodegenerative disorders caused by gene mutations in which gene testing can be performed in at-risk populations, such as HD or SCAs, presymptomatic diagnosis already occurs. Once disease modifying therapies are available, the initiation of therapies that slow or stop the neurodegenerative process may prevent patients at risk for the disease from ever developing the clinical features of the disorder.

References

Al-Chalabi, A., Jones, A., Troakes, C., King, A., Al-Sarraj, S., van den Berg, L.H., 2012. The genetics and neuropathology of amyotrophic lateral sclerosis. Acta Neuropathol. 124 (3), 339–352. http://dx.doi.org/10.1007/s00401-012-1022-4.

Alam, Z.I., Jenner, A., Daniel, S.E., Lees, A.J., Cairns, N., Marsden, C.D., et al., 1997. Oxidative DNA damage in the parkinsonian brain: an apparent selective increase in 8-hydroxyguanine levels in substantia nigra. J. Neurochem. 69 (3), 1196–1203.

Almer, G., Vukosavic, S., Romero, N., Przedborski, S., 1999. Inducible nitric oxide synthase up-regulation in a transgenic mouse model of familial amyotrophic lateral sclerosis. J. Neurochem. 72 (6), 2415–2425.

Alzheimer's Association, 2014. 2014 Alzheimer's disease facts and figures. Alzheimer's Dement. 10 (2).

Anglade, P., Vyas, S., Javoy-Agid, F., Herrero, M.T., Michel, P.P., Marquez, J., et al., 1997. Apoptosis and autophagy in nigral neurons of patients with Parkinson's disease. Histol. Histopathol. 12 (1), 25–31.

Arai, H., Terajima, M., Miura, M., Higuchi, S., Muramatsu, T., Machida, N., et al., 1995. Tau in cerebrospinal fluid: a potential diagnostic marker in Alzheimer's disease. Ann. Neurol. 38 (4), 649–652. http://dx.doi.org/10.1002/ana.410380414.

Balch, W.E., Morimoto, R.I., Dillin, A., Kelly, J.W., 2008. Adapting proteostasis for disease intervention. Science 319 (5865), 916–919. http://dx.doi.org/10.1126/science.1141448.

Baltazar, M.T., Dinis-Oliveira, R.J., de Lourdes Bastos, M., Tsatsakis, A.M., Duarte, J.A., Carvalho, F., 2014. Pesticides exposure as etiological factors of Parkinson's disease and other neurodegenerative diseases—a mechanistic approach. Toxicol. Lett. 230 (2), 85–103. http://dx.doi.org/10.1016/j.toxlet.2014.01.039.

Bamberger, M.E., Harris, M.E., McDonald, D.R., Husemann, J., Landreth, G.E., 2003. A cell surface receptor complex for fibrillar beta-amyloid mediates microglial activation. J. Neurosci. 23 (7), 2665–2674.

Bedford, L., Hay, D., Devoy, A., Paine, S., Powe, D.G., Seth, R., et al., 2008. Depletion of 26S proteasomes in mouse brain neurons causes neurodegeneration and Lewy-like inclusions resembling human pale bodies. J. Neurosci. 28 (33), 8189–8198. http://dx.doi.org/10.1523/JNEUROSCI.2218-08.2008.

Beers, D.R., Henkel, J.S., Xiao, Q., Zhao, W., Wang, J., Yen, A.A., et al., 2006. Wild-type microglia extend survival in PU.1 knockout mice with familial amyotrophic lateral sclerosis. Proc. Natl. Acad. Sci. U.S.A. 103 (43), 16021–16026. http://dx.doi.org/10.1073/pnas.0607423103.

Benner, E.J., Banerjee, R., Reynolds, A.D., Sherman, S., Pisarev, V.M., Tsiperson, V., et al., 2008. Nitrated alpha-synuclein immunity accelerates degeneration of nigral dopaminergic neurons. PLoS One 3 (1), e1376. http://dx.doi.org/10.1371/journal.pone.0001376.

Betarbet, R., Sherer, T.B., MacKenzie, G., Garcia-Osuna, M., Panov, A.V., Greenamyre, J.T., 2000. Chronic systemic pesticide exposure reproduces features of Parkinson's disease. Nat. Neurosci. 3 (12), 1301–1306. http://dx.doi.org/10.1038/81834.

Boillee, S., Yamanaka, K., Lobsiger, C.S., Copeland, N.G., Jenkins, N.A., Kassiotis, G., et al., 2006. Onset and progression in inherited ALS determined by motor neurons and microglia. Science 312 (5778), 1389–1392. http://dx.doi.org/10.1126/science.1123511.

Borghi, R., Marchese, R., Negro, A., Marinelli, L., Forloni, G., Zaccheo, D., et al., 2000. Full length alpha-synuclein is present in cerebrospinal fluid from Parkinson's disease and normal subjects. Neurosci. Lett. 287 (1), 65–67.

Bower, J.H., Maraganore, D.M., Peterson, B.J., Ahlskog, J.E., Rocca, W.A., 2006. Immunologic diseases, anti-inflammatory drugs, and Parkinson disease: a case-control study. Neurology 67 (3), 494–496. http://dx.doi.org/10.1212/01.wnl.0000227906.99570.cc.

Braak, H., Braak, E., 1991. Neuropathological stageing of Alzheimer-related changes. Acta Neuropathol. 82 (4), 239–259.

Braak, H., Braak, E., 1995. Staging of Alzheimer's disease-related neurofibrillary changes. Neurobiol. Aging 16 (3), 271–278 (Discussion 278–284).

Braak, H., Del Tredici, K., Rub, U., de Vos, R.A., Jansen Steur, E.N., Braak, E., 2003. Staging of brain pathology related to sporadic Parkinson's disease. Neurobiol. Aging 24 (2), 197–211.

Bradford, J., Shin, J.Y., Roberts, M., Wang, C.E., Li, X.J., Li, S., 2009. Expression of mutant huntingtin in mouse brain astrocytes causes age-dependent neurological symptoms. Proc. Natl. Acad. Sci. U.S.A. 106 (52), 22480–22485. http://dx.doi.org/10.1073/pnas.0911503106.

Brochard, V., Combadiere, B., Prigent, A., Laouar, Y., Perrin, A., Beray-Berthat, V., et al., 2009. Infiltration of $CD4^+$ lymphocytes into the brain contributes to neurodegeneration in a mouse model of Parkinson disease. J. Clin. Invest. 119 (1), 182–192. http://dx.doi.org/10.1172/JCI36470.

Brouillet, E., Conde, F., Beal, M.F., Hantraye, P., 1999. Replicating Huntington's disease phenotype in experimental animals. Prog. Neurobiol. 59 (5), 427–468.

Brundin, P., Melki, R., Kopito, R., 2010. Prion-like transmission of protein aggregates in neurodegenerative diseases. Nat. Rev. Mol. Cell Biol. 11 (4), 301–307. http://dx.doi.org/10.1038/nrm2873.

Chao, Y., Wong, S.C., Tan, E.K., 2014. Evidence of inflammatory system involvement in Parkinson's disease. Biomed. Res. Int. 2014, 308654. http://dx.doi.org/10.1155/2014/308654.

Chen, H., Jacobs, E., Schwarzschild, M.A., McCullough, M.L., Calle, E.E., Thun, M.J., Ascherio, A., 2005. Nonsteroidal antiinflammatory drug use and the risk for Parkinson's disease. Ann. Neurol. 58 (6), 963–967. http://dx.doi.org/10.1002/ana.20682.

Chen, H., Zhang, S.M., Hernan, M.A., Schwarzschild, M.A., Willett, W.C., Colditz, G.A., et al., 2003. Nonsteroidal anti-inflammatory drugs and the risk of Parkinson disease. Arch. Neurol. 60 (8), 1059–1064. http://dx.doi.org/10.1001/archneur.60.8.1059.

Clark, I.E., Dodson, M.W., Jiang, C., Cao, J.H., Huh, J.R., Seol, J.H., et al., 2006. Drosophila pink1 is required for mitochondrial function and interacts genetically with parkin. Nature 441 (7097), 1162–1166. http://dx.doi.org/10.1038/nature04779.

Costanzo, M., Abounit, S., Marzo, L., Danckaert, A., Chamoun, Z., Roux, P., Zurzolo, C., 2013. Transfer of polyglutamine aggregates in neuronal cells occurs in tunneling nanotubes. J. Cell Sci. 126 (Pt 16), 3678–3685. http://dx.doi.org/10.1242/jcs.126086.

Costanzo, M., Zurzolo, C., 2013. The cell biology of prion-like spread of protein aggregates: mechanisms and implication in neurodegeneration. Biochem. J. 452 (1), 1–17. http://dx.doi.org/10.1042/BJ20121898.

Crotti, A., Benner, C., Kerman, B.E., Gosselin, D., Lagier-Tourenne, C., Zuccato, C., et al., 2014. Mutant Huntingtin promotes autonomous microglia activation via myeloid lineage-determining factors. Nat. Neurosci. 17 (4), 513–521. http://dx.doi.org/10.1038/nn.3668.

Crotti, A., Glass, C.K., 2015. The choreography of neuroinflammation in Huntington's disease. Trends Immunol. http://dx.doi.org/10.1016/j.it.2015.04.007.

Cuervo, A.M., Stefanis, L., Fredenburg, R., Lansbury, P.T., Sulzer, D., 2004. Impaired degradation of mutant alpha-synuclein by chaperone-mediated autophagy. Science 305 (5688), 1292–1295. http://dx.doi.org/10.1126/science.1101738.

de Calignon, A., Polydoro, M., Suarez-Calvet, M., William, C., Adamowicz, D.H., Kopeikina, K.J., et al., 2012. Propagation of tau pathology in a model of early Alzheimer's disease. Neuron 73 (4), 685–697. http://dx.doi.org/10.1016/j.neuron.2011.11.033.

Desplats, P., Lee, H.J., Bae, E.J., Patrick, C., Rockenstein, E., Crews, L., et al., 2009. Inclusion formation and neuronal cell death through neuron-to-neuron transmission of alpha-synuclein. Proc. Natl. Acad. Sci. U.S.A. 106 (31), 13010–13015. http://dx.doi.org/10.1073/pnas.0903691106.

Dexter, D.T., Holley, A.E., Flitter, W.D., Slater, T.F., Wells, F.R., Daniel, S.E., et al., 1994. Increased levels of lipid hydroperoxides in the parkinsonian substantia nigra: an HPLC and ESR study. Mov. Disord. 9 (1), 92–97. http://dx.doi.org/10.1002/mds.870090115.

Dorsey, E.R., Constantinescu, R., Thompson, J.P., Biglan, K.M., Holloway, R.G., Kieburtz, K., et al., 2007. Projected number of people with Parkinson disease in the most populous nations, 2005 through 2030. Neurology 68 (5), 384–386. http://dx.doi.org/10.1212/01.wnl.0000247740.47667.03.

El-Agnaf, O.M., Salem, S.A., Paleologou, K.E., Cooper, L.J., Fullwood, N.J., Gibson, M.J., et al., 2003. Alpha-synuclein implicated in Parkinson's disease is present in extracellular biological fluids, including human plasma. FASEB J. 17 (13), 1945–1947. http://dx.doi.org/10.1096/fj.03-0098fje.

El Khoury, J.B., Moore, K.J., Means, T.K., Leung, J., Terada, K., Toft, M., et al., 2003. CD36 mediates the innate host response to beta-amyloid. J. Exp. Med. 197 (12), 1657–1666. http://dx.doi.org/10.1084/jem.20021546.
Engelhardt, J.I., Tajti, J., Appel, S.H., 1993. Lymphocytic infiltrates in the spinal cord in amyotrophic lateral sclerosis. Arch. Neurol. 50 (1), 30–36.
Gillardon, F., Schmid, R., Draheim, H., 2012. Parkinson's disease-linked leucine-rich repeat kinase 2(R1441G) mutation increases proinflammatory cytokine release from activated primary microglial cells and resultant neurotoxicity. Neuroscience 208, 41–48. http://dx.doi.org/10.1016/j.neuroscience.2012.02.001.
Gu, M., Gash, M.T., Mann, V.M., Javoy-Agid, F., Cooper, J.M., Schapira, A.H., 1996. Mitochondrial defect in Huntington's disease caudate nucleus. Ann. Neurol. 39 (3), 385–389. http://dx.doi.org/10.1002/ana.410390317.
Guerreiro, R., Wojtas, A., Bras, J., Carrasquillo, M., Rogaeva, E., Majounie, E., et al., 2013. TREM2 variants in Alzheimer's disease. N. Engl. J. Med. 368 (2), 117–127. http://dx.doi.org/10.1056/NEJMoa1211851.
Hall, E.D., Oostveen, J.A., Gurney, M.E., 1998. Relationship of microglial and astrocytic activation to disease onset and progression in a transgenic model of familial ALS. Glia 23 (3), 249–256.
Hansen, C., Angot, E., Bergstrom, A.L., Steiner, J.A., Pieri, L., Paul, G., et al., 2011. alpha-Synuclein propagates from mouse brain to grafted dopaminergic neurons and seeds aggregation in cultured human cells. J. Clin. Invest. 121 (2), 715–725. http://dx.doi.org/10.1172/JCI43366.
Hara, T., Nakamura, K., Matsui, M., Yamamoto, A., Nakahara, Y., Suzuki-Migishima, R., et al., 2006. Suppression of basal autophagy in neural cells causes neurodegenerative disease in mice. Nature 441 (7095), 885–889. http://dx.doi.org/10.1038/nature04724.
Hebert, L.E., Weuve, J., Scherr, P.A., Evans, D.A., 2013. Alzheimer disease in the United States (2010–2050) estimated using the 2010 census. Neurology 80 (19), 1778–1783. http://dx.doi.org/10.1212/WNL.0b013e31828726f5.
Hely, M.A., Reid, W.G., Adena, M.A., Halliday, G.M., Morris, J.G., 2008. The Sydney multicenter study of Parkinson's disease: the inevitability of dementia at 20 years. Mov. Disord. 23 (6), 837–844. http://dx.doi.org/10.1002/mds.21956.
Heneka, M.T., Carson, M.J., El Khoury, J., Landreth, G.E., Brosseron, F., Feinstein, D.L., et al., 2015. Neuroinflammation in Alzheimer's disease. Lancet Neurol. 14 (4), 388–405. http://dx.doi.org/10.1016/S1474-4422(15)70016-5.
Heng, M.Y., Duong, D.K., Albin, R.L., Tallaksen-Greene, S.J., Hunter, J.M., Lesort, M.J., et al., 2010. Early autophagic response in a novel knock-in model of Huntington disease. Hum. Mol. Genet. 19 (19), 3702–3720. http://dx.doi.org/10.1093/hmg/ddq285.
Henkel, J.S., Beers, D.R., Zhao, W., Appel, S.H., 2009. Microglia in ALS: the good, the bad, and the resting. J. Neuroimmune Pharmacol. 4 (4), 389–398. http://dx.doi.org/10.1007/s11481-009-9171-5.
Hensley, K., Hall, N., Subramaniam, R., Cole, P., Harris, M., Aksenov, M., et al., 1995. Brain regional correspondence between Alzheimer's disease histopathology and biomarkers of protein oxidation. J. Neurochem. 65 (5), 2146–2156.
Hernan, M.A., Logroscino, G., Garcia Rodriguez, L.A., 2006. Nonsteroidal anti-inflammatory drugs and the incidence of Parkinson disease. Neurology 66 (7), 1097–1099. http://dx.doi.org/10.1212/01.wnl.0000204446.82823.28.
Hirtz, D., Thurman, D.J., Gwinn-Hardy, K., Mohamed, M., Chaudhuri, A.R., Zalutsky, R., 2007. How common are the "common" neurologic disorders? Neurology 68 (5), 326–337. http://dx.doi.org/10.1212/01.wnl.0000252807.38124.a3.
Hollingworth, P., Harold, D., Sims, R., Gerrish, A., Lambert, J.C., Carrasquillo, M.M., et al., 2011. Common variants at ABCA7, MS4A6A/MS4A4E, EPHA1, CD33 and CD2AP are associated with Alzheimer's disease. Nat. Genet. 43 (5), 429–435. http://dx.doi.org/10.1038/ng.803.
Hsiao, H.Y., Chen, Y.C., Chen, H.M., Tu, P.H., Chern, Y., 2013. A critical role of astrocyte-mediated nuclear factor-kappaB-dependent inflammation in Huntington's disease. Hum. Mol. Genet. 22 (9), 1826–1842. http://dx.doi.org/10.1093/hmg/ddt036.
Jick, H., Zornberg, G.L., Jick, S.S., Seshadri, S., Drachman, D.A., 2000. Statins and the risk of dementia. Lancet 356 (9242), 1627–1631.
Kegel, K.B., Kim, M., Sapp, E., McIntyre, C., Castano, J.G., Aronin, N., DiFiglia, M., 2000. Huntingtin expression stimulates endosomal-lysosomal activity, endosome tubulation, and autophagy. J. Neurosci. 20 (19), 7268–7278.
Kfoury, N., Holmes, B.B., Jiang, H., Holtzman, D.M., Diamond, M.I., 2012. Trans-cellular propagation of Tau aggregation by fibrillar species. J. Biol. Chem. 287 (23), 19440–19451. http://dx.doi.org/10.1074/jbc.M112.346072.
Kim, R.H., Smith, P.D., Aleyasin, H., Hayley, S., Mount, M.P., Pownall, S., et al., 2005. Hypersensitivity of DJ-1-deficient mice to 1-methyl-4-phenyl-1,2,3,6-tetrahydropyrindine (MPTP) and oxidative stress. Proc. Natl. Acad. Sci. U.S.A. 102 (14), 5215–5220. http://dx.doi.org/10.1073/pnas.0501282102.

Komatsu, M., Waguri, S., Chiba, T., Murata, S., Iwata, J., Tanida, I., et al., 2006. Loss of autophagy in the central nervous system causes neurodegeneration in mice. Nature 441 (7095), 880–884. http://dx.doi.org/10.1038/nature04723.

Kowal, S.L., Dall, T.M., Chakrabarti, R., Storm, M.V., Jain, A., 2013. The current and projected economic burden of Parkinson's disease in the United States. Mov. Disord. 28 (3), 311–318. http://dx.doi.org/10.1002/mds.25292.

Langston, J.W., Ballard, P., Tetrud, J.W., Irwin, I., 1983. Chronic Parkinsonism in humans due to a product of meperidine-analog synthesis. Science 219 (4587), 979–980.

Langston, J.W., Forno, L.S., Rebert, C.S., Irwin, I., 1984. Selective nigral toxicity after systemic administration of 1-methyl-4-phenyl-1,2,5,6-tetrahydropyrine (MPTP) in the squirrel monkey. Brain Res. 292 (2), 390–394.

Launer, L., 2003. Nonsteroidal anti-inflammatory drug use and the risk for Alzheimer's disease: dissecting the epidemiological evidence. Drugs 63 (8), 731–739.

Lee, J.H., Yu, W.H., Kumar, A., Lee, S., Mohan, P.S., Peterhoff, C.M., et al., 2010. Lysosomal proteolysis and autophagy require presenilin 1 and are disrupted by Alzheimer-related PS1 mutations. Cell 141 (7), 1146–1158. http://dx.doi.org/10.1016/j.cell.2010.05.008.

Lee, M., Hyun, D., Jenner, P., Halliwell, B., 2001. Effect of overexpression of wild-type and mutant Cu/Zn-superoxide dismutases on oxidative damage and antioxidant defences: relevance to Down's syndrome and familial amyotrophic lateral sclerosis. J. Neurochem. 76 (4), 957–965.

Lee, S., Kim, H.J., 2015. Prion-like mechanism in amyotrophic lateral sclerosis: are protein aggregates the key? Exp. Neurobiol. 24 (1), 1–7. http://dx.doi.org/10.5607/en.2015.24.1.1.

Lievens, J.C., Woodman, B., Mahal, A., Spasic-Boscovic, O., Samuel, D., Kerkerian-Le Goff, L., Bates, G.P., 2001. Impaired glutamate uptake in the R6 Huntington's disease transgenic mice. Neurobiol. Dis. 8 (5), 807–821. http://dx.doi.org/10.1006/nbdi.2001.0430.

Lim, J., Yue, Z., 2015. Neuronal aggregates: formation, clearance, and spreading. Dev. Cell 32 (4), 491–501. http://dx.doi.org/10.1016/j.devcel.2015.02.002.

Liu, L., Drouet, V., Wu, J.W., Witter, M.P., Small, S.A., Clelland, C., Duff, K., 2012. Trans-synaptic spread of tau pathology in vivo. PLoS One 7 (2), e31302. http://dx.doi.org/10.1371/journal.pone.0031302.

Louis, E.D., Marder, K., Cote, L., Tang, M., Mayeux, R., 1997. Mortality from Parkinson disease. Arch. Neurol. 54 (3), 260–264.

Luk, K.C., Kehm, V., Carroll, J., Zhang, B., O'Brien, P., Trojanowski, J.Q., Lee, V.M., 2012. Pathological alpha-synuclein transmission initiates Parkinson-like neurodegeneration in nontransgenic mice. Science 338 (6109), 949–953. http://dx.doi.org/10.1126/science.1227157.

Marcus, D.L., Thomas, C., Rodriguez, C., Simberkoff, K., Tsai, J.S., Strafaci, J.A., Freedman, M.L., 1998. Increased peroxidation and reduced antioxidant enzyme activity in Alzheimer's disease. Exp. Neurol. 150 (1), 40–44. http://dx.doi.org/10.1006/exnr.1997.6750.

Markesbery, W.R., Lovell, M.A., 1998. Four-hydroxynonenal, a product of lipid peroxidation, is increased in the brain in Alzheimer's disease. Neurobiol. Aging 19 (1), 33–36.

Martinez-Vicente, M., 2015. Autophagy in neurodegenerative diseases: from pathogenic dysfunction to therapeutic modulation. Semin. Cell Dev. Biol. 40, 115–126. http://dx.doi.org/10.1016/j.semcdb.2015.03.005.

Martinez-Vicente, M., Talloczy, Z., Wong, E., Tang, G., Koga, H., Kaushik, S., et al., 2010. Cargo recognition failure is responsible for inefficient autophagy in Huntington's disease. Nat. Neurosci. 13 (5), 567–576. http://dx.doi.org/10.1038/nn.2528.

McNaught, K.S., Perl, D.P., Brownell, A.L., Olanow, C.W., 2004. Systemic exposure to proteasome inhibitors causes a progressive model of Parkinson's disease. Ann. Neurol. 56 (1), 149–162. http://dx.doi.org/10.1002/ana.20186.

Miller, R.G., Jackson, C.E., Kasarskis, E.J., England, J.D., Forshew, D., Johnston, W., et al., 2009. Practice parameter update: the care of the patient with amyotrophic lateral sclerosis: drug, nutritional, and respiratory therapies (an evidence-based review): report of the Quality Standards Subcommittee of the American Academy of Neurology. Neurology 73 (15), 1218–1226. http://dx.doi.org/10.1212/WNL.0b013e3181bc0141.

Morens, D.M., Davis, J.W., Grandinetti, A., Ross, G.W., Popper, J.S., White, L.R., 1996. Epidemiologic observations on Parkinson's disease: incidence and mortality in a prospective study of middle-aged men. Neurology 46 (4), 1044–1050.

Morgante, L., Salemi, G., Meneghini, F., Di Rosa, A.E., Epifanio, A., Grigoletto, F., et al., 2000. Parkinson disease survival: a population-based study. Arch. Neurol. 57 (4), 507–512.

Morimoto, R.I., 2008. Proteotoxic stress and inducible chaperone networks in neurodegenerative disease and aging. Genes Dev. 22 (11), 1427–1438. http://dx.doi.org/10.1101/gad.1657108.

Murphy, S.L., Xu, J., Kochanek, K.D., 2013. Deaths: final data for 2010. Natl. Vital Stat. Rep. 61 (4), 1–117.
Naj, A.C., Jun, G., Beecham, G.W., Wang, L.S., Vardarajan, B.N., Buros, J., et al., 2011. Common variants at MS4A4/MS4A6E, CD2AP, CD33 and EPHA1 are associated with late-onset Alzheimer's disease. Nat. Genet. 43 (5), 436–441. http://dx.doi.org/10.1038/ng.801.
Nixon, R.A., Wegiel, J., Kumar, A., Yu, W.H., Peterhoff, C., Cataldo, A., Cuervo, A.M., 2005. Extensive involvement of autophagy in Alzheimer disease: an immuno-electron microscopy study. J. Neuropathol. Exp. Neurol. 64 (2), 113–122.
Noyes, K., Liu, H., Li, Y., Holloway, R., Dick, A.W., 2006. Economic burden associated with Parkinson's disease on elderly Medicare beneficiaries. Mov. Disord. 21 (3), 362–372. http://dx.doi.org/10.1002/mds.20727.
Omar, R.A., Chyan, Y.J., Andorn, A.C., Poeggeler, B., Robakis, N.K., Pappolla, M.A., 1999. Increased expression but reduced activity of antioxidant enzymes in Alzheimer's disease. J. Alzheimers Dis. 1 (3), 139–145.
Panov, A.V., Gutekunst, C.A., Leavitt, B.R., Hayden, M.R., Burke, J.R., Strittmatter, W.J., Greenamyre, J.T., 2002. Early mitochondrial calcium defects in Huntington's disease are a direct effect of polyglutamines. Nat. Neurosci. 5 (8), 731–736. http://dx.doi.org/10.1038/nn884.
Paresce, D.M., Ghosh, R.N., Maxfield, F.R., 1996. Microglial cells internalize aggregates of the Alzheimer's disease amyloid beta-protein via a scavenger receptor. Neuron 17 (3), 553–565.
Park, J., Lee, S.B., Lee, S., Kim, Y., Song, S., Kim, S., et al., 2006. Mitochondrial dysfunction in Drosophila PINK1 mutants is complemented by parkin. Nature 441 (7097), 1157–1161. http://dx.doi.org/10.1038/nature04788.
Perry, T.L., Yong, V.W., 1986. Idiopathic Parkinson's disease, progressive supranuclear palsy and glutathione metabolism in the substantia nigra of patients. Neurosci. Lett. 67 (3), 269–274.
Phukan, J., Pender, N.P., Hardiman, O., 2007. Cognitive impairment in amyotrophic lateral sclerosis. Lancet Neurol. 6 (11), 994–1003. http://dx.doi.org/10.1016/S1474-4422(07)70265-X.
Pickford, F., Masliah, E., Britschgi, M., Lucin, K., Narasimhan, R., Jaeger, P.A., et al., 2008. The autophagy-related protein beclin 1 shows reduced expression in early Alzheimer disease and regulates amyloid beta accumulation in mice. J. Clin. Invest. 118 (6), 2190–2199. http://dx.doi.org/10.1172/JCI33585.
Polymenidou, M., Cleveland, D.W., 2012. Prion-like spread of protein aggregates in neurodegeneration. J. Exp. Med. 209 (5), 889–893. http://dx.doi.org/10.1084/jem.20120741.
Prahlad, V., Morimoto, R.I., 2009. Integrating the stress response: lessons for neurodegenerative diseases from *C. elegans*. Trends Cell Biol. 19 (2), 52–61. http://dx.doi.org/10.1016/j.tcb.2008.11.002.
Recasens, A., Dehay, B., Bove, J., Carballo-Carbajal, I., Dovero, S., Perez-Villalba, A., et al., 2014. Lewy body extracts from Parkinson disease brains trigger alpha-synuclein pathology and neurodegeneration in mice and monkeys. Ann. Neurol. 75 (3), 351–362. http://dx.doi.org/10.1002/ana.24066.
Reisberg, B., Doody, R., Stoffler, A., Schmitt, F., Ferris, S., Mobius, H.J., Memantine Study Group, 2003. Memantine in moderate-to-severe Alzheimer's disease. N. Engl. J. Med. 348 (14), 1333–1341. http://dx.doi.org/10.1056/NEJMoa013128.
Reynolds, A.D., Glanzer, J.G., Kadiu, I., Ricardo-Dukelow, M., Chaudhuri, A., Ciborowski, P., et al., 2008a. Nitrated alpha-synuclein-activated microglial profiling for Parkinson's disease. J. Neurochem. 104 (6), 1504–1525. http://dx.doi.org/10.1111/j.1471-4159.2007.05087.x.
Reynolds, A.D., Kadiu, I., Garg, S.K., Glanzer, J.G., Nordgren, T., Ciborowski, P., et al., 2008b. Nitrated alpha-synuclein and microglial neuroregulatory activities. J. Neuroimmune Pharmacol. 3 (2), 59–74. http://dx.doi.org/10.1007/s11481-008-9100-z.
Ringholz, G.M., Appel, S.H., Bradshaw, M., Cooke, N.A., Mosnik, D.M., Schulz, P.E., 2005. Prevalence and patterns of cognitive impairment in sporadic ALS. Neurology 65 (4), 586–590. http://dx.doi.org/10.1212/01.wnl.0000172911.39167.b6.
Rogers, S.L., Farlow, M.R., Doody, R.S., Mohs, R., Friedhoff, L.T., 1998. A 24-week, double-blind, placebo-controlled trial of donepezil in patients with Alzheimer's disease. Donepezil Study Group. Neurology 50 (1), 136–145.
Sanders, D.W., Kaufman, S.K., DeVos, S.L., Sharma, A.M., Mirbaha, H., Li, A., et al., 2014. Distinct tau prion strains propagate in cells and mice and define different tauopathies. Neuron 82 (6), 1271–1288. http://dx.doi.org/10.1016/j.neuron.2014.04.047.
Schapira, A.H., Cooper, J.M., Dexter, D., Jenner, P., Clark, J.B., Marsden, C.D., 1989. Mitochondrial complex I deficiency in Parkinson's disease. Lancet 1 (8649), 1269.
Schapira, A.H., Olanow, C.W., Greenamyre, J.T., Bezard, E., 2014. Slowing of neurodegeneration in Parkinson's disease and Huntington's disease: future therapeutic perspectives. Lancet 384 (9942), 545–555. http://dx.doi.org/10.1016/S0140-6736(14)61010-2.

Shin, J.Y., Fang, Z.H., Yu, Z.X., Wang, C.E., Li, S.H., Li, X.J., 2005. Expression of mutant huntingtin in glial cells contributes to neuronal excitotoxicity. J. Cell Biol. 171 (6), 1001–1012. http://dx.doi.org/10.1083/jcb.200508072.

Sian, J., Dexter, D.T., Lees, A.J., Daniel, S., Agid, Y., Javoy-Agid, F., et al., 1994. Alterations in glutathione levels in Parkinson's disease and other neurodegenerative disorders affecting basal ganglia. Ann. Neurol. 36 (3), 348–355. http://dx.doi.org/10.1002/ana.410360305.

Sofic, E., Lange, K.W., Jellinger, K., Riederer, P., 1992. Reduced and oxidized glutathione in the substantia nigra of patients with Parkinson's disease. Neurosci. Lett. 142 (2), 128–130. http://dx.doi.org/10.1016/0304-3940(92)90355-B.

Song, W., Chen, J., Petrilli, A., Liot, G., Klinglmayr, E., Zhou, Y., et al., 2011. Mutant huntingtin binds the mitochondrial fission GTPase dynamin-related protein-1 and increases its enzymatic activity. Nat. Med. 17 (3), 377–382. http://dx.doi.org/10.1038/nm.2313.

Spillantini, M.G., Schmidt, M.L., Lee, V.M., Trojanowski, J.Q., Jakes, R., Goedert, M., 1997. Alpha-synuclein in Lewy bodies. Nature 388 (6645), 839–840. http://dx.doi.org/10.1038/42166.

Tariot, P.N., Farlow, M.R., Grossberg, G.T., Graham, S.M., McDonald, S., Gergel, I., Memantine Study Group, 2004. Memantine treatment in patients with moderate to severe Alzheimer disease already receiving donepezil: a randomized controlled trial. JAMA 291 (3), 317–324. http://dx.doi.org/10.1001/jama.291.3.317.

Tashiro, Y., Urushitani, M., Inoue, H., Koike, M., Uchiyama, Y., Komatsu, M., et al., 2012. Motor neuron-specific disruption of proteasomes, but not autophagy, replicates amyotrophic lateral sclerosis. J. Biol. Chem. 287 (51), 42984–42994. http://dx.doi.org/10.1074/jbc.M112.417600.

Theodore, S., Cao, S., McLean, P.J., Standaert, D.G., 2008. Targeted overexpression of human alpha-synuclein triggers microglial activation and an adaptive immune response in a mouse model of Parkinson disease. J. Neuropathol. Exp. Neurol. 67 (12), 1149–1158. http://dx.doi.org/10.1097/NEN.0b013e31818e5e99.

Ton, T.G., Heckbert, S.R., Longstreth Jr., W.T., Rossing, M.A., Kukull, W.A., Franklin, G.M., et al., 2006. Nonsteroidal anti-inflammatory drugs and risk of Parkinson's disease. Mov Disord. 21 (7), 964–969. http://dx.doi.org/10.1002/mds.20856.

Tonoki, A., Kuranaga, E., Tomioka, T., Hamazaki, J., Murata, S., Tanaka, K., Miura, M., 2009. Genetic evidence linking age-dependent attenuation of the 26S proteasome with the aging process. Mol. Cell Biol. 29 (4), 1095–1106. http://dx.doi.org/10.1128/MCB.01227-08.

Wahner, A.D., Bronstein, J.M., Bordelon, Y.M., Ritz, B., 2008. Statin use and the risk of Parkinson disease. Neurology 70 (16 Pt 2), 1418–1422. http://dx.doi.org/10.1212/01.wnl.0000286942.14552.51.

Wang, X., Wang, W., Li, L., Perry, G., Lee, H.G., Zhu, X., 2014. Oxidative stress and mitochondrial dysfunction in Alzheimer's disease. Biochim. Biophys. Acta 1842 (8), 1240–1247. http://dx.doi.org/10.1016/j.bbadis.2013.10.015.

Watts, J.C., Giles, K., Oehler, A., Middleton, L., Dexter, D.T., Gentleman, S.M., et al., 2013. Transmission of multiple system atrophy prions to transgenic mice. Proc. Natl. Acad. Sci. U.S.A. 110 (48), 19555–19560. http://dx.doi.org/10.1073/pnas.1318268110.

Weintraub, D., Comella, C.L., Horn, S., 2008. Parkinson's disease—Part 1: Pathophysiology, symptoms, burden, diagnosis, and assessment. Am. J. Manag. Care 14 (2 Suppl.), S40–S48.

Winslow, A.R., Chen, C.W., Corrochano, S., Acevedo-Arozena, A., Gordon, D.E., Peden, A.A., et al., 2010. alpha-Synuclein impairs macroautophagy: implications for Parkinson's disease. J. Cell Biol. 190 (6), 1023–1037. http://dx.doi.org/10.1083/jcb.201003122.

Witgert, M., Salamone, A.R., Strutt, A.M., Jawaid, A., Massman, P.J., Bradshaw, M., et al., 2010. Frontal-lobe mediated behavioral dysfunction in amyotrophic lateral sclerosis. Eur. J. Neurol. 17 (1), 103–110. http://dx.doi.org/10.1111/j.1468-1331.2009.02801.x.

Wolozin, B., Kellman, W., Ruosseau, P., Celesia, G.G., Siegel, G., 2000. Decreased prevalence of Alzheimer disease associated with 3-hydroxy-3-methyglutaryl coenzyme A reductase inhibitors. Arch. Neurol. 57 (10), 1439–1443.

Wolozin, B., Wang, S.W., Li, N.C., Lee, A., Lee, T.A., Kazis, L.E., 2007. Simvastatin is associated with a reduced incidence of dementia and Parkinson's disease. BMC Med. 5, 20. http://dx.doi.org/10.1186/1741-7015-5-20.

Yamaguchi, O., Otsu, K., 2012. Role of autophagy in aging. J. Cardiovasc. Pharmacol. 60 (3), 242–247. http://dx.doi.org/10.1097/FJC.0b013e31824cc31c.

Yokota, T., Sugawara, K., Ito, K., Takahashi, R., Ariga, H., Mizusawa, H., 2003. Down regulation of DJ-1 enhances cell death by oxidative stress, ER stress, and proteasome inhibition. Biochem. Biophys. Res. Commun. 312 (4), 1342–1348. pii:S0006291X03024008.

Zetterstrom, P., Andersen, P.M., Brannstrom, T., Marklund, S.L., 2011. Misfolded superoxide dismutase-1 in CSF from amyotrophic lateral sclerosis patients. J. Neurochem. 117 (1), 91–99. http://dx.doi.org/10.1111/j.1471-4159.2011.07177.x.

Zhang, W., Wang, T., Pei, Z., Miller, D.S., Wu, X., Block, M.L., et al., 2005. Aggregated alpha-synuclein activates microglia: a process leading to disease progression in Parkinson's disease. FASEB J. 19 (6), 533–542. http://dx.doi.org/10.1096/fj.04-2751com.

CHAPTER

2

Cognitive and Functional Considerations in Alzheimer's Disease Diagnosis

M.A. Glenn, L.C. Mace, S.T. Moelter

OUTLINE

Alzheimer's disease (AD) is a neurodegenerative condition that primarily impacts older adults and manifests as a gradual onset and progressive worsening of cognitive and functional impairment (Alzheimer's Association, 2014; McKhann et al., 2011). It is the most common form of dementia, accounting for approximately 60–80% of cases (Alzheimer's Association, 2014). The most significant risk factor for AD is age, with individuals over the age of 65 bearing the greatest risk for developing the disease and comprising 5 million out of the 5.2 million affected persons in the United States (Hebert et al., 2013). A notable increase in the population of individuals over the age of 65 is occurring in the United States, because of the aging of the large generation of baby boomers (individuals born between 1946 and 1964), as well as innovations in medical knowledge and intervention strategies.

Drug Discovery Approaches for the Treatment of Neurodegenerative Disorders
http://dx.doi.org/10.1016/B978-0-12-802810-0.00002-7

By 2030, older adults over the age of 65 may constitute an estimated 20% of the total population in America, compared to 13% in 2010 (Vincent and Velkof, 2010). In turn, it is predicted that approximately 8.4 million of these individuals will have a diagnosis of AD, a 68% increase from 2014 prevalence rates. By 2050, the number of individuals with AD could reach 13.8 million, or three times the 2014 prevalence rate (Alzheimer's Association, 2014; Herbert et al., 2013). The aging population combined with increased awareness and improved diagnostic procedures will result in an exponential increase in the number of older adults diagnosed with AD in the upcoming decades. This is a looming public health crisis, especially given the debilitating nature of the disease, significant social and economic costs to society, and growing disparity between the number of geriatric health care specialists and those in need of care (Alzheimer's Association, 2014). Therefore it is imperative for investigators to continue to elucidate the clinical and pathological disease continuum, with the ultimate goal of uncovering a successful disease-modifying treatment for AD—the only major cause of death that, as of yet, has none (Sperling et al., 2013b).

Patients, caregivers, and even some health care providers, may mistake early symptoms of AD as normal aging. Common examples include labels such as "just old age," "just senility," or "old age depression" (Small et al., 1997). AD—or dementia—and old age, however, are not synonymous. Although change in cognitive performance may be expected with the aging process, progressively disabling functional and cognitive symptoms are not part of conventional aging models. When such symptoms do progress, older adults and their caregivers often rely on health care experts to provide symptom evaluation, health education, and referral for specialized care (Holzer et al., 2013). As such, good clinical practice and clinical trials management demand close attention to guidelines for how AD is diagnosed, especially as the potential for diagnosis is pushed to earlier disease stages. These early stages may predate the onset of even very early cognitive and functional decline (ie, "preclinical AD") and incorporate pathophysiological [eg, amyloid imaging, cerebrospinal fluid (CSF) Aβ and CSF tau] and topographic [eg, magnetic resonance imaging (MRI), fluorodeoxyglucose-positron emission tomography, and single photon emission computed tomography] biomarkers. This chapter provides an overview of current diagnostic approaches to AD and offers specific examples of how particular cognitive and functional measures may be implemented to aid in diagnosis.

DIAGNOSIS OF ALZHEIMER'S DISEASE

In a living person, the diagnosis of AD is largely based on the presence of *cognitive deficits* in two or more domains severe enough to *interfere with normal daily functioning*. These standards are well known in the AD community as the National Institute of Neurological and Communicative Disorders and Stroke–Alzheimer's Disease and Related Disorders Association (NINCDS-ADRDA) criteria (McKhann et al., 1984). These criteria have been very successful—standing as the primary AD diagnostic guidelines for more than a quarter century and achieving sensitivity for detecting AD greater than 80% and specificity distinguishing AD from other conditions of approximately 70% (Knopman et al., 2001). Lower specificity is expected because AD shares clinical features with other forms of dementia, including vascular dementia, dementia with Lewy bodies, and behavioral variant frontotemporal dementia.

In response to the more recent advances in our understanding of and ability to detect the pathophysiological changes that occur in the clinical spectrum of AD, a joint National Institute on Aging/Alzheimer's Association (NIA-AA) Work Group revised the NINCDS-ADRDA criteria for Probable AD in 2011. In that revision, the criteria for Probable AD were essentially unchanged—leaving in place Probable AD requirements for evidence of functional decline and cognitive performance below normative expectations. The NIA-AA guidelines added diagnostic criteria that emphasized the need for evidence of gradual onset and progression of cognitive symptoms, and recognized variations in presentation as either amnestic or non-amnestic variants. Furthermore, clinicians and scientists applying the criteria are expected to confirm the absence of core symptom criteria from other dementia diagnoses, such as vascular dementia or Lewy body disease, to specify the diagnosis (McKhann et al., 2011).

DIAGNOSIS OF MILD COGNITIVE IMPAIRMENT

Recent NIA-AA working group guidelines (Albert et al., 2011) have also recalibrated the diagnostic process for mild cognitive impairment (MCI). These guidelines recognize the presence of significant cognitive impairment that is beyond what is expected in normal aging, but has not yet caused significant functional decline. The NIA-AA MCI diagnosis is meant to identify people who have a high likelihood of progressing to Probable AD, with the presence of AD pathophysiology (ie, *MCI due to underlying AD pathology*). Core clinical criteria for the diagnosis of MCI includes (1) concern regarding a change in memory or cognition by the patient or an informant; (2) impairment in one or more cognitive domains greater than expected for age and education, often including memory; (3) preservation of independence in functional abilities or very mild functional impairment; and (4) general cognition and functional performance must be sufficiently preserved such that a diagnosis of AD is not likely. Furthermore, it should be emphasized that the cognitive diagnostic requirements of MCI require evidence of intraindividual change. Therefore serial evaluations are optimal, but may not be feasible in some circumstances (Albert et al., 2011).

Functional Measures and Alzheimer's Disease and Mild Cognitive Impairment Diagnosis

As indicated in the NINCDS-ADRDA and NIA-AA criteria, functional assessment remains an indispensable component of AD evaluations for clinical and research purposes. Functional evaluations are necessary to differentiate normal aging from MCI and MCI from AD, and to track AD progression (Desai et al., 2004). While cognitive test performance is a necessary part of the diagnostic process, functional measures may have higher ecological validity, better reveal decline or gain from previous levels of ability, and be less sensitive to the effects of education and premorbid intelligence (Jorm, 2003; Morris, 1997). Functional assessment is improved by the careful selection of instruments that guide the evaluation.

The Clinical Dementia Rating Scale (CDR), a commonly used dementia staging instrument, employs a semistructured interview to collect detailed information from both patient and informant regarding the patient's ability to function in various domains. The instrument incorporates items that measure the ability to perform both instrumental activities of daily living and basic activities of daily living, as well as cognitively mediated tasks. The CDR offers a global characterization of everyday functions that may be affected by neurodegenerative disease (Morris, 1997; Hughes et al., 1982), though the value of global characterizations during the assessment of MCI has been questioned (Chang et al., 2011).

Recent evidence suggests that the wider range of scores available when CDR sum of boxes (CDR-SB) scoring is employed may provide a more refined analysis of subtle changes associated with very mild disease or evaluating changes between stages in later AD (Lynch et al., 2006; O'Bryant, 2011). This improved sensitivity to subtle changes suggests that the CDR-SB may be suitable as a coprimary endpoint in clinical trials (Cedarbaum et al., 2012; Coley et al., 2011). In addition, functional decline, as measured by the CDR-SB, is associated with abnormal levels of CSF biomarkers of AD (Okonkwo et al., 2011; Snider et al., 2009). Such findings suggest that scores on the CDR are sensitive to and reflective of the accumulation of AD biomarkers and pathology.

Although the CDR is the most well-known, well-studied, dementia staging instrument (Rikkert et al., 2011), the scale is not without limitations. Primary concerns include a lengthy rater certification process, 30-min administration time, and clinical judgment required during both administration and scoring (Morris, 1997). The Dementia Severity Rating Scale (DSRS) (also known as the Functional Rating Scale) is a brief informant-rated, multiple-choice questionnaire made up of 12 items that measure functional abilities and parallels CDR content (Clark and Ewbank, 1996). The DSRS requires minimal staff training to administer, takes 5 min to complete, and can be completed via mail, online, or phone. Similar to the CDR-SB, the DSRS incorporates a broad range of scores, making this instrument useful for quantifying all levels of functional impairment, and permitting the detection of fine increments of change over time (Xie et al., 2009). DSRS total scores of 0–11 may be used as a screening boundary as scores in that range have predicted CDR-SB scores ≤4, suggesting no or only very mild impairment (Moelter et al., 2014) and are consistent with CDR global scores of 0–0.5, a range that appears consistent with the preclinical or MCI phase of AD. A DSRS score of 10 or 11 may be optimal for distinguishing the transition from MCI to AD (Moelter et al., 2014; Roalf et al., 2012). While there are other functional measures that may be applied when arriving at a diagnostic decision, CDR-Global, CDR-SB, and DSRS scores are common functional assessment measures for the classification of Alzheimer's disease, mild cognitive impairment and, healthy aging.

Cognitive Measures and Alzheimer's Disease and Mild Cognitive Impairment Diagnosis

Episodic memory impairment is the hallmark symptom of AD and typical among the earliest detectable signs of the disease (Bateman et al., 2012; Rentz et al., 2013; Salmon, 2012). Indeed, CSF biomarkers of AD (ie, reduced CSF Aβ42 and/or increased CSF tau) have been associated with reduced global cognitive functioning in individuals with MCI. The most severe disruptions, however, have been observed in memory among individuals with both abnormal CSF tau *and* Aβ42 (Nordlund et al., 2008). When comparing both MRI and CSF biomarkers among participants with MCI and AD, episodic memory was associated with cortical thickness in 7 of 10 brain regions associated with AD (Fjell et al., 2008). This finding fits well with results of PET neuroimaging of β-amyloid cortical burden, measured by Pittsburgh

Compound B (C-PIB), showing that memory performance is associated with C-PIB binding, particularly in nondemented, healthy, and MCI older adults (Pike et al., 2007). In a later meta-analytic study, Hedden et al. (2013) assessed the relationship between amyloid deposition and neuropsychological functioning in 3495 cognitively normal older adults across 34 studies, finding that memory had the strongest and most consistent relationship with amyloid, suggesting that memory performance is the first to change, even in the very earliest stages of AD (ie, AD-P).

Global cognitive abilities, and memory performance in particular, appear aligned with the pathophysiological progression of AD; as such the NINCDS-ADRDA and NIA-AA diagnostic criteria emphasize cognitive assessment as a critical component of most AD evaluations. For many investigators and clinicians, a brief cognitive screening metric will be among the earliest diagnostic steps. We describe here two potential measures. First, the *Telephone Interview for Cognitive Status Modified* (TICSm) is an instrument with established reliability and validity for telephone screening for cognitive impairment associated with mild cognitive impairment and AD (Brandt et al., 1988; Knopman et al., 2010). The TICSm provides a total score from 0 to 50 with higher performances indicating more intact cognitive ability. Education adjusted cutoff scores for distinguishing MCI participants from normal controls are provided by Knopman et al. Such cut scores offer clinicians the opportunity to make decisions appropriate to the clinical or research study context. For example, an education-adjusted TICSm cutoff score of ≤35 may be used to identify those who are likely to have MCI. Subjects who score ≥36 may be excluded, because these participants are unlikely to meet diagnostic criteria for MCI. This approach will capture 93% of MCI/AD (ie, sensitivity) but will necessarily include healthy participants who will not later meet criteria for MCI (ie, lower specificity). An education adjusted TICSm cutoff score of ≤27 may be used to exclude subjects with high likelihood of dementia.

An alternative to the TICSm for in-person cognitive screening is the *Montreal Cognitive Assessment* (MoCA) (Nasreddine et al., 2005). The MoCA is a 30-point test with higher scores indicating better performance. The MoCA was developed to detect the earliest cognitive symptoms of AD when evidence began to accumulate that the widely used mini-mental state examination (MMSE) was not sufficiently sensitive to early cognitive changes. If judged by its assimilation as a preferred cognitive screening metric since its introduction in 2005, the MoCA is unquestionably a success, having been used in more than 200 published studies, multiple countries, and many clinical settings beyond memory disorders clinics (see "references" at www.mocatest.org). The MoCA is superior to the MMSE for detecting subtle cognitive impairment associated with onset of MCI (Roalf et al., 2012). MoCA scores of 25 showed optimal diagnostic classification for distinguishing between healthy aging and MCI, while a score of 19 best marked the transition between MCI and AD. Roalf et al. also showed that combining the MoCA or MMSE cut points with a functional metric, such as the DSRS, improved diagnostic accuracy by 9–12% for distinguishing between healthy aging and MCI.

Following preliminary screening, follow-up with a more comprehensive neuropsychological battery is often required. Comprehensive batteries characterize neuropsychological function in multiple domains and are a core component of a sound diagnostic approach (eg, Bennett et al., 2006; Morris et al., 1989). Cognitive assessment is necessary to determine whether memory is impaired and which, if any, other cognitive domains are disrupted. For example, most MCI criteria emphasize that the diagnosis of MCI requires no or very mild functional impairment (CDR 0–0.5) *but* cognitive impairment greater than expected for age and education in at least one cognitive domain as objectively measured (Albert et al., 2011; Petersen et al., 1999, 2014; Alzheimer's Disease Neuroimaging Initiative 2 (ADNI2) 2007/2008). Thus in MCI, global cognition *and* functional performance are sufficiently preserved to preclude a diagnosis of AD. Episodic memory measures, such as paired associate learning and free and cued list learning, establish the AD clinical phenotype necessary for sound diagnostic decision making (see Dubois et al., 2014). The Procedures Manual defines abnormal memory function as a score below the education-adjusted cutoff on the Logical Memory II subscale (Delayed Paragraph Recall) from the Wechsler Memory Scale—Revised.

DIAGNOSIS OF PRECLINICAL ALZHEIMER'S DISEASE

The continuum of AD stages has expanded to include a preclinical phase (AD-P) that precedes the subsequent stages of MCI and AD. During AD-P, cognitive and functional abilities remain within normal limits (Jack and Holtzman, 2013; Salmon, 2012; Sperling et al., 2011a,b). AD-P emerged because a substantial portion of the AD pathological processes begins one to two decades, or more, prior to the emergence of cognitive and functional impairment; approximately one-third of cognitively normal older adults harbor substantial levels of AD pathology (Braak et al., 2011; Fagan, 2014; Landau et al., 2012). Thus it is posited that the preclinical phase of AD may be the optimal time to intervene with disease-modifying treatments to prevent or postpone the onset of cognitive decline.

Furthermore, the lack of success thus far in clinical trials of pharmacotherapies for AD may be because of the recruitment of subjects at the stages of MCI or AD dementia, when the pathology of the disease has already damaged the brain irreparably (Cash et al., 2014; Golde et al., 2011; Sperling et al., 2013a,b). Also in early clinical trials technology was not advanced enough to enable biomarker-based verification of AD pathology in study participants, perhaps leading to the inclusion of individuals with other underlying causes of cognitive changes (Lemere, 2013; Vassar, 2014). As such, secondary prevention trials (ie, Anti-Amyloid Treatment in Asymptomatic Alzheimer's study "A4 study") enroll cognitively normal older adults deemed to be in the preclinical phase of AD based on biomarker evidence of AD pathology, specifically elevated levels of amyloid on positron emission tomography (PET) (Donohue et al., 2014; Vassar, 2014; Rentz et al., 2013).

According to NIA-AA guidelines, AD-P occurs in three stages that are ordered in terms of the progression of biomarker-based disease pathology and increased likelihood of conversion to MCI or AD (Knopman et al., 2012; Sperling et al., 2011a,b; Vos et al., 2013). The first stage is marked by abnormalities in biomarkers of β-amyloid, as measured in the CSF or on PET imaging, indicating increased accumulation of brain amyloid. The second stage of preclinical AD is marked by abnormalities in biomarkers of neurodegeneration, including the so-called "downstream" pathological events of AD, such as accumulation of neurofibrillary tangles as measured by CSF or PET, synaptic dysfunction as measured by functional neuroimaging, or cerebral atrophy as measured by structural neuroimaging. In the third stage of AD-P, the accumulation of biomarker abnormalities is believed to reach a threshold at which the onset of subtle cognitive deterioration begins to occur (Sperling et al., 2011a,b; Knopman et al., 2012).

With the prominence of biomarker-based diagnostic approaches, neuropsychological techniques that can reliably detect cognitive decline have also started to emerge. Cognitive decline from baseline on standard neuropsychological measures may be detectable 7–18 years prior to a diagnosis of AD dementia, with an increased likelihood of detection occurring approximately 3–4 years prior to a diagnosis of MCI (Grober et al., 2008; Howieson et al., 2008; Rajan et al., 2015; Salmon, 2012). A growing number of studies have found that cognitively normal older adults with biomarkers of AD, or those examined retrospectively with postmortem AD histopathology, have a higher likelihood of demonstrating cognitive decline on neuropsychological measures than those without such pathological indices (Bennett et al., 2012; Sperling et al., 2014).

FUTURE DIRECTIONS FOR DIAGNOSIS

Currently, there are two major definitions that dictate diagnostic criteria for AD. The International Working Group (IWG) was the first to develop guidelines that moved diagnosis of AD from a clinically expressed disorder with cognitive, behavioral, and neuropsychiatric features to a biologically expressed disorder (Dubois et al., 2007, 2010, 2014). The IWG guidelines are consistent with, but not the same as, the guidelines developed by NIA-AA (Jack et al., 2011) and a number of papers highlight the differences (eg, Cummings, 2012; Morris et al., 2012).

Some of the major differences between these definitions can be found in how they determine what merits an AD diagnosis. The IWG suggests that AD refers only to the symptomatic stage and thus requires objective impairment in memory and the presence of biomarker abnormality. The IWG defines episodic memory impairment as the core cognitive risk factor for AD, while the NIA-AA allows for impairment in memory and/or nonmemory domains such as language, visuospatial, and executive abilities. In the IWG guidelines, the absence of memory impairment classifies the individual as either normal, asymptomatic at risk for AD (with a positive biomarker), or presymptomatic AD (with the presence of a genetic determinant of AD) (Dubois et al., 2014). In this way, the MCI diagnostic category is abandoned by the IWG criteria, which instead uses the concept of "typical" AD to characterize symptomatic individuals with a positive pathophysiological or topographic marker of AD (Cummings, 2012; Dubois et al., 2014). A current limitation of the IWG approach may be the loss of the MCI option in clinical contexts where biomarkers are not available.

In summary, multiple diagnostic procedures are confusing to clinicians, scientists, patients, and families and carry substantial risk of slowing progress in diagnostic and treatment development. Recommendations to harmonize the IWG and NIA-AA guidelines (Morris et al., 2014) emphasize that (1) AD is a brain disorder regardless of clinical status; (2) symptomatic AD represents a clinically expressed disorder that spans from very mild (ie, MCI to AD) to severe; (3) biomarkers are currently not required for clinical diagnosis but may be used to support diagnosis when they are available; and (4) amnestic/memory cognitive impairment is the typical presentation of AD but the diagnosis can be made in the absence of memory impairment, especially with biomarker support. Bringing together these approaches is one of the most pressing of current challenges in AD diagnosis.

References

Albert, M.S., DeKosky, S.T., Dickson, D., et al., 2011. The diagnosis of mild cognitive impairment due to Alzheimer disease: recommendations from the national institute on aging-Alzheimer's association workgroups on diagnostic guidelines for Alzheimer's disease. Alzheimers Dement. 7, 270–279.

Alzheimer's Disease Neuroimaging Initiative 2, 2007/2008. ADNI2 Procedures Manual. http://adni.loni.usc.edu/wp-content/uploads/2008/07/adni2-procedures-manual.pdf.

Alzheimer's Association, 2014. 2014 Alzheimer's disease facts and figures. Alzheimers Dement. 10 (2), e47–92. Retrieved from: http://www.ncbi.nlm.nih.gov/pubmed/24818261.

Bateman, R.J., Xiong, C., Benzinger, T.L.S., Fagan, A.M., Goate, A., Fox, N.C., Marcus, D.S., Morris, J.C., 2012. Clinical and biomarker changes in dominantly inherited Alzheimer's disease. N. Engl. J. Med. 367 (9), 795–804.

Bennett, D.A., Schneider, J.A., Aggarwal, N.T., et al., 2006. Decision rules guiding the clinical diagnosis of Alzheimer's disease in two community-based cohort studies compared to standard practice in a clinic-based cohort study. Methods Neuroepidemiol. 27, 169–176.

Bennett, D.A., Wilson, R.S., Boyle, P.A., Buchman, A.S., Schneider, J.A., 2012. Relation of neuropathology to cognition in persons without cognitive impairment. Annals of Neurology 72 (4), 599–609.

Braak, H., Thal, D.R., Ghebremedhin, E., Del Tredici, K., 2011. Stages of the pathologic process in Alzheimer disease: age categories from 1 to 100 years. J. Neuropathol. Exp. Neurol. 70 (11), 960–969.

Brandt, J., Spencer, M., Folstein, M., 1988. The telephone interview for cognitive status. Neuropsychiatry Neuropsychol. Behav. Neurol. 1, 111–117.

Cash, D.M., Rohrer, J.D., Ryan, N.S., Ourselin, S., Fox, N.C., 2014. Imaging endpoints for clinical trials in Alzheimer's disease. Alzheimer's Research & Therapy 6 (9), 87.

Cedarbaum, J.M., Jaros, M., Hernandez, C., et al., May 31, 2012. Rationale for use of the Clinical Dementia Rating Sum of Boxes as a primary outcome measure for Alzheimer's disease clinical trials. Alzheimers Dement. 9.

Chang, Y.L., Bondi, M.W., McEvoy, L.K., et al., February 15, 2011. Global clinical dementia rating of 0.5 in MCI masks variability related to level of function. Neurology 76 (7), 652–659.

Clark, C.M., Ewbank, D.C., Spring 1996. Performance of the dementia severity rating scale: a caregiver questionnaire for rating severity in Alzheimer disease. Alzheimer Dis. Assoc. Disord. 10 (1), 31–39.

Coley, N., Andrieu, S., Jaros, M., Weiner, M., Cedarbaum, J., Vellas, B., November 2011. Suitability of the Clinical Dementia Rating-Sum of Boxes as a single primary endpoint for Alzheimer's disease trials. Alzheimers Dement. 7 (6), 602–610 e602.

Cummings, J., 2012. Alzheimer's disease diagnostic criteria: practical applications. Alzheimer's Research & Therapy 4, 35.

Desai, A.K., Grossberg, G.T., Sheth, D.N., 2004. Activities of daily living in patients with dementia: clinical relevance, methods of assessment and effects of treatment. CNS Drugs 18 (13), 853–875.

Donohue, M.C., Sperling, R.A., Salmon, D.P., Rentz, D.M., Raman, R., Thomas, R.G., Weiner, M., Aisen, P.S., 2014. The preclinical Alzheimer cognitive composite measuring amyloid-related decline. JAMA Neurol. 71 (8), 961–970.

Dubois, B., Feldman, H.H., Jacova, C., et al., 2007. Research criteria for the diagnosis of Alzheimer's disease: revising the NINCDS-ADRDA criteria. Lancet Neurol. 6, 734–746.

Dubois, B., Feldman, H., Jacova, C., et al., 2010. Revising the definition of Alzheimer's disease: a new lexicon. Lancet Neurol. 9, 1118–1127.

Dubois, B., Feldman, H.H., Jacova, C., Hampel, H., Molinuevo, J.L., Blennow, K., DeKosky, S.T., Gauthier, S., Selkoe, D., Bateman, R., et al., 2014. Advancing research diagnostic criteria for Alzheimer's disease: the IWG-2 criteria. Lancet Neurol. 13 (6), 614–629. http://www.ncbi.nlm.nih.gov/pubmed/24849862.

Fagan, A., 2014. CSF biomarkers of Alzheimer's disease: impact on disease concept, diagnosis, and clinical trial design. Adv. Geriatr. 2014, 1–14. http://dx.doi.org/10.1155/2014/302712.

Fjell, A.M., Walhovd, K.B., Amlien, I., Bjornerud, A., Reinvang, I., Gjerstad, L., Cappelen, T., Willoch, F., Due-Tonnessen, P., Grambaite, R., Skinningsrud, A., Stenset, V., Fladby, T., 2008. Morphometric changes in the episodic memory network and tau pathologic features correlate with memory performance in patients with mild cognitive impairment. Am. J. Neuroradiol. 29, 1183–1189.

Golde, T.E., Schneider, L.S., Koo, E.H., 2011. Anti-AB therapeutics in Alzheimer's disease: the need for a paradigm shift. Neuron 69 (2), 203–213.

Grober, E., Hall, C.B., Lipton, R.B., Zonderman, A.B., Resnick, S.M., Kawas, C., 2008. Memory impairment, executive dysfunction, and intellectual decline in preclinical Alzheimer's disease. J. Int. Neuropsychol. Soc. 14 (2), 266–278.

Hebert, L.E., Weuve, J., Scherr, P.A., Evans, D.A., 2013. Alzheimer disease in the United States (2010–2050) estimated using the 2010 census. Neurology 80 (19), 1778–1783. http://dx.doi.org/10.1212/WNL.0b013e31828726f5.

Hedden, T., Oh, H., Younger, A.P., Patel, T.A., 2013. Meta-analysis of amyloid-cognition relations in cognitively normal older adults. Neurology 80 (14), 1341–1348.

Holzer, S., Warner, J.P., Iliffe, S., 2013. Diagnosis and management of the patient with suspected dementia in primary care. Drugs Aging 30 (9), 667–676. http://dx.doi.org/10.1007/s40266-013-0098-4.

Howieson, D.B., Carlson, N.E., Moore, M.M., Wasserman, D., Abendroth, C.D., Payne-Murphey, J., Kaye, J.A., 2008. Progressive impairment on neuropsychological tasks in a longitudinal study of preclinical Alzheimer's disease. J. Int. Neuropsychol. Soc. 14 (2), 192–198.

Hughes, C.P., Berg, L., Danziger, W.L., Coben, L.A., Martin, R.L., June 1982. A new clinical scale for the staging of dementia. Br. J. Psychiatry 140, 566–572.

Jack, C.R., Albert, M.S., Knopman, D.S., McKhann, G.M., Sperling, R.a, Carrillo, M.C., et al., 2011. Introduction to the recommendations from the National Institute on Aging-Alzheimer's Association workgroups on diagnostic guidelines for Alzheimer's disease. Alzheimers Dement. 7 (3), 257–262. http://dx.doi.org/10.1016/j.jalz.2011.03.004.

Jack, C.R., Holtzman, D.M., 2013. Biomarker modeling of Alzheimer's disease. Neuron 80 (6), 1347–1358.

Jorm, A.F., June 2003. The value of informant reports for assessment and prediction of dementia. J. Am. Geriatr. Soc. 51 (6), 881–882.

Knopman, D.S., DeKosky, S.T., Cummings, J.L., Chuit, H., Corey-Bloom, J., Relkin, N., et al., 2001. Practice parameter: diagnosis of dementia (an evidence-based review). Neurology 56, 1143–1153.

Knopman, D.S., Jack, C.R., Wiste, H.J., Weigand, S.D., Vemuri, P., Lowe, V., Kantarci, K., et al., 2012. Short-term clinical outcomes for stages of NIA-AA preclinical Alzheimer disease. Neurology 78 (20), 1576–1582.

Knopman, D.S., Jack, C.R., Wiste, H.J., Weigand, S.D., Vemuri, P., Kantarci, K., et al., 2013. Brain injury biomarkers are not dependent on β-amyloid in normal elderly. Ann. Neurol. 73 (4), 472–480.

Knopman, D.S., Roberts, R.O., Geda, Y.E., Pankratz, V.S., Christianson, T.J.H., Petersen, R.C., Rocca, W.A., 2010. Validation of the telephone interview for cognitive status-modified in subjects with normal cognition, mild cognitive impairment, or dementia. Neuroepidemiology 34, 34–42.

Landau, S.M., Mintun, M.A., Joshi, A.D., Koeppe, R.A., Petersen, R.C., Aisen, P.S., Weiner, M.W., Jagust, W.J., 2012. Amyloid deposition, hypometabolism, and longitudinal cognitive decline. Ann. Neurol. 72 (4), 578–586.

Lemere, C.A., 2013. Immunotherapy for Alzheimer's disease: hoops and hurdles. Mol. Neurodegener. 8 (36), 1–6.

Lynch, C.A., Walsh, C., Blanco, A., et al., 2006. The clinical dementia rating sum of box score in mild dementia. Dement. Geriatr. Cogn. Disord. 21 (1), 40–43.

McKhann, G., Drachman, D., Folstein, M., Katzman, R., Price, D., Stadlan, E.M., July 1984. Clinical diagnosis of Alzheimer's disease: report of the NINCDS-ADRDA Work Group under the auspices of department of health and human services task force on Alzheimer's disease. Neurology 34 (7), 939–944.

McKhann, G.M., Knopman, D.S., Chertkow, H., et al., May 2011. The diagnosis of dementia due to Alzheimer's disease: recommendations from the National Institute on Aging-Alzheimer's Association workgroups on diagnostic guidelines for Alzheimer's disease. Alzheimers Dement. 7 (3), 263–269.

Moelter, S.T., Glenn, M.A., Xie, S.X., Chittams, J., Clark, C.M., Watson, M., Arnold, S.E., 2014. The dementia severity rating scale predicts clinical dementia rating sum of boxes scores. Alzheimer Dis. Assoc. Disord. 1.

Morris, J.C., Heyman, A., Mohs, R.C., Hugues, J.P., van Belle, G., Fillenbaum, G., Mellits, E.D., Clark, C., 1989. The Consortium to Establish a Registry for Alzheimer's Disease (CERAD). Part I. Clinical and neuropsychological assessment of Alzheimer's disease. Neurology 39 (9), 1159–1165.

Morris, J.C., 1997. Clinical dementia rating: a reliable and valid diagnostic and staging measure for dementia of the Alzheimer type. Int. Psychogeriatr. 9 (Suppl. 1), 173–176 discussion 177–178.

Morris, J.C., 2012. Revised criteria for mild cognitive impairment may compromise the diagnosis of Alzheimer Disease Dementia. Arch. Neurol. 69 (6), 700–708.

Nasreddine, Z.S., Phillips, N.A., Bedirian, V., Charbonneau, S., Whitehead, V., Collin, I., Cummings, J.L., Chertkow, H., 2005. The Montreal Cognitive Assessment (MoCA): a brief screening tool for mild cognitive impairment. J. Am. Geriatr. Soc. 53 (4), 695–699.

Nordlund, A., Rolstad, S., Klang, O., Lind, K., Pedersen, M., Blennow, K., Edman, A., Hansen, S., Wallin, A., 2008. Episodic memory and speed/attention deficits are associated with Alzheimer-typical CSF abnormalities in MCI. J. Int. Neuropsychol. Soc. 14, 582–590.

Okonkwo, O.C., Mielke, M.M., Griffith, H.R., et al., January 2011. Cerebrospinal fluid profiles and prospective course and outcome in patients with amnestic mild cognitive impairment. Arch. Neurol. 68 (1), 113–119.

Petersen, R.C., Caracciolo, B., Brayne, C., Gauthier, S., Jelic, V., Fratiglioni, L., 2014. Mild cognitive impairment: a concept in evolution. (Key Symposium). J. Intern. Med. 275, 214–228.

Petersen, R.C., Smith, G.E., Waring, S.C., Ivnik, R.J., Tangalos, E.G., Kokmen, E., March 1999. Mild cognitive impairment: clinical characterization and outcome. Arch. Neurol. 56 (3), 303–308.

Pike, K.E., Savage, G., Villemagne, V.L., Ng, S., Moss, S.A., Maruff, P., Mathis, C.A., Klunk, W.E., Masters, C.L., Rowe, C.C., 2007. β-amyloid imaging and memory in non-demented individuals: evidence for preclinical Alzheimer's disease. Brain 130, 2837–2844.

Rajan, K., Wilson, R., Weueve, J., Barnes, L.L., Evans, D.A., 2015. Cognitive impairment 18 years before clinical diagnosis of Alzheimer disease dementia. Neurology 85 (10), 898–904.

Rentz, D.M., Parra Rodriguez, M.A., Amariglia, R., Stern, Y., Sperling, R., Ferris, S., 2013. Promising developments in neuropsychological approaches for the detection of preclinical Alzheimer's disease: a selective review. Alzheimers Res. Ther. 5 (6), 1–10.

Rikkert, M.G., Tona, K.D., Janssen, L., et al., August 2011. Validity, reliability, and feasibility of clinical staging scales in dementia: a systematic review. Am. J. Alzheimers Dis. Other Demen. 26 (5), 357–365.

Roalf, D.R., Moberg, P.J., Xie, S.X., Wolk, D.A., Moelter, S.T., Arnold, S.E., 2012. Comparative accuracies of two common screening instruments for the classification of Alzheimer's disease, mild cognitive impairment, and healthy aging. Alzheimer's & Dementia 9 (5), 529–537.

Salmon, D.P., 2012. Neuropsychological features of mild cognitive impairment and preclinical Alzheimer's disease. Curr. Top. Behav. Neurosci. 10, 187–212.

Small, G.W., Rabins, P.V., Barry, P.P., Buckholtz, N.S., DeKosky, S.T., Ferris, S.H., Finkel, S.I., Gwyther, L.P., Khachaturian, Z.S., Lebowitz, B.D., McRae, T.D., Morris, J.C., Oakley, F., Schneider, L.S., Streim, J.E., Sunderland, T., Teri, L.A., Tune, L.E., 1997. Diagnosis and treatment of Alzheimer disease and related disorders. Consensus statement of the American Association for Geriatric Psychiatry, the Alzheimer's Association, and the American Geriatrics Society. JAMA 278 (16), 1363–1371.

Snider, B.J., Fagan, A.M., Roe, C., et al., May 2009. Cerebrospinal fluid biomarkers and rate of cognitive decline in very mild dementia of the Alzheimer type. Arch. Neurol. 66 (5), 638–645.

Sperling, R.A., Aisen, P.S., Beckett, L.A., 2011a. Toward defining the preclinical stages of Alzheimer's disease: recommendations from the national institute on aging-Alzheimer's association workgroups on diagnostic guidelines for Alzheimer's disease. Alzheimers Dement. 2011 (7), 280–292.

Sperling, R.A., Jack Jr., C.R., Aisen, P.S., 2011b. Testing the right target and the right drug at the right stage. Sci. Transl. Med. 3 (111), 111cm33.

Sperling, R.A., Johnson, K.A., Doraiswamy, P.M., Reiman, E.M., Fleisher, A.S., Sabbagh, M.N., Sadowsky, C.H., et al., 2013a. Amyloid deposition detected with florbetapir F 18 (^{18}F-AV-45) is related to lower episodic memory performance in clinically normal older individuals. Neurobiol. Aging 34 (3), 822–831.

Sperling, R.A., Karlawish, J., Johnson, K.A., 2013b. Preclinical Alzheimer disease-the challenges ahead. Nat. Rev. Neurol. 9 (1), 54–58.

Sperling, R.A., Mormino, E., Johnson, K., 2014. The evolution of preclinical Alzheimer's disease: implications for prevention trials. Neuron 84 (3), 608–622.

Vassar, R., 2014. BACE1 inhibitor drugs in clinical trials for Alzheimer's disease. Alzheimers Res. Ther. 6 (9), 1.

Vincent, G.K., Velkof, V.A., 2010. The Next Four Decades: The Older Population in the United States: 2010 to 2050. Census Bureau, Washington, DC, US.

Vos, S.J.B., Xiong, C., Visser, P.J., Jasielec, M.S., Hassenstab, J., Grant, E.A., Cairns, N.J., Fagan, A.M., 2013. Preclinical Alzheimer's disease and its outcome: a longitudinal cohort study. Lancet Neurol. 12 (10), 957–965.

Xie, S.X., Ewbank, D.C., Chittams, J., Karlawish, J.H., Arnold, S.E., Clark, C.M., July–September 2009. Rate of decline in Alzheimer disease measured by a dementia severity rating scale. Alzheimer Dis. Assoc. Disord. 23 (3), 268–274.

CHAPTER

3

National Plan and Resources to Address Alzheimer's Disease

M. Alamri, A. Adejare

OUTLINE

Drug Discovery Approaches for the Treatment of Neurodegenerative Disorders
http://dx.doi.org/10.1016/B978-0-12-802810-0.00003-9

Alzheimer's disease (AD) remains a major health concern for the public and care providers alike. With debilitating effects on patients and increasing costs for health care, AD continues to attract more attention. The demographics also show that cases of AD will only continue to increase in the foreseeable future unless drastic measures are taken with immediate effects. The major nonprofit driving force against AD is undoubtedly the National Institutes of Health (NIH, www.nih.gov), mainly the National Institute of Mental Health (NIMH, www.nimh.nih.gov), the National Institute of Neurological Disorders and Stroke (NINDS, www.ninds.nih.gov), and the National Institute on Aging (NIA, www.nia.nih.gov). While these institutes are well known for addressing AD through research funding and providing various related services and infrastructures, other less known efforts, initiatives, and associations are also doing their part in fighting AD. Given the huge AD market, many private efforts are also ongoing with companies searching for different treatment modalities. Many public–private partnerships are also being formed. In this chapter we list important efforts, centers, infrastructures, and resources that provide support against AD, ranging from research funding and services all the way to basic information for patients and care providers. Individual investigators, both nonprofit and for-profit institutions, may find this chapter useful in understanding the National Plan and addressing resource needs.

The chapter begins with efforts by the Department of Health and Human Services under which NIH falls and which crafted the National Plan, to efforts by NIH including summits, centers, and studies funded to consortia, which range from international to state levels to associations, advocacy groups, and finally social media. Apart from the Arizona consortium, which claims to be the state model, the focus is on national resources, though each state and county may also have programs. Appropriate links and/or references are provided for each resource for more information as desired.

NATIONAL ALZHEIMER'S PROJECT ACT

National Alzheimer's Project Act (NAPA) was established in 2012 by the US Department of Health and Human Services to:

1. Create the National Plan to overcome AD.
2. Improve coordination of AD research and services between federal agencies.

3. Develop treatments to prevent or reverse AD.
4. Improve diagnosis and care for AD patients.
5. Fight AD globally by coordinating with international agencies/organizations.

NAPA is guided by three principles:

1. Optimize and coordinate existing resources.
2. Improve public–private partnerships.
3. Innovate and transform approaches to Alzheimer's Disease-Related Dementias (ADRD) treatment.

NAPA has five ambitious goals:

1. Prevent and treat AD by 2025.
2. Improve care quality.
3. Expand support for AD patients and their families.
4. Increase public awareness and involvement.
5. Facilitate progress tracking by enhancing data collection, organization, and access.

Sources: http://aspe.hhs.gov/daltcp/napa/NatlPlan2015.shtml and http://aspe.hhs.gov/daltcp/napa/reports.shtml.

NIH MEETING: ALZHEIMER'S DISEASE RESEARCH SUMMIT 2012: PATH TO TREATMENT AND PREVENTION (MAY 14–15, 2012)

This summit was hosted by the Department of Health and Human Services and the NIA at NIH, with support from the Foundation for NIH (FNIH). The goal of the Alzheimer's Disease Research Summit 2012 was to accelerate the development of therapies for AD via a multidisciplinary research agenda. This goal includes identification of the various infrastructure, resources, and public–private partnerships that are vital to implement the agenda.

Summit recommendations were organized by a group of speakers and panelists and were based on summit discussions. The general recommendations are:

1. Acknowledge multifactorial disease aspects.
2. Support new research perspectives (eg, network pharmacology and systems biology).
3. Promote sharing of data and biological samples.
4. Establish multidisciplinary teams.
5. Overcome AD drug development issues related to intellectual property laws.
6. Support AD research through new public–private partnerships.
7. Form a National Institutional Review Board for AD clinical research.

The specific recommendations are covered in the following six sessions:

1. "Interdisciplinary Approach to Discovering and Validating the Next Generation of Therapeutic Targets for Alzheimer's Disease":
   a. Increase efforts and probe new targets to understand AD pathology using systems biology approaches and stem cell technology.

   b. Develop better understanding of how the different discoveries (genetic, pathological, biochemical, etc.) are related.
   c. Use genomic sequencing to identify rare genetic variants of large functional effect.
   d. Develop experimental models that better simulate AD and use these models to identify disease modulators and insure that these models are accessible.
   e. Generate in vivo imaging agents [positron emission tomography (PET) tracers] to aid in assessment of pathology and therapies.
   f. Promote biomarker development for diagnosis and prognosis, as well as disease subtypes.
   g. Enable sharing of data via web-based resources with the capacity to use these data for testing different models or hypotheses at the computational level.
   h. Facilitate analysis of new data before they are published via collaboration with scientists.
   i. Increase awareness to existing infrastructure and resources (eg, biobanks, research centers, and repositories) by advertising their availability.
   j. Promote creation of translational research teams to accelerate discovery of new targets through collaboration.
2. "Challenges in Preclinical Therapy Development":
   a. Develop infrastructure and resources to increase preclinical therapeutic development success, including assembling advisory committees and establishing open-access resources for publishing negative and discrepant findings.
   b. Increase the reliability of preclinical testing in animals by having standards for developing and characterizing animal models, as well as ensuring the availability of these models to researchers. Also establish guidelines for testing and reporting of both positive and negative results.
3. "Whom to Treat, When to Treat, and What Outcomes to Measure":
   a. Initiate therapy trials in asymptomatic individuals at risk such as genetically predisposed or old individuals with positive biomarkers.
   b. Develop and standardize neuropsychological and behavioral measures for early detection of AD.
   c. Develop biomarkers for monitoring disease progression and predict long-term clinical outcomes.
   d. Individualize treatments according to the heterogeneity of patients' symptoms.
   e. Facilitate infrastructure alterations that may accelerate and improve prevention initiatives.
4. "Drug Repurposing and Combination Therapy":
   a. Expand libraries of drugs and AD tissues and publicize their availability to the research community.
   b. Support the development of combination therapies by developing translational workgroups with experts in biology and pharmacology.
5. "Nonpharmacological Interventions":
   a. Employ epidemiological data to better understand underlying factors that contribute to AD.

   b. Identify the mechanisms by which nonpharmacological measures affect the disease status.
   c. Examine the combination of nonpharmacological with pharmacological measures to potentiate therapeutic benefit.
   d. Develop standards for outcomes to facilitate comparison of data across studies. These standards should cover quality of life and cognitive and physical function.
   e. Examine the effects of behavioral changes as a nonpharmacological intervention.
6. "New Models of Public–Private Partnerships":
   a. Promote partnerships between all sectors concerned with basic, translational, and clinical research to make integrated translational research possible.
   b. Enable partnerships for data sharing, as well as creating and sharing tools for translational research (eg, biomarkers, instruments, high-throughput screening, and animal models).

Source: https://www.nia.nih.gov/newsroom/announcements/2012/05/alzheimers-disease-research-summit-offers-research-recommendations.

NIH MEETING: ALZHEIMER'S DISEASE-RELATED DEMENTIAS: RESEARCH CHALLENGES AND OPPORTUNITIES (MAY 1–2, 2013)

This meeting was sponsored by the NINDS in collaboration with the NIA. This workshop falls under the "2012 National Plan to Address Alzheimer's Disease." Its general goal was to better understand the fundamentals of the nervous system and utilize that knowledge to address neurological disorders.

The research recommendations were focused on five arching topics:

- Topic 1: Multiple Etiology Dementias: The Public Health Problem and Improving Recognition Across the Spectrum.
- Topic 2: Health Disparities.
- Topic 3: Lewy Body Dementias: Dementia with Lewy Bodies and Parkinson's Disease Dementia.
- Topic 4: Frontotemporal dementia (FTD) and Related Tauopathies.
- Topic 5: Vascular Contributions to ADRD: Focus on Small Vessel Disease and AD/Vascular Interactions.

The specific recommendations were categorized into three classes: high, intermediate, and additional. The high priority recommendations are listed in Table 3.1 and are stratified based on the timeline target for completion into the 1–3 years group and the 3–7 years group.

Sources: http://www.ninds.nih.gov/funding/areas/neurodegeneration/workshops/adrd2013/ and the ADRD 2013 report.

TABLE 3.1 High Priority Recommendations From the Alzheimer's Disease-Related Dementias National Institutes of Health (ADRD NIH) 2013 Meeting

Topic	Focus	Recommendation
HIGH PRIORITY RECOMMENDATIONS (1–3-YEAR TIMELINE)		
Topic 1: MED	Differential diagnosis	Develop algorithms detecting dementia and VCI in (1) primary care, (2) general neurology, and (3) general psychiatry settings; and algorithms for specialist referrals.
	Epidemiology	Conduct studies of dementia incidence and prevalence within different ethnicities and age groups using imaging and biomarkers.
Topic 3: LBD	Establish longitudinal cohorts with common measures	Examine the efficacy of current symptomatic therapies in treating DLB and PDD.
		Create resources for clinical, biological, and imaging assessment of DLB and PDD from the early stages to autopsy to improve disease diagnosis and detection in patients with high risk factors.
Topic 4: FTD	Clinical science	Support genotyping of FTD patients and identifying new genes.
Topic 5: VAS	Human-based studies	Identify noninvasive biomarkers of vascular changes related to cognitive and neurological impairment.
HIGH PRIORITY RECOMMENDATIONS (3–7-YEAR TIMELINE)		
Topic 2: HD	Recruitment	Initiate studies of incident dementia in different populations using imaging, biomarkers, and autopsies.
	Treatment and prevention	Optimize trials of vascular health interventions for increased application to different populations.
Topic 4: FTD	Basic science	Further probe tau pathogenesis and its effect on neurodegeneration.
Topic 5: VAS	Mechanisms and models	Develop new experiment models of VCI and VAD.
	Human-based studies	Further identify biomarkers of vascular changes related to cognitive and neurological impairment.

DLB, dementia with Lewy bodies; *FTD*, frontotemporal dementia; *HD*, health disparities; *LBD*, Lewy body dementias; *MED*, multiple etiology dementias; *PDD*, Parkinson's disease dementia; *VAD*, vascular cognitive dementia; *VAS*, vascular contributions to ADRD; *VCI*, vascular cognitive impairment.

NIH MEETING: ALZHEIMER'S DISEASE RESEARCH SUMMIT 2015: PATH TO TREATMENT AND PREVENTION (FEBRUARY 9–10, 2015)

This summit was hosted by the Department of Health and Human Services and the NIA at the NIH, with support from the FNIH. The goal of the AD Research Summit 2015 was continuous with the agenda that was set in prior summits and addresses discovery of treatments for AD patients in the different stages of the disease. This goal was attempted by identifying the resources and infrastructure necessary to implement this research agenda. The summit recommendations were generated by over 60 experts from industry, academia, nonprofit organizations, and advocacy groups. These recommendations can be summarized into:

1. Improve AD prevention strategies by having a better understanding of normal brain aging and resilience to disease.
2. Maximize the potential of approaches such as systems pharmacology and biology.
3. Develop infrastructure and tools to store and analyze biological and other patient-relevant data.
4. Make use of mobile sensors and other technologies to inform AD research.
5. Facilitate open science in clinical and basic research.
6. Promote collaboration, transparency, and reproducibility in research using incentives.
7. Support and advance translational and data science workforce.
8. Involve citizens, caregivers, and patients as collaborates in AD research.

The summit sessions and their specific recommendations were:

1. "Interdisciplinary Research to Understand the Heterogeneity and Multifactorial Etiology of Disease":
   a. Fill in the gaps in human data needed to formulate better hypotheses on AD heterogeneity using phenotyping of established cohorts that are genetically, epigenetically, or caused by other factors at risk.
   b. Develop new cohorts for phenotyping (eg, exposome, imaging, cognitive, etc.) that better represent gender and population diversity.
   c. Optimize and improve existing NIA/NIH infrastructure and facilitate sharing and integration of data needed to develop predictive AD models.
   d. Develop new programs to better understand AD by integrating AD research with neurobiology and aging research.
   e. Develop new in vivo models that are based on human data and examine the biology and physiology of the different AD risk factors.
   f. Integrate new technologies (eg, genome editing, brain stimulation, and in vivo imaging) to improve assessment of human studies.
   g. Acknowledge shortcomings of rodent models and use biochemical and physiological endpoints instead of behavioral endpoints as measures of treatment efficacy.
   h. Generate biomarkers that probe efficacy early in the development of a drug.
   i. Support the translational aspect of AD research by developing integrative training programs that cover data science, bioinformatics, software engineering, and drug discovery disciplines.
   j. Improve reproducibility in AD research by implementing new policies. These should cover the reward systems in academia, fund providers, and journals.
2. "Transforming AD Therapy Development: From Targets to Trials":
   a. Probe the interaction between the different aspects of AD (eg, tau filaments, inflammation, amyloid, metabolism, oxidative stress, etc.).
   b. Expand efforts focused on generation and integration of molecular, cellular, and physiological data to develop better AD models.
   c. Examine synergy and additivity of therapeutics (including synergy between drugs and nonpharmacological actions) using quantitative methods.

   d. Advance drug repurposing and drug combinations development by leveraging the network concept of drug targets and phenotype screening.
   e. Develop high-throughput methods to isolate neural cells for further assessment (eg, for drug screening).
   f. Develop new biomarkers that are indicative of incipient disease (ie, ocular or olfactory biomarkers) as well as biomarkers for detection of synaptic dysfunction.
   g. Develop clinical tools to assess disease progression to evaluate meaningful clinical outcomes of therapies.
   h. Support education and training in drug discovery disciplines and develop and bring together academic and industry experts using research programs.
3. "New Strategies for Prevention":
   a. Liberate data funded by the public into the public domain and facilitate its usability.
   b. Enhance community-driven studies to generate molecular and physiological measurements that can be utilized in systems biology. These measurements can be done by collecting quantitative data using technologies such as actigraphy.
   c. Develop cohorts with participants from different races to identify genomic and other risk and protective factors that underline heterogeneity of dementias.
   d. Examine how lifestyle impacts risk of AD using an ecological perspective. This perspective should cover physical, social, and environmental factors.
   e. Test epigenetic regulators as targets for treatment or prevention.
   f. Focus on the pathological and protective role of apolipoprotein E (APOE) on pharmacological as well as nonpharmacological interventions.
   g. Probe how peripheral systems (eg, immune and metabolic) impact brain aging and AD using new research programs.
   h. Elucidate the consequences of sleep disruption and optimization on AD.
4. "Innovating Disease Monitoring, Assessment, and Care":
   a. Develop technologies for patients monitoring throughout the disease stages.
   b. Standardize measures of study outcomes to compress data across studies.
   c. Utilize cross-disciplinary expertise to develop new monitoring technologies.
   d. Utilize mobile health technologies in monitoring and assessing disease formally.
   e. Determine the hurdles of early dementia diagnosis.
5. "Empowering Patients, Engaging Citizens":
   a. Create public education programs by networking and creating relationships with community leaders.
   b. Involve communities in determining how to measure meaningful impact of treatments and appropriate return from participation in research.
   c. Optimize collaboration between federally funded programs such as the Patient-Centered Outcomes Research Institute and the Clinical and Translational Science Awards to lower the cost of community involvement.
   d. Initiate new research platforms that accelerate collecting data while providing public education.
   e. Empower participant control using methods and policies for collecting and sharing data such as electronic consent forms that give the option to share data.
   f. Facilitate patient consent and data sharing by having an accordance between innovative technologies and policy.

6. "Enabling Partnerships for Open Innovation":
   a. Incentivize data sharing by creating partnerships across funding agencies.
   b. Promote participation of early-career researchers in large-scale studies through incentives from academia, funding agencies, and journals.
   c. Support novel research on nonmainstream ideas.
   d. Tailor intellectual properties laws to promote additional research in the field and not to block others from the same area of interest.

Source: https://www.nia.nih.gov/research/recommendations-nih-ad-research-summit-2015.

ALZHEIMER'S DISEASE CENTERS

Funded by the NIA, these centers (34 currently) are located in major medical institutes across the country and are tasked to translate AD research advances into enhanced diagnosis and treatment of AD patients (Fig. 3.1). Research is focused on basic pathology and disease management using basic, behavioral, and clinical studies. Alzheimer's Disease Centers (ADCs) offer support to patients and their families in the form of diagnosis, medical management, and information on the disease and related resources and services. These centers also give the opportunity for patients to take part in clinical trials and studies.

Source: http://www.nia.nih.gov/alzheimers/alzheimers-disease-research-centers.

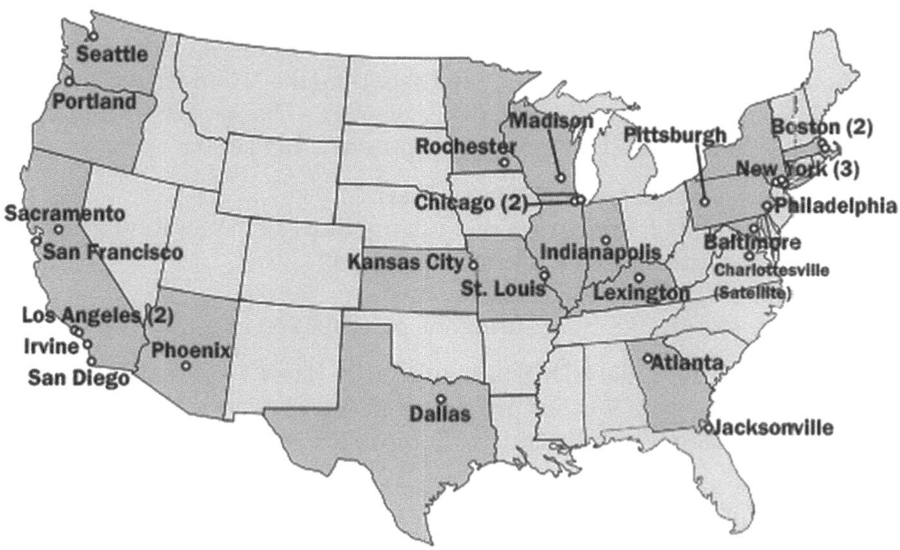

FIGURE 3.1 ADC locations. Number in parentheses indicates the number of centers in that city. *Source: https://www.nia.nih.gov.*

NATIONAL ALZHEIMER'S COORDINATING CENTER

The National Alzheimer's Coordinating Center (NACC) was established in 1999 as part of the NIA's Alzheimer's Disease Centers (ADCs). It operates in partnership with the Alzheimer's Disease Genetics Consortium (ADGC) and the National Cell Repository for Alzheimer's Disease (NCRAD) to facilitate AD research by providing a comprehensive database that includes clinical and neuropathological data as well as magnetic resonance images (MRI). The data are collected from ADCs and provided to the research community free of charge and with no NIA affiliation requirements. Consultation is also provided to help researchers identify the most relevant data to their research. The NACC is one of the most comprehensive databases of its kind and its data have been utilized in over 450 different studies.

Source: http://www.alz.washington.edu.

NATIONAL CELL REPOSITORY FOR ALZHEIMER'S DISEASE

Located at Indiana University Medical Center in Indianapolis, Indiana. The goal of the National Cell Repository for Alzheimer's Disease (NCRAD) is to advance AD research by helping researchers identify genetic factors that influence AD and dementia. Since 1990, NCRAD was funded by the NIA to help researchers by providing biological samples (DNA, RNA, serum, plasma, and brain tissue) as well as data. NCRAD accepts subject referrals to participate in projects as well as brain tissue samples.

Source: http://ncrad.iu.edu.

ALZHEIMER'S DISEASE COOPERATIVE STUDY

The Alzheimer's Disease Cooperative Study (ADCS) was formed as a cooperative agreement between the University of California, San Diego, and the NIA as an initiative to advance research on AD treatment. It is part of both the Alzheimer's Disease Prevention Initiative and the NIA Division of Neuroscience program. This program focuses on:

1. Improving cognition and delaying the onset of AD.
2. Conducting studies on potential drugs that can minimize behavioral symptoms.
3. Developing new instruments to aid in clinical studies.
4. Innovation in clinical studies design and analysis.
5. Enhancing AD clinical studies by ensuring the participation of minority groups.

Since its formation in 1991, the ADCS has initiated 30 Phase I to Phase III research studies with participants ranging from 9 to 800 people per study. These studies had many key highlights and have generated many publications. Some of these key highlights include:

1. Facilitating abilities of AD centers to carry out studies in the United States and Canada.
2. Development of the first Activities of Daily Living Scale as an important instrument for AD patients assessment.
3. Standardization of worksheets used in the Clinical Dementia Rating Scale.
4. Testing vitamin E and selegiline, which showed that both drugs can delay disease progression in moderately advanced AD patients.

5. Completion of studies with major public health impact, such as the demonstration of lack of benefit from the use of B vitamins, estrogen, nonsteroidal antiinflammatory drugs, and statins in AD patients.

The ADCS continues to run major AD studies such as the ADNI-D Study, the Connect Study, the Noble Study, the A4 Study, and the Dominantly Inherited Alzheimer Network (DIAN) Study.

Source: http://www.adcs.org/.

ALZHEIMER'S DISEASE EDUCATION AND REFERRAL CENTER

The Alzheimer's Disease Education and Referral Center (ADEAR) is one of NIA's AD-related service providers. It was created in 1990 by the US Congress with the aim to compile, archive, and share AD information with health professionals as well as the public.

ADEAR has a staff of information specialists that can assist with the following:

1. Specific AD questions.
2. Providing publications regarding AD (symptoms, diagnosis, risk factors, and treatment) free of charge.
3. Assisting with referrals to other AD services and centers for research or diagnosis purposes.
4. Providing resources in Spanish.
5. Providing information on clinical trials, training manuals, and news updates.

Source: https://www.nia.nih.gov/alzheimers/about-adear-center.

ALZHEIMER'S DISEASE GENETICS STUDY

This study is a collaboration between Indiana University and the NIA with the purpose of identifying the genes that are involved in AD. Genetic materials and clinical data were collected and analyzed from 1000 or more families in the United States with three qualifying members over the span of 3years. Participating centers included the NIA's Alzheimer's Disease Centers, which helped with collecting blood and DNA samples. While clinical and demographic data were sent to NCRAD, these data and biological samples will be made available to the research community.

Source: http://www.nia.nih.gov/alzheimers/clinical-trials/alzheimers-disease-genetics-study.

ALZHEIMER'S DISEASE GENETICS CONSORTIUM

Funded by a grant from the NIA, the Alzheimer's Disease Genetics Consortium (ADGC) aim is to identify genetic variants associated with AD. This identification is done through collaboration between the University of Pennsylvania, NCRAD, and NACC (National Alzheimer's Coordinating Center and National Cell Repository for Alzheimer's Disease, respectively) to conduct genome-wide association studies (GWAS) using over 10,000 samples from families around the globe.

Source: http://alois.med.upenn.edu/adgc/.

NIA GENETICS OF ALZHEIMER'S DISEASE DATA STORAGE SITE

The NIA's policies require that genetic data from NIA-funded AD studies be deposited at the NIA Genetics of Alzheimer's Disease Data Storage (NIAGADS). NIAGADS provides investigators with different kinds of data ranging from genome studies of AD, such as high-density genotyping and sequencing, and statistics from genetic studies. In addition to data, NIAGADS also provides software packages (eg, DNA-SEQ and RNA-SEQ), web-based tools, and online resources that can help analyze and interpret large-scale genomic data. NIAGADS is heavily involved with two major studies: the ADGC, and the Alzheimer's Disease Sequence Project (ADSP). Funds are provided from NIH/NIA grants.

Source: https://www.niagads.org/.

ALZHEIMER'S DISEASE SEQUENCE PROJECT

The Alzheimer's Disease Sequence Project (ADSP) is supported by the NIA and the National Human Genome Research Institute. It is composed mainly of five groups, some of which provide DNA and phenotypes, while others perform sequencing and data processing. Other institutes provide auxiliary support in the form of coordination and sample handling.

The ADSP's database provides researchers with detailed sequencing data. The goals of this program are:

1. Identify genetic factors related to late-onset AD.
2. Identify genes involved in protection from AD.
3. Investigate why some high-risk individuals do not develop AD.
4. Examine risk factors in populations with different ethnicities and search for pathways for preventing AD.

Source: https://www.niagads.org/adsp/content/home.

INVESTIGATIONAL NEW DRUG TOXICOLOGY PROGRAM

The Investigational New Drug Toxicology Program is sponsored by the NIA with the purpose of treating symptoms of AD and aging-related conditions. Services are provided to academia as well as independent investigators with potential AD medicines. The program also provides toxicology evaluations required by the Food and Drug Administration (FDA) for clinical studies.

The services provided fall under four categories:

1. Analytical chemistry.
2. Pharmacokinetics.
3. Preliminary toxicity screens.
4. Toxicology studies and safety pharmacology.

Source: http://www.nia.nih.gov/research/dn/investigational-new-drug-toxicology-program.

ALZHEIMER'S DISEASE NEUROIMAGING INITIATIVE

Alzheimer's Disease Neuroimaging Initiative (ADNI) is a global collaboration to investigate treatments for AD. It is funded by both NIA and National Institute of Bioimaging and Bioengineering (parts of the NIH) as well as pharmaceutical companies and other foundations. It was initiated over a decade ago with the goal being to study normal cognitive aging, mild impairment, and early AD. ADNI aims to use neuroimaging and biomarkers for detecting the onset and progression of such conditions.

ADNI collects and utilizes imaging data (eg, MRI and PET images) as well as genetic data, cognitive tests, and fluid biomarkers to identify correlations with disease onset and progression. Access to such data is available and the website also provides tools for PET and MRI analyses.

Sources: http://www.nia.nih.gov/research/dn/alzheimers-disease-neuroimaging-initiative-adni, http://adni.loni.usc.edu/ and http://www.adni-info.org/Scientists/ADNIStudyProcedures.aspx.

GENOME-WIDE ASSOCIATION STUDIES

Genome-Wide Association Studies (GWAS) contribute to understanding the genetics involved in AD (Table 3.2). This area of research aims to understand genes that influence late-onset AD. Identification of genes that are involved in susceptibility have shown that amyloid precursor protein and tau metabolism remain important in AD. Large-scale GWAS

TABLE 3.2 Genome-Wide Association Studies (GWAS) and Alzheimer's Disease (AD)

Major Pathways Identified by GWAS Studies	
Pathway	**Gene**
Amyloid pathway	*APOE, SORL1, CLU, CR1. PICALM, BIN1, ABCA7*
Immune system/inflammation	*CLU, CR1, EPHA1, ABCA7, MS4A4A/MS4A6E, CD33, CD2AP*
Lipid transport and metabolism	*APOE, CLU, ABCA7*
Synaptic cell functioning/endocytosis	*CLU, PICALM, BIN1, EPHA1, MS4A4A/MS4A6E, CD33 CD2AP*
Major AD GWAS Studies Performed	
Study	**Genes Identified Outside *APOE* Region**
Lambert et al. (2009)	*CLU, CRI*
Harold et al. (2009)	*CLU, PICALM*
Seshadri et al. (2010)	*BIN1, XOC3L2/BLOC1S3/MARK4, CLU, PICALM*
Naj et al. (2011)	*MS4A4A, CD2AP, CD33, EPHA1, CRI, CLU, BIN1, PICALM*
Hollingworth et al. (2011)	*ABCA7, MS4A6A/MS4A4E, EPHAI, CD33, CD2AP*
Lee et al. (2011)	*CLU, PICALM, BIN1, CUGBP2*, loci on 2p25.1; 3q25.2; 7p21.1; 10q23.1
Reitz et al. (2013)	*ABCA7*, intergenic locus on 5q35.2

and genome sequencing studies can potentially identify harmful variants in these genes, as well as targets for genetic testing for AD. While GWAS identified some susceptibility genes, sequencing studies provided strong evidence for the involvement of genetic variants in AD, ending the debate of whether genetic factors had anything to do with the disease.

Major pathways identified by GWAS:

1. Amyloid pathway (genes: *APOE*, *SORL1*, etc.).
2. Immunity and inflammation pathway (genes: *CLU*, *CR1*, etc.).
3. Lipid transport and metabolism (genes: *APOE*, *ABCA7*, etc.).
4. Synapse function and endocytosis (genes: *BINI*, *CD33*, etc.).

Source: Tosto, G., Reitz, C., 2013. Genome-wide Association Studies in Alzheimer's Disease: A Review. Curr. Neurol. Neurosci. Rep. 13, 381. Lambert, J.C., et al., 2009. Genome-wide association study identifies variants at CLU and CR1 associated with Alzheimer's disease. Nat. Genet. 41, 1094–1099. Harold, D., et al., 2009. Genome-wide association study identifies variants at CLU and PICALM associated with Alzheimer's disease. Nat. Genet. 41, 1088–1093. Seshadri, S., et al., 2010. Genome-wide analysis of genetic loci associated with Alzheimer disease. JAMA. 303, 1832–1840. Naj, A.C., et al., 2011. Common variants at MS4A4/MS4A6E, CD2AP, CD33 and EPHA1 are associated with late-onset Alzheimer's disease. Nat. Genet. 43, 436–441. Hollingworth, P., et al., 2011. Common variants at ABCA7, MS4A6A/ MS4A4E, EPHA1, CD33 and CD2AP are associated with Alzheimer's disease. Nat. Genet. 43, 429–435. Lee, J.H., et al., 2011. Identification of novel loci for Alzheimer disease and replication of CLU, PICALM, and BIN1 in Caribbean Hispanic individuals. Arch. Neurol. 68, 320–328. Reitz, C., et al., 2013. Variants in the ATP-binding cassette transporter (ABCA7), apolipoprotein E ε4, and the risk of late-onset Alzheimer disease in African Americans. JAMA. 309, 1483–1492. https://www.genome.gov.

ACCELERATING MEDICINES PARTNERSHIP-ALZHEIMER'S DISEASE

Accelerating Medicines Partnership-Alzheimer's Disease (AMP-AD) is an initiative from the Accelerating Medicines Partnership, which is a collaboration between the NIH, 10 biopharmaceutical companies, and various nonprofit organizations aiming to accelerate the development of new medicines by transforming the current model for drug development by identifying and validating novel and relevant therapeutic targets, and discovering biomarkers to validate current therapeutic targets.

AMP-AD projects:

1. Biomarkers project: concerned with tau imaging and discovering novel fluid biomarkers to assess disease progression and treatment efficacy. This project is being run by three NIA-supported clinical studies: A4 Trial, DIAN, and Alzheimer's Prevention Initiative (API) APOE.
2. AMP-AD Target Discovery and Preclinical Validation Project: to accelerate the discovery of drugs and drug targets for AD by the integration, analyses, and validation of large-scale data from human brain samples. The project also focuses on understanding genes, proteins, and pathways within which these novel targets reside.

Source: http://www.nia.nih.gov/alzheimers/amp-ad.

AD TRANSLATIONAL INITIATIVES

Since its launch in 2004, the AD Translational Initiative has been supporting drug discovery and development for AD by academia and small companies. The focus is on steps in translational research that tend to be overlooked by pharmaceutical companies. The NIA provided funding for two initiatives for drug discovery and preclinical drug development from 2009 through 2012 (Fig. 3.2).

Source: http://www.nia.nih.gov/research/dn/ad-translational-initiatives.

THE DOMINANTLY INHERITED ALZHEIMER NETWORK

DIAN is an international research collaboration focusing on early-onset familial AD in adults with parents who have mutated genes. It is funded by the NIA and is conducted across 13 institutions in the United States, Europe, and Australia. These studies are currently enrolling participants.

Source: http://dian-info.org/.

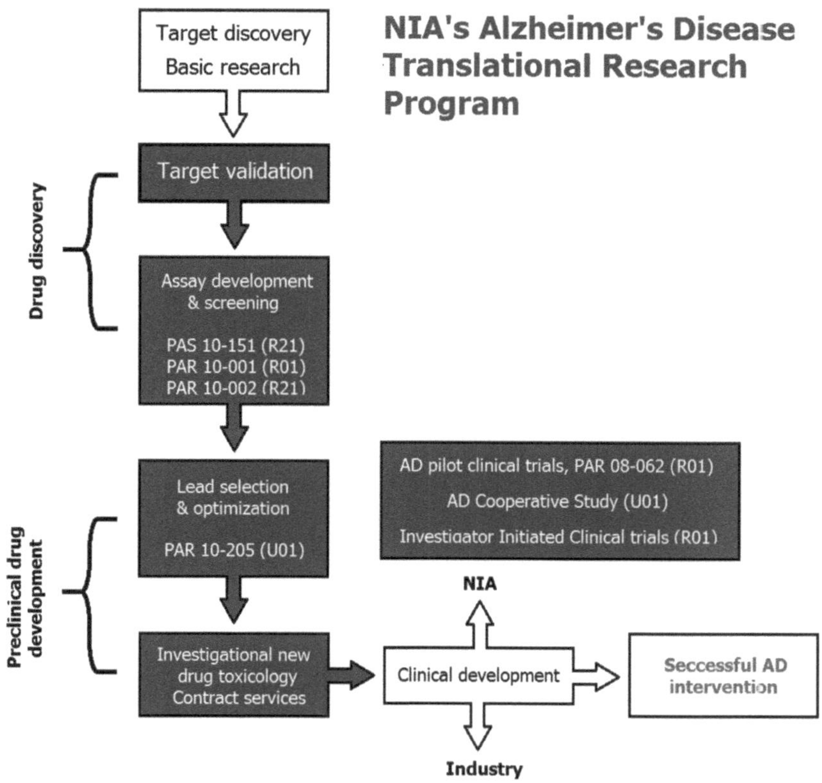

FIGURE 3.2 Overview of the AD Translational Initiatives by the National Institute on Aging (NIA). The numbers signify specific grant mechanisms used to fund the program. *Adapted from: http://www.nia.nih.gov/research/dn/ad-translational-initiatives.*

CLINICAL TRIALS

There are many clinical trials revolving around AD (over 1300). These trials cover many aspects of research such as genetics, drug safety and efficacy, effects of other conditions on disease (eg, sleep apnea), neuroimaging, diagnosis-related studies, and much more.

For more details: https://www.clinicaltrials.gov.

ALZHEIMER'S PREVENTION INITIATIVE

The Alzheimer's Prevention Initiative (API) was established in 2012, and is supported by the NIA. It is a collaborative effort that is led by the Banner Alzheimer's Institute (BAI—Phoenix, Arizona). Its goal is to prevent or slow the onset of AD. This goal is addressed by evaluating therapies in normal people at high risk. Physicians, scientists, and industry and regulatory agency representatives work together to achieve this goal. The API focuses on clinical trials as well as biomarker studies. It also enables participation in studies through the Alzheimer's Prevention Registry (Fig. 3.3).

The API has a number of ongoing studies, including:

1. Alzheimer's Prevention Initiative Autosomal Dominant Alzheimer's Disease Treatment Trial.
2. Alzheimer's Prevention Initiative APOE4 Treatment Trial.

Source: http://banneralz.org/research-plus-discovery/alzheimers-prevention-initiative.aspx.

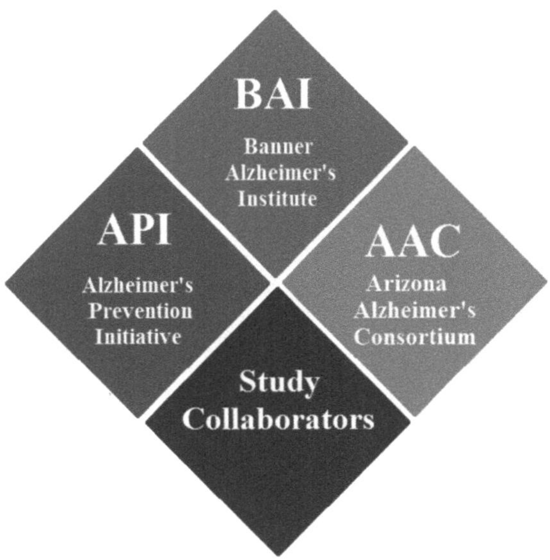

FIGURE 3.3 The Banner Alzheimer's Institute (BAI), Alzheimer's Prevention Initiative (API), and Arizona Alzheimer's Consortium (AAC) work in conjunction with other collaborators to address the challenges of AD. *Adapted from: http://azalz.org/.*

ARIZONA ALZHEIMER'S CONSORTIUM

The Consortium was established in 1998 to focus on different aspects of AD research such as imaging, genetics, computer science, cognition, as well as clinical and neuropathological research. It is a nonprofit organization. The Arizona Alzheimer's Consortium (AAC) aims to effectively treat and prevent the onset of AD within 12 years. The Consortium consists of Arizona State University, Banner Sun Health Research Institute, BAI, Mayo Clinic Arizona, the Translational Genomics Research Institute, Barrow Neurological Institute, and the University of Arizona. The Consortium claims to be "the nation's leading model of statewide collaboration in Alzheimer's disease research".

PHARMACEUTICAL RESEARCH AND MANUFACTURERS OF AMERICA

Established in 1958, Pharmaceutical Research and Manufacturers of America (PhRMA) is composed of pharmaceutical and biotechnology companies, and biopharmaceutical researchers. PhRMA's aims are to encourage discovery of novel therapies for patients by advocating for policies that facilitate research and improve incentives. PhRMA is focused on achieving these goals in the United States and the world by:

1. Facilitating patient access to safe and effective therapies through a free market, with no price controls.
2. Improved incentives for intellectual property.
3. Effective regulation and availability of information to patients.

PhRMA members are currently developing 93 medicines for AD and dementias, all of which are in either clinical trials or review by the FDA (81 for AD, 2 for dementias, and 11 for cognition disorders). PhRMA also interacts with the public by supporting over 90 science, technology, engineering, and math programs that focus on students and teachers.

Sources: http://www.phrma.org/research/medicines-development-alzheimers-disease and http://www.phrma.org/about.

ADVISORY COUNCIL ON ALZHEIMER'S RESEARCH, CARE, AND SERVICES

The council consists of over 22 members and meets every 3 months to examine and assess government programs for AD. The Advisory Council influences the National Plan for AD by making recommendations for actions and assessing the implementation of such recommendations. Members of the Council span the federal government, patient advocates, caregivers, health care providers, state health departments, researchers, and health association representatives.

Source: http://aspe.hhs.gov/daltcp/napa/#Council.

ALZHEIMER'S DRUG DISCOVERY FOUNDATION

Founded in 1998, the Alzheimer's Drug Discovery Foundation (ADDF)'s mission is to support drug discovery for AD prevention and treatment. The foundation funds promising and innovative AD research globally. The ADDF has funded over 450 AD studies ranging from drug discovery to clinical trials.

The categories of research funded are:

1. Drug discovery and preclinical development.
2. Early detection.
3. Clinical trials.
4. Prevention.

The ADDF holds and participates in many conferences for the purpose of sharing ideas, results, and collaboration, some of which are:

1. The Annual Drug Discovery for Neurodegeneration Conference.
2. The International Conference on Alzheimer's Drug Discovery.
3. The Biology of Aging: Novel Drug Targets for Neurodegenerative Disease.

Source: http://www.alzdiscovery.org and http://alzdiscovery.org/events/conferences/past.

ALZHEIMER'S ASSOCIATION

The association prides itself as a global leader in AD care, support, and research. It provides support on many levels such as information and advice for patients and caregivers in the forms of symposia, 24/7 helpline, and online message boards. The association also helps individuals who desire to participate in clinical studies. It houses Alzheimer's Association Green-Field Library, a large resource center for AD. The Alzheimer's Association is a major fund provider for researchers. The association also promotes the sharing of research findings through the annual Alzheimer's Association International Conference (AAIC) and its journal "Alzheimer's & Dementia". The AAIC is the world's largest forum for AD research where researchers, clinicians, and caregivers meet and discuss recent findings and theories.

Source: http://www.alz.org/.

ALZHEIMER'S FOUNDATION OF AMERICA

Uniting more than 2400 national organizations, the Alzheimer's Foundation of America (AFA) aims to raise awareness on AD and related illnesses by educating the public and care providers through a host of efforts such as a toll-free helpline, conferences, and publications as well as meeting the "educational, social, emotional and practical needs of individuals with Alzheimer's disease and related illnesses, and their caregivers and families". As part of the AFA's educational effort, events such as the National Memory Screening Day are held to educate the public and raise awareness of dementias. AFA's efforts extend to providing several research grants to its members with the purpose of improving social and educational services.

Source: http://www.alzfdn.org/.

ALZFORUM

Since 1996, Alzforum has been providing information and news to researchers to help facilitate research in drug discovery and diagnosis for AD and related disorders. Alzforum improves scientific communication by reporting and analyzing recent findings and industry news. Alzforum also helps researchers by providing open-access databases. The forum covers grant news and major AD conferences. It also has access to several databases such as AlzBiomarker, AlzPedia, and AlzRisk. Alzforum also helps job seekers by allowing the posting of jobs and career opportunities.

Source: http://www.alzforum.org/.

INTERNATIONAL SOCIETY TO ADVANCE ALZHEIMER'S RESEARCH AND TREATMENT

The International Society to Advance Alzheimer's Research and Treatment (ISTAART) was created by the Alzheimer's Association in 2008 to further support international AD research by facilitating networking and collaboration between scientists as well as sponsoring students to attend the annual Alzheimer's Association International Conference (AAIC). Members enjoy benefits such as access to some journals (eg, *Alzheimer's & Dementia: The Journal of the Alzheimer's Association* and *Neurobiology of Aging*). They also get access to other professional networks and discounts on some conferences fees.

Source: https://act.alz.org/site/SPageServer?pagename=ISTAART_about.

ALZHEIMER'S IMPACT MOVEMENT

The Alzheimer's Impact Movement (AIM) is a nonprofit organization. AIM works with the Alzheimer's Association to advocate the importance of AD research and to make it a national priority. This advocacy is done by supporting congressional candidates who have AD high in their priorities list. AIM makes sure the AD community stays relevant in congress. AIM also has a corporate program that helps build beneficial partnerships and networks between industry parties that are involved in AD research.

AIM's goals are:

1. Increase AD research commitment.
2. Make diagnosis and care more accessible.

Source: http://alzimpact.org/.

RESEARCHERS AGAINST ALZHEIMER'S/USAGAINST ALZHEIMER'S

These organizations collect donations and provide tools for researchers interested in AD. Their websites have access to resources, clinical trial data, and talks on AD. They are also involved in global events such as the Leaders Engaged on Alzheimer's Disease Coalition and the Global CEO Initiative on Alzheimer's Disease.

Researchers Against Alzheimer's goals are:

1. Focusing the research community's effort to stop AD by 2025.
2. Investing in AD research resources to match the scale of the epidemic.
3. Reforming the drug development and approval pipeline to make it fast and efficient.

USAgainst Alzheimer's goal is to stop AD by 2020. It hopes to achieve this goal by increasing investments in AD research from both public and private sectors. The organization helped in securing more than $200 million to fund AD research. It also helped form a network of more than 70 organizations and corporations concerned with AD and networks for AD activists such as the "Activists Against Alzheimer's" and "Women Against Alzheimer's." The organization also facilitates enrollment in major AD clinical trials such as A4 Trial, SNIFF, NCA&T Study, and EXERT Study.

Sources: http://www.usagainstalzheimers.org/networks/researchers and http://www.usagainstalzheimers.org/.

SOCIAL MEDIA

Social networks can help the research community by increasing accessibility to professional advice, job listings, and networking between researchers, industry representatives, students, and legislators. While there are many social networks, some tend to be more profession oriented:

1. ResearchGate: Founded in 2008, ResearchGate prides itself as a "by scientists for scientists" social network. Today ResearchGate members exceed 6 million. Their goal is to improve research by facilitating the sharing of data and expertise. This goal is done by:
   a. Enabling data publishing and access.
   b. Providing statistics about citations and views.
   c. Posting and viewing job listings.
   d. Discussing research problems with other members.
   e. Collaboration with fellow scientists in the field.

   Source: http://www.researchgate.net/.

2. LinkedIn: LinkedIn is a large social network for professionals with 300 million members. This social network aims to globally connect professionals from different fields to increase productivity. Members can contact other members, post and view job listings, and get news and updates of various fields and interests. There is a subdivision that focuses on job opportunities and employers by categorizing them in a directory where a member can search either by name or interest (eg, pharmaceuticals). Also the website provides a directory for academic institutes. Summary of resources provided by various organizations to address AD, from research funding to educational services, are given in Table 3.3.

   Source: https://www.linkedin.com/nhome.

TABLE 3.3 Summary of Resources to Address Alzheimer's Disease

Provider	Resource Provided
National Institutes of Health (NIA, NIMH, and NINDS)	• Research funding • Information for the public • Data and services for researchers • National strategy and coordination against AD
Alzheimer's Disease Centers	• Information on disease and related services • Diagnosis and medical management • Patient participation in clinical trials
National Alzheimer's Coordinating Center	• Database (MRI images, and clinical and neuropathological data)
National Cell Repository for Alzheimer's Disease	• Biological samples for researchers (DNA, RNA, serum, plasma, and brain tissue) as well as data • Patient participation in projects • Accept brain tissue samples for autopsy
Alzheimer's Disease Education and Referral Center	• Publications on disease information and treatments • Assists patients with referrals to other centers for diagnosis or research participation • Information on clinical trials
NIA Genetics of Alzheimer's Disease Data Storage Site	• Provides genomic data to researchers (genotyping, sequencing, and statistics) • Provides software for genomic data (DNA-SEQ and RNA-SEQ)
Investigational New Drug Toxicology Program	• Analytical chemistry • Pharmacokinetic studies • Preliminary toxicity screens
Alzheimer's Disease Neuroimaging Initiative	• Genetic and imaging data (MRI and PET images) • Data on fluid biomarkers and correlations with disease onset and progression • Tools for PET and MRI image analysis
Alzheimer's Drug Discovery Foundation	• Provides research funding for AD drug discovery, early detection, and clinical trials
Alzheimer's Association	• Provides information to caregivers and patients (symposia, telephone helpline, *Alzheimer's & Dementia* journal, and online forums) • Patient clinical trial participation • Research grants
Alzheimer's Foundation of America	• Education through conferences, publications, and social events • Telephone helpline • Grants for AFA member organizations
The International Society to Advance Alzheimer's Research and Treatment	• Student sponsorship for AAIC attendance • Grants members journal access
Alzforum	• General information and news to researchers (recent findings, grants, and conferences) • Access to databases (AlzBiomarker, AlzPedia, and AlzRisk) • Helps job seekers by allowing job postings
Researchers Against Alzheimer's and USAgainst Alzheimer's	• Access to clinical trials data • Patient enrollment in clinical trials

Source: https://www.linkedin.com/nhome.

References

Harold, D., et al., 2009. Genome-wide association study identifies variants at CLU and PICALM associated with Alzheimer's disease. Nat. Genet. 41, 1088–1093.

Hollingworth, P., et al., 2011. Common variants at ABCA7, MS4A6A/ MS4A4E, EPHA1, CD33 and CD2AP are associated with Alzheimer's disease. Nat. Genet. 43, 429–435. https://www.genome.gov.

Lambert, J.C., et al., 2009. Genome-wide association study identifies variants at CLU and CR1 associated with Alzheimer's disease. Nat. Genet. 41, 1094–1099.

Lee, J.H., et al., 2011. Identification of novel loci for Alzheimer disease and replication of CLU, PICALM, and BIN1 in Caribbean Hispanic individuals. Arch. Neurol. 68, 320–328.

Naj, A.C., et al., 2011. Common variants at MS4A4/MS4A6E, CD2AP, CD33 and EPHA1 are associated with late-onset Alzheimer's disease. Nat. Genet. 43, 436–441.

Reitz, C., et al., 2013. Variants in the ATP-binding cassette transporter (ABCA7), apolipoprotein E ε4, and the risk of late-onset Alzheimer disease in African Americans. JAMA 309, 1483–1492.

Seshadri, S., et al., 2010. Genome-wide analysis of genetic loci associated with Alzheimer disease. JAMA 303, 1832–1840.

Tosto, G., Reitz, C., 2013. Genome-wide Association Studies in Alzheimer's Disease: A Review. Curr. Neurol. Neurosci. Rep. 13, 381.

CHAPTER

4

Current Medications for the Treatment of Alzheimer's Disease: Acetylcholinesterase Inhibitors and NMDA Receptor Antagonist

L.A. Finn

OUTLINE

INTRODUCTION

Alzheimer's disease (AD) treatment strategies build upon generally recognized goals of pharmacotherapy in the older adult, which include maintaining the highest level of functional independence and improving overall health-related quality of life. Current Food and Drug Administration (FDA)-approved pharmacologic options for AD do not reverse pathology associated with AD and are not initiated with the goal of cure (National Institute of Aging, 2014). Medicinal foods have also been approved by the FDA and numerous pharmaceuticals are under investigation in clinical trials for AD.

Drug Discovery Approaches for the Treatment of Neurodegenerative Disorders
http://dx.doi.org/10.1016/B978-0-12-802810-0.00004-0

Several medications approved for other indications are being studied for efficacy in AD (Cummings et al., 2015).

Goals for treatment of AD include treating the symptoms of deteriorating cognition and delaying the progression of functional loss along with managing the behavioral and psychological symptoms of dementia (BPSD) (Geldmacher, 2007; Sadowsky et al., 2012). The course of treatment follows a predictable direction from treatment of mild to moderate to severe AD although patients vary in the rapidity of progression and the emergence of BPSD. In practice, both pharmacologic and nonpharmacologic options are initiated and maintained to enable patients to have active engagement with their family members with least progressive loss of independence, thus delaying placement into more restrictive living environments. Because current therapy offers no cure or reversal of AD pathology, there is a significant need for continued research. Patient and family education on the use of FDA-approved medications focuses on the early initiation of drug therapy and realistic goals including the limited benefits and potential adverse effects of medication. AD educational topics including the course of the disease, resolution of legal matters, availability of clinical trials, and end of life care should be addressed early in the disease while patient cognition is highest (California Workshop, 2008; Hort et al., 2010; Lindstrom et al., 2006).

Geriatric patients experiencing AD often have multiple comorbid conditions and geriatric syndromes, which may involve drug therapy (Doraiswamy et al., 2002). Clinicians aim to maximize benefits of pharmacologic treatment and nondrug interventions for these comorbid conditions to improve overall health status including cognitive and functional abilities (Duthie et al., 2011). Since cardiovascular risk factors of hypertension, hyperlipidemia, and diabetes are associated with more rapid progression of AD, their optimal management is a priority early in AD treatment (Nelson et al., 2009; Wysocki et al., 2012). Patients diagnosed with AD should also be screened for depression, which may occur concurrently in up to a third of patients presenting with AD and can affect cognition (Williams et al., 2010). In addition to optimal treatment of risk factors and comorbid conditions, a comprehensive medication review is important to assess for potentially inappropriate medications, particularly those that may cause further impairment of cognition or increase risk for falls and injury to the patient with AD (California Workshop, 2008).

FDA-approved pharmacologic management of AD includes the cholinesterase inhibitors (ChEIs) and *N*-methyl-D-aspartate (NMDA) glutamate receptor antagonist. Since 1993, the FDA has approved four ChEIs although the first ChEI, tacrine, is no longer marketed because of the disadvantages of hepatic adverse effects and lack of tolerability with four times a day dosing. The currently available ChEIs, donepezil, galantamine and rivastigmine, are each available in oral dosage forms with rivastigmine also available as a transdermal patch (Table 4.1). The only NMDA antagonist currently approved is oral memantine. These medications are available in a variety of doses and dosage forms, including a recently approved combination product to provide options to clinicians based on the patient's changing condition and functional needs. Choice of ChEI is based upon patient-specific factors as no agent shows clear evidence of superiority (Birks, 2006; Quirion, 1993).

TABLE 4.1 Approved Cholinesterase Inhibitors for Treatment of Alzheimer's Disease

	Donepezil (Aricept, Aricept ODT)	Rivastigmine (Exelon, Exelon Patch)	Galantamine (Razadyne, Razadyne ER)
FDA approval	1996	2000	2001
Mechanisms	AChEI	AChEI + BuChEI	AChEI + nicotinic modulation
Indication	Mild to moderate AD Moderate to severe AD	Mild to moderate AD Moderate to severe AD Dementia of Parkinson's disease	Mild to moderate AD
Dosage form	Per os tablet, orally dissolving tablet	Per os capsules, oral solution, transdermal patch	Per os tablets, oral solution, extended release capsules
Frequency of administration	Once daily	Twice daily per os	Tablets and solution twice daily with food
		Patch application every 24h	Extended release capsules once daily in am with food
Initial dose	5mg per os daily	1.5mg per os twice daily 4.6mg patch once daily	4mg per os twice daily or 8mg extended release capsule once daily
Titration schedule	Increase to 10mg daily after 4–6 weeks May increase to 23mg daily after additional 3 months for severe AD	Increase per os by 3mg/day at 2 week intervals with target of 6mg twice daily Increase patch to 9.5mg after 4 weeks then may increase to 13.3mg after additional 4 weeks for severe AD	Increase by 8mg/day at 4 week intervals to maximum of 12mg per os twice daily or 24mg extended release capsule once daily

AChEI, acetylcholinesterase inhibitor; *BuChEI*, butyrylcholinesterase inhibitor.

ACETYLCHOLINESTERASE INHIBITORS

FDA-approved treatment of AD reflects the brain pathology thought to be associated with the neurodegenerative symptoms and neuronal changes. As cholinergic neuronal pathways are destroyed, there is a decrease in activity of acetylcholine-synthesizing enzyme and loss of cholinergic neurotransmission in the cerebral cortex (Quirion, 1993). ChEIs boost the available acetylcholine for improved cholinergic transmission at the neuronal synapse. It is unknown to what extent rivastigmine's additional inhibition of butyrylcholinesterase (BuChE) and galantamine's modulating effect on nicotinic receptors provide clinical benefits to AD patients. The ChEIs are first-line agents with all three indicated for treatment of mild to moderate AD and the higher doses of donepezil (10 and 23mg tablets) along with rivastigmine (13.3mg/24h patch) indicated for moderate to severe disease (Donepezil US Prescribing Information, 2015; Galantamine US Prescribing Information, 2013; Rivastigmine US Prescribing Information, 2015a,b).

Relative contraindications and cautions to the use of ChEI include bradycardia, sick sinus syndrome, chronic obstructive pulmonary disease, asthma, seizure disorder, ulcer disease, bladder outlet obstruction, and history of an excessive response to succinylcholine anesthetic muscle relaxants. Caution is also advised when used in patients with low body weight <50–55 kg. The three agents, donepezil, rivastigmine, and galantamine, have similar efficacy results on cognition, global status, and ability to perform activities of daily living (ADLs) with some variation in adverse effect profile and pharmacokinetic characteristics. Common adverse effects include gastrointestinal complaints of nausea, vomiting, diarrhea, decreased appetite occurring in 5–20% of patients along with reports of insomnia, dizziness, and headache. Systemic effects associated with excessive peripheral cholinergic activity include urinary frequency, bradycardia, and syncope. Because of the risk of falls with syncope, close monitoring may be advised to prevent injury. Each of the ChEIs has a recommended titration schedule, which allows time for the body to adjust to potential adverse effects. When gaps occur in ChEI therapy, restarting at initial dose is advised (Donepezil US Prescribing Information, 2015; Galantamine US Prescribing Information, 2013; Rivastigmine US Prescribing Information, 2015a,b).

Donepezil, brand name Aricept, was approved in 1996 and is often chosen as ChEI upon initial diagnosis as it is indicated for use from mild to severe AD treatment. Donepezil binds to the enzyme acetylcholinesterase (AChE) in a noncompetitive means and is hydrolyzed instead of acetylcholine (Herrmann et al., 2011). Donepezil has limited peripheral effects and a long half-life, which allow once daily dosing. The initial dose of 5 mg by mouth daily may be increased to 10 mg daily after 4–6 weeks. Both 5 and 10 mg doses are considered maintenance dosing for mild to moderate disease. For moderate to severe AD, a further dose titration to 23 mg is possible after 3 months at 10 mg daily dose, although the limited clinical benefits of this higher dose must be balanced with the increased risk for adverse effects (Farlow et al., 2010). If therapy is interrupted for more than 7 days, the patient is advised to return to the starting dose of 5 mg daily (Donepezil US Prescribing Information, 2015).

Rivastigmine, brand name Exelon, was approved in 2000 and is available in immediate release capsules, oral liquid, and a daily patch formulation. All dosage forms are indicated for mild to moderate AD and the highest patch dose of 13.3 mg/24 h is indicated for moderate to severe AD. This agent remains bound to AChE after hydrolysis resulting in a pseudo-irreversible effect (Herrmann et al., 2011). Titration for capsules takes place at 2-week intervals from 1.5 mg twice a day (bid) to 3 mg bid to 4.5 mg bid to a maximum of 6 mg bid. The patch dose increases at 4-week intervals from 4.6 mg/24 h to 9.5 mg/24 h and finally to 13.3 mg/24 h for moderate-to-severe disease. In patients with moderate to severe renal or hepatic disease or low body weight <50 kg, a maximum dose of 4.6 mg/24 h is advised. Special instructions with the patch include rotating to a different application site with no site used twice in a 14-day period. Removal of a patch prior to application of a new patch is an important patient/caregiver counseling point as the simultaneous use of more than one patch can lead to significant adverse effects including death. The patch cannot be cut and detailed directions for administration must be followed for both safe and efficacious use. If patch therapy is interrupted for more than 3 days, the patient may be advised to return to starting patch dose. Oral capsules and solution are administered with food twice a day. Rivastigmine is also indicated for mild and moderate dementia associated with Parkinson's disease (Rivastigmine US Prescribing Information, 2015a,b).

Galantamine, brand name Razadyne, was approved in 2001 and is available in 4, 8, and 12 mg immediate release tablets along with extended release capsules in 8, 16, and 24 mg doses and an oral solution. It is indicated for mild-to-moderate disease with dosage increased every 4 weeks to maximally tolerated dose. In addition to the reversible and competitive inhibition of AChE, galantamine exhibits a modulation of nicotinic receptors (Herrmann et al., 2011). The manufacturer recommends administration of all dosage forms with food to decrease gastrointestinal (GI) adverse effects and there are dose restrictions for moderate renal and hepatic impairment. Daily extended release capsules are recommended for morning administration. Twice daily dosage forms are recommended to be given at the time of morning and evening meals. If treatment is interrupted for more than 3 days, the patient should be retitrated from the initial dose (Galantamine US Prescribing Information, 2013).

PRACTICAL USE OF ACETYLCHOLINESTERASE INHIBITORS

In practice, the various dosage forms present practical solutions as well as obstacles for individual patients' appropriate use and adherence to treatment. Practitioners may choose the Aricept 10 mg ODT (orally dissolving tablet) as a convenient dosage form for a patient who needs extensive cueing to swallow. For the same patient, however, the Aricept 23 mg oral tablet, which cannot be chewed, crushed, or broken, might create difficulty in swallowing whole. As the ability to adhere to strict administration requirements may be impaired with disease progression, tablets that must be swallowed whole might be challenging in patients with significant difficulty in swallowing. Oral solutions, transdermal patches, sustained release capsules, which may be opened and sprinkled on applesauce, are all examples of patient-friendly dosage forms for specific populations. Once-daily products are associated with greater adherence and extended release products also may avoid increased side effects seen with higher peak serum levels of immediate release products. Adherence to proper patch application and removal may be more complicated in a patient receiving other medications in transdermal patch dosage form with differing frequency of application. Ease of adherence, frequency of administration, storage requirements, and cost are also considerations for the practitioner and necessary topics for patient, family, and caregiver discussions (California Workshop, 2008).

How do the medication factors apply to a patient living with AD? (a fictional example based on typical experiences) *Patient JR is an 83-year-old widower experiencing mild-moderate AD and resides in an assisted living unit of a continuing care community. He has progressed from living independently to a more structured environment with some assistance with activities of daily living but is not confined to a locked, memory support environment. His health care is provided with a team approach of nurses, nursing assistants, attending physician, nurse practitioners, dietician, social worker, recreational therapist, and a pharmacist quarterly review. Here is the Nurse Practitioner Progress Note from the Sep. 7 encounter: "Asked to see patient JR by daughter who is concerned with worsening memory and weight loss. JR cooks own breakfast, lunches in the dining room and receives a premade dinner. He goes to sleep about 6 pm nightly. Vital signs within normal limits, physical exam unremarkable except for a weight decrease of 4 lbs in past 3 months. MMSE is 19/30 today—down from 25/30 in April. Assessment/Plan: 1. Weight Loss—agrees to take a supplement shake with breakfast 2. AD—continue donepezil 10 mg daily and start memantine 5 mg bid and titrate up—daughter in agreement."*

9/22 Medical Progress Note: "Asked to see JR secondary to confusion/forgetfulness. Patient is pleasant and cooperative with appropriate responses to questions. Medication non-compliance is noted as it appears JR is forgetting to take pm meds. Agrees to assisted medication packaging system with each dose individually labeled with date and time. Donepezil had not been refilled or taken in past month so dose decreased to 5 mg daily × 4 weeks to retitrate."

11/2 Nurse Progress Note: "Nursing assistant found 3 days of medications lying in trash can. Prior days were missing. JR stated, 'I had too many of them' when asked why medications were thrown away."

11/5 Nurse Progress Note: "Nurse observed resident taking all am and pm medications in the morning. Nurse explained importance of taking medications at the correct time and keeping time between medications scheduled for am and pm."

Adherence can become more difficult with memory impairment and institutionalization may occur as difficulty in medication management progresses. Among prescribers, the different titration schedules for AD treatment can cause confusion with too rapid dose escalation potentially increasing initial adverse effects. However, if a patient remains on the initial ChEI dose and is not titrated to a maintenance dose, ineffective therapeutic outcomes may result. Packaging the medication into titration packets and use of computerized templates for ordering in electronic prescribing systems can avoid these pitfalls of incorrect titration. A pitfall with electronic records is the documentation of intolerance to a specific product as an allergy or intolerance to the entire class.

Prescribing information provides limitations to the use of ChEIs including the potential for drug interactions when ChEIs are used with aspirin and nonsteroidal antiinflammatory drugs increasing the risk of GI adverse effects including bleeding and vomiting. Warnings include caution for use of ChEIs because of synergistic effects with other medications/classes that increase seizure potential or decrease heart rate. ChEIs may increase the skeletal muscle relaxation of succinylcholine anesthetics. Antagonistic interactions may occur with medications having anticholinergic effects. Individual agents have the potential for drug interactions involving the cytochrome P450 enzyme system such as donepezil whose clearance may be decreased by CYP 2D6 inhibitors. Rivastigmine prescribing information instructs that use with metoclopramide, beta blockers, cholinomimetics, and anticholinergic medications is not recommended (Donepezil US Prescribing Information, 2015; Rivastigmine US Prescribing Information, 2015a,b; Galantamine US Prescribing Information, 2013).

NMDA ANTAGONIST USE

As AD progresses to moderate to severe disease, the NMDA antagonist memantine may be added to a ChEI or used alone. Memantine reduces overexcitation of the glutamate receptors to retain their function in cognition. This overexcitation may be more commonly expressed with disease progression, thus the indication for use in moderate to severe AD. Memantine is generally well tolerated without the common GI adverse effects of ChEIs. Its adverse effects include constipation, dizziness, confusion, headache, cough, and somnolence (Robinson and Keating, 2006). Memantine is available in immediate release tablets, extended release capsules, an oral solution, and in a combination product with donepezil. Initial memantine dosing is titrated weekly to a maximum dose of 10 mg bid for tablets or 28 mg daily for extended release capsules. Efficacy, safety, and tolerability have been demonstrated in the use of 28 mg extended release capsules in combination with ChEIs for moderate to severe AD with the advantage of once-daily memantine dosing (Grossberg et al., 2013). A maximum dose of 5 mg bid or 14 mg extended release capsule daily is recommended for renal impairment when creatinine clearance is 5–29 mL/min. Medications that increase urinary pH may reduce the tubular reabsorption of memantine resulting in increased levels of memantine in the blood stream. Caution is advised when therapy is combined with other NMDA antagonists used for different indications, ketamine, amantadine, or dextromethorphan (Memantine US Prescribing Information, 2014, 2013). Memantine in combination therapy with donepezil has shown outcome benefits on cognition, global outcomes, ADLs, and behavior when compared to donepezil plus a placebo (Tariot et al., 2004).

TREATMENT GUIDELINES AND DISEASE MANAGEMENT

Recommended guidelines from the American College of Physicians and the American Academy of Family Physicians for treatment of AD include initiation of ChEIs for mild to moderate AD with titration to maintenance dose as tolerated (Qaseem et al., 2008). Patients are monitored at 2–4 weeks for potential adverse effects and closely followed during dose titrations. Therapeutic effectiveness can be assessed in 3–6 months after drug initiation with a variety of cognition scales and caregiver questionnaires (California Workshop, 2008). The patient's ability to adhere to a titration schedule and consistent dose administration may influence the effectiveness of treatment. If patients experience intolerable adverse effects or lack of efficacy such as a drop in mini-mental status exam (MMSE) score of more than 2–4 points/year, clinicians may choose to switch to an alternate ChEI and retitrate to maintenance dose. With disease progression, ChEI dose maximization and changes in pharmacologic agent can be made. For moderate to severe AD, the ChEI should be maintained or initiated and antiglutamergic therapy with NMDA antagonist can be added and titrated to maintenance dose as tolerated. With disease progression, ChEI use may significantly decrease caregiver burden and lower the risk of institutional care. Greatest benefit is expected when pharmacologic treatment begins early and is maintained over the course of disease although expectations for cognitive improvement may not be observed (Geldmacher, 2007; Geldmacher et al., 2003). Outcome measures of minimally improved or stable cognitive testing status may differ from the caregiver's perception of improved ability to complete ADLs and patient's functional behavioral status. Patient and caregiver goal-setting may differ from that which is measured in standardized assessment scales. For example, a patient-specific goal may be less reliance on reminder lists and calendars in early AD compared to an objective clinician's goal of improved 5-min recall per MMSE testing. Caregivers may look for a reduction in repetitive questions or improvement in behavior for moderate AD versus change in attention and cognition scales.

To maximize therapeutic outcomes with currently approved medications, counseling is important. When initiating AD therapy, patients and caregivers should be counseled on potential adverse effects and self-care to minimize those effects. Taking ChEIs in the evening and/or with food may minimize the initial GI adverse effects. Patients experiencing insomnia associated with the introduction of daily ChEIs may move an evening administration time to morning. Proper patch rotation may decrease local dermatologic effects. The ability to choose a dosage form compatible with an individual patient may also influence ChEI choice.

With introduction of ChEI therapy, new or worsening urinary incontinence may be the result of the peripheral cholinergic effects. If an anticholinergic medication is added for treatment of urinary frequency because of cholinergic effects of AD treatment, this prescribing cascade may have detrimental effects on cognition. A Canadian study enrolling over 44,000 patients with dementia demonstrated this increased risk for use of anticholinergic medication to treat new or worsening urinary incontinence, which may have been associated with a ChEI prescribed for dementia treatment (Gill et al., 2005). An Archives of Internal Medicine study of 19,000 dementia patients noted an association with syncope risk and use of ChEIs. Syncope-related complications of hospitalization for treatment of hip fracture, bradycardia, and pacemaker insertion were serious measured outcomes (Gill et al., 2009). Medications with anticholinergic properties are often considered potentially inappropriate pharmacologic agents for the elderly population (AGS Beers, 2015). When anticholinergic medications are used for more than 2 months, there is an increased risk for cognitive impairment and potentially more rapid progression of dementia (Cai et al., 2013).

Patients being treated for AD may benefit at all stages of disease from proper management of comorbid conditions and attention to fall prevention. Hospitalization from exacerbated comorbid conditions or treatment of falls with injury can lead to agitation, confusion, and disorientation for patients with AD. If misinterpreted, a patient with AD may be ordered medication to control behaviors associated with confusion from a change in living location or could be treated for agitated behavior when pain relief was indicated. There is currently no FDA-approved medication to treat BPSD. ChEIs have been studied in the treatment of BPSD with limited effectiveness noted (Rodda et al., 2009). Antipsychotics used outside FDA approval for the treatment of BPSD have resulted in a Black Box warning for this medication class for increased risk of mortality (Maust et al., 2015). There is a potential for misinterpretation of symptoms of other medical conditions, geriatric syndromes, or age-related impairments as progression of the cognitive decline associated with AD. For example, a patient with AD may inappropriately answer a question during cognitive assessment. The inappropriate response may be considered an expression of their worsening cognitive deficit directly caused by AD. However, upon further exploration, it may be discovered that the patient is experiencing sensory impairment and needs pharmacologic treatment to remove excessive wax in the ear, which was distorting hearing, or perhaps the addition of an assistive hearing device. CNS adverse effects of an inappropriate drug used in the treatment of a comorbid condition may also be misinterpreted as AD symptom progression. Therefore optimizing treatment of other medical conditions and impairments and minimizing the use of potentially inappropriate medications, particularly those with CNS adverse effects, should be addressed early in the treatment of AD. A comprehensive medication review assessing both prescription and nonprescription medications can be helpful to reduce use of medications that worsen cognition or increase potential for falls and their disabling consequences. These in-depth medication reviews can identify the potential for polypharmacy and should continue throughout AD treatment to reduce the risk for drug-induced cognitive loss or misidentification of a drug adverse effect as AD progression. When practitioners add new medications regardless of indication, there is the potential for drug interactions and difficulty in maintaining compliance to a more complicated drug regimen (Cummings et al., 2015). Identification of potentially inappropriate medications in this aged population includes a benefit/risk assessment for all medications to minimize likelihood of adverse effects detrimental to cognition (AGS, 2015).

TREATMENT DISCONTINUATION

The decision of when to discontinue AD pharmacologic therapy can be difficult to make in the absence of significant demonstration of efficacy or absence of adverse effects. Therapeutic treatment plans are individualized to patient response and family and caregiver needs as well as emerging clinical practice guidelines. The benefit to risk ratio changes with advancing disease burden and routinely needs evaluation by the collaborative team. Clinical trials demonstrate some benefit up to 4 years of ChEI treatment (Lyle et al., 2008). Clinicians may choose to stop therapy when the patient reaches a stage of little cognitive or functional ability or when the risks of treatment exceed potential benefits. With end-stage disease, it may be difficult for patients to comply with medication administration, thus prompting discontinuation. Hospice and palliative care may be initiated during terminal stages of AD per patient or family wishes. These consultations may involve decisions to stop ChEI and NMDA antagonist therapy as there are limited data to support use in end-stage AD. With the decision to stop AD therapy, tapering of dose and patient monitoring for significant deterioration are advised (Herrmann et al., 2013). There remains a need for additional research into the optimal duration of ChEI and memantine therapy along with more intensive studies comparing ChEI agents both alone and in combination with memantine (Qaseem et al., 2008). Because patients respond as individuals to AD treatment, practitioners should be prepared to adjust pharmacologic therapy to promote quality of life for each individual patient and caregiver. Research into more effective means of treatment, disease reversal, and a cure are hopes for the future.

References

AGS 2015 Beers Criteria Update Expert Panel, 2015. American Geriatrics Society 2015 Updated Beers Criteria for Potentially Inappropriate Medication Use in Older Adults. J. Am. Geriatr. Soc. 63, 2227–2246.

Birks, J., 2006. Cholinesterase inhibitors for Alzheimer's disease. Cochrane Database Syst. Rev. 1, CD005593.

Cai, X., Cambell, N., et al., 2013. Long-term anticholinergic use and the aging brain. Alzheimers Dement. 9, 377–385.

California Workshop on Guidelines for Alzheimer's Disease Management, 2008. Guidelines for Alzheimer's Disease Management. Final Report.

Cummings, J.L., Isaacson, R.S., Schmitt, F.A., Velting, D.M., 2015. A practical algorithm for managing Alzheimer's disease: what, when, and why? Ann. Clin. Transl. Neurol. 2, 307–323.

Donepezil (Aricept®) US Prescribing Information, 2015. Available at: http://www.aricept.com/docs/pdf/aricept_PI.pdf.

Doraiswamy, P.M., Leon, J., Cummings, J.L., et al., 2002. Prevalence and impact of medical comorbidity in Alzheimer's disease. J. Gerontol. A Biol. Sci. Med. Sci. 57, M173–M177.

Duthie, A., Chew, D., Soiza, R.I., 2011. Non-psychiatric comorbidity associated with Alzheimer's disease. QJM 104, 913–920.

Farlow, M.R., Salloway, S., Tariot, P.N., et al., 2010. Effectiveness and tolerability of high-dose (23 mg/d) versus standard-dose (10 mg/d) donepezil in moderate to severe Alzheimer's disease: a 24-week, randomized, double-blind study. Clin. Ther. 32, 1234–1251.

Galantamine (Razadyne®, Razadyne ER®) US Prescribing Information, 2013. Available at: http://www.janssenpharmaceuticalsinc.com/assets/razadyne_er.pdf.
Geldmacher, D.S., 2007. Treatment guidelines for Alzheimer's disease: redefining perceptions in primary care. Prim. Care Companion J. Clin. Psychiatry 9, 113–121.
Geldmacher, D.S., Provenzano, G., McRae, R., Mastey, V., Leni, J.R., 2003. Donepezil is associated with delayed nursing home placement in patients with Alzheimer's disease. J. Am. Geriatr. Soc. 51 (7), 937–944.
Gill, S.S., et al., 2009. Syncope and its consequences in patients with dementia receiving cholinesterase inhibitors – a population-based cohort study. Arch. Intern. Med. 169 (9), 867–873.
Gill, S.S., et al., 2005. Prescribing cascade involving cholinesterase inhibitors and anticholinergic drugs. Arch. Intern. Med. 165, 808–813.
Grossberg, G.T., Manes, F., Allegri, R.F., et al., 2013. The safety, tolerability, and efficacy of once-daily memantine (28 mg): a multinational, randomized, double-blind, placebo-controlled trial in patients with moderate-to-severe Alzheimer's disease taking cholinesterase inhibitors. CNS Drugs 27, 469–478.
Herrmann, N., Lanctôt, K.L., Hogan, D.B., 2013. Pharmacological recommendations for the symptomatic treatment of dementia: the Canadian Consensus Conference on the diagnosis and treatment of dementia 2012. Alzheimers Res. Ther. (Suppl. 1), S5.
Herrmann, N., Chau, S.A., Kircanski, I., et al., 2011. Current and emerging drug treatment options for Alzheimer's disease: a systematic review. Drugs 71 (15), 2013–2065.
Hort, J., O'Brien, J.T., Gainotti, G., et al., 2010. EFNS 2010 guidelines for the diagnosis and management of Alzheimer's disease. Eur. J. Neurol. 17, 1236–1248.
Lindstrom, H.A., Smyth, K.A., Sami, S.A., et al., 2006. Medication use to treat memory loss in dementia: perspectives of persons with dementia and their caregivers. Dementia 5, 27–50.
Lyle, S., Grizzell, M., Willmott, S., et al., 2008. Treatment of a whole population sample of Alzheimer's disease with donepezil over a 4-year period: lessons learned. Dement. Geriatr. Cogn. Disord. 25, 226–231.
Maust, D.T., Kim, H., Seyfried, L.S., et al., March 18, 2015. Antipsychotics, other psychotropics, and the risk of death in patients with dementia: number needed to harm. JAMA Psychiatry. 72(5), 438–445.
Memantine (Namenda®) US Prescribing Information, 2013. Available at: http://pi.actavis.com/data_stream.asp?product_group=1901&p=pi&language=E.
Memantine (Namenda XR®) US Prescribing Information, 2014. Available at: http://pi.actavis.com/data_stream.asp?product_group=1902&p=pi&language=E.
National Institute of Aging 2014 Alzheimer's Disease medications fact sheet, 2014. National Institute on Aging Website. http://www.nia.nih.gov/alzheimers/publication/alzheimers-disease-medications-fact-sheet.
Nelson, P.T., Smith, C.D., Abner, E.A., et al., 2009. Human cerebral neuropathology of Type 2 diabetes mellitus. Biochim. Biophys. Acta 1792 (5), 454–469.
Qaseem, A., Snow, V., Cross, J.T., Forciea, M.A., Hopkins, R., Shekelle, P., et al., 2008. Current pharmacologic treatment of dementia: a clinical practice guideline from the American College of physicians and the American Academy of family physicians. Ann. Intern. Med. 148, 370–378.
Quirion, R., 1993. Cholinergic markers in Alzheimer's disease and the auto-regulation of acetylcholine release. J. Psychiatry Neurosci. 18 (5), 226–234.
Rivastigmine (Exelon® Oral) US Prescribing Information, 2015a. Available at: http://pharma.us.novartis.com/product/pi/pdf/exelon.pdf.
Rivastigmine (Exelon® Patch®) US Prescribing Information, 2015b. Available at: http://www.pharma.us.novartis.com/product/pi/pdf/exelonpatch.pdf.
Robinson, D.M., Keating, G.M., 2006. Memantine: a review of its use in Alzheimer's disease. Drugs 66, 1515–1534.
Rodda, J., Morgan, S., Walker, A., 2009. Are cholinesterase inhibitors effective in the management of behavioral and psychological symptoms of dementia in AD? A systematic review of randomized, placebo-controlled trials of donepezil, rivastigmine and galantamine. Int. Psychogeriatr. 21 (5), 813–824.
Sadowsky, C.H., Galvin, J.E., et al., 2012. Guidelines for the management of cognitive and behavioral problems in dementia. J. Am. Board Fam. Med. 25, 350–366.
Tariot, P.N., Farlow, M.R., Grossberg, G.T., et al., 2004. Memantine treatment in patients with moderate to severe Alzheimer disease already receiving donepezil: a randomized controlled trial. JAMA 291, 317–324.
Williams, J.W., Plassman, B.L., Burke, J., et al., 2010. Preventing Alzheimer's Disease and Cognitive Decline. In: Rockville, M.D. (Ed.). Agency for Healthcare Research and Quality, U.S. Dept of HHS. Publication No.: 10-E005.
Wysocki, M., Luo, X., Schmeidler, J., et al., 2012. Hypertension is associated with cognitive decline in elderly people at high risk for dementia. Am. J. Geriatr. Psychiatry 20, 179–187.

CHAPTER

5

Physicochemical Properties for Potential Alzheimer's Disease Drugs

Z. Ates-Alagoz, A. Adejare

OUTLINE

INTRODUCTION

Alzheimer's disease (AD) is a neurodegenerative disorder that results in loss of cognitive function and is eventually fatal (Pettersson et al., 2012). It is increasingly diagnosed in all countries where the number of patients rises exponentially with life expectancy (Florent-Béchard et al., 2007; Cummings, 2004; Forsyth and Ritzline, 1998). It is related to progressive cognitive decline, deficits in memory and executive functions, along with significant neuropsychiatric symptoms (Wilson et al., 2013; Chamberlain et al., 2011; Lyketsos et al., 2011). AD represents a significant unmet medical need since no disease-modifying therapy is yet available with more than 35 million people affected worldwide. To better understand the causes of AD, which can lead to the development of safe and effective pharmacological treatments, has been one of the foremost challenges in health research during the past decades (Sahni et al., 2011).

AD is characterized by extracellular amyloid plaques and intracellular neurofibrillary tangles composed of aggregates of misfolded amyloid-β-peptide (Aβ) and hyperphosphorylated tau proteins, respectively, in brain areas such as the hippocampus and basal forebrain

Drug Discovery Approaches for the Treatment of Neurodegenerative Disorders
http://dx.doi.org/10.1016/B978-0-12-802810-0.00005-2

(Tolnay and Probst, 1999; Gandy, 2005; Walsh et al., 2002). The loss of neurons in brain areas associated with learning process and memory consolidation results in the symptoms associated with AD. Aβ peptides are produced by the proteolytic processing of a type 1 transmembrane protein: the amyloid precursor protein (APP) by β- and γ-secretase enzymes, both of which are aspartyl proteases (Walsh et al., 2002). β-Secretase, also called β-site of APP cleaving enzyme, cleaves APP at the extracellular domain to generate a membrane spanning C terminal fragment β (C99), which is subsequently processed by γ-secretase to liberate Aβ40/42. Altered metabolism of the APP causing overproduction of Aβ peptides, more importantly the longer and hydrophobic Aβ42, has been implicated as a key player in the series of neuropathological changes that result in the disease. The ensuing pathological aggregation process may proceed via seed "precipitation" with a higher risk of such events with increasing peptide concentration (Adeniji, 2010).

The main agents prescribed nowadays are acetylcholinesterase inhibitors (AChEIs), but they are only useful for treating patients with mild-to-moderate AD. Tacrine (THA) was the first drug approved by the Food and Drug Administration for the treatment of AD (Brasnjevic et al., 2009; Farlow, 2002). However, this drug was withdrawn from the market because it exhibited side effects like hepatotoxicity and high dosing frequency (Forsyth et al., 1989; Watkins et al., 1994). Donezapil, galantamine (Kryger et al., 1998; Greenblatt et al., 1999), and rivastigmine (Farlow, 2002) are a second generation of AChEI drugs. Compared to THA, they have small but statistically significant benefits on cognitive measures relevant to dementia with improved safety profiles. Since their effects are neither long lasting nor substantially altering the progression of AD, it becomes obvious that AChEIs are far from ideal therapeutics to combat AD (Brasnjevic et al., 2009). Another approach to the treatment of AD is to block glutamatergic neurotransmission. Glutamate is one of the principal excitatory neurotransmitters in the mammalian CNS. A major function of glutamate is control of ion flow at excitatory synapses. Glutamate receptors are subdivided into two, namely, metabotropic and ionotropic. Three ionotropic receptor types have been identified based on ligand selectivity: α-amino-3-hydroxy-5-methyl-4-isoxazolepropionic acid (AMPA), *N*-methyl-D-aspartate (NMDA), and kainate. In addition to ionotropic receptors, three classes of metabotropic receptors are acknowledged (Madden, 2002). The ionotropic NMDA receptor (NMDAR) is noteworthy in that it requires binding by agonist glutamate and coagonist D-serine or glycine for it to be activated (open state). NMDAR is also distinct in that it exhibits slow kinetics, is permeable to Na^+, K^+, and Ca^{2+} (Dingledine et al., 1999; Liu and Zhang, 2000; Cull-Candy, 2001), and is both ligand and voltage gated (Schiller et al., 1998; Yuste et al., 1999). It is a complex made up of distinct binding sites including sites for amino acids L-glutamate, glycine, and D-serine. In addition to these sites, allosteric modulatory sites for Mg^{2+}, phencyclidine (PCP), polyamines, and Zn^{2+} are known (Iversen et al., 2009). While glutamate, glycine, and polyamine sites are found outside the ion channel, the sites for Mg^{2+} and PCP are located within the channel itself (Javitt and Zukin, 1989). The NMDAR has been implicated in the pathophysiology of a variety of neurological and neuropsychiatric diseases including AD (Cacabelos, 1999), epilepsy, chronic pain syndrome, schizophrenia, Parkinson's disease, Huntington's disease (Raymond, 2003; Fan and Raymond, 2007), major depression, addiction, and anxiety (Parsons, 1998). Excessive glutamate and subsequent overstimulation of NMDARs leading to excessive Ca^{2+} influx has been implicated in the pathophysiology of these disease states (Mody and MacDonald,

1995; Sattler and Tymianski, 2000). Several preclinical paradigms have found that noncompetitive NMDA antagonism can effectively reduce NMDAR-mediated neurotoxicity (Rothman and Olney, 1987). A major limitation for therapeutically available NMDA antagonists is the essential role of NMDAR in neurophysiology. While blockade of excessive NMDAR activity is desirable, it must be achieved without complete amelioration of normal glutamate function. As a result of this dichotomy, many competitive antagonists have failed in clinical trials (Chen and Lipton, 2006). Utilization of noncompetitive antagonists working through open-channel blockade has been proposed as an attractive alternative, as this mechanism requires initial activation of the channel for inhibition to occur, possibly leading to a higher likelihood of channel blockade in the presence of excessive levels of glutamate and a lower likelihood of antagonism with normal physiological levels of glutamate (Chen and Lipton, 2006).

Current methods for the treatment of AD provide temporary relief, improve cognitive function, but do not slow the progression of this disorder (Bullock and Dengiz, 2005). Therefore there is an urgent need to develop strategies to improve the efficacy, bioavailability, transport across the blood–brain barrier (BBB), and subsequently to limit the adverse effects of pharmaceutical compounds for the treatment of AD.

THE BLOOD–BRAIN BARRIER

Brain and spinal cord are completely separated from the blood by the BBB and the blood–spinal cord barrier. BBB hinders entry from blood to brain of nearly all molecules, except those that are small and lipophilic or those that enter the brain through an active transport mechanism, particularly with essential nutrients, precursors, and cofactors (Alavijeh et al., 2005). Significant progress has been made in understanding the molecular basis of neurodegeneration for many years (Rowinska-Zyreka et al., 2015), but the BBB remains a big obstacle to exploiting this knowledge and developing drugs to treat diseases of the CNS. The BBB controls the exchange of molecules between the blood and brain with anatomical, physicochemical, and biochemical mechanisms (Nag, 2003). These mechanisms make the BBB virtually impermeable to drugs developed for the treatment of neurodegenerative diseases.

Eukaryotic ATP binding cassette (ABC) transporters are efflux pumps, and are found in tissues and organs with secretory and barrier functions. They are also found at the BBB, and they play direct and indirect roles in many neurological disorders. There is reasonable evidence that the BBB becomes increasingly permeable with increasing age, in the presence of AD (Farrall and Wardlaw, 2009). It was also suggested that the ABC transporters, especially ABCB1, may have a significant effect on the pathogenesis of AD. Lam et al. (2001) showed that ABCB1 serves as an Aβ efflux pump, but they also showed a significant decrease of ABCB1 function in the elderly brains (Pahnke et al., 2009). Age-related neurodegenerative disorders have in common the accumulation of insoluble neurotoxic proteins (Johnson, 2000; Walker and LeVine, 2000). Involvement of the BBB in the accumulation of Aβ peptides has been considered for a number of years. It was showed that Aβ in plasma and cerebrospinal fluid exists at equilibrium, controlled by an unknown mechanism that shifts the concentration toward the brain during plaque development (Pahnke et al., 2009; DeMattos et al., 2002).

PHYSICOCHEMICAL PROPERTIES OF ALZHEIMER'S DISEASE DRUGS

If a drug has a high metabolic clearance, it could be subject to an extensive first-pass effect, resulting in low bioavailability. In addition to membrane permeability, lipophilic compounds tend to have a greater affinity for metabolic enzymes so the lipophilicity of a drug also affects metabolic activity. The greater the lipophilicity of a drug, the higher permeability and greater metabolic clearance (Riley et al., 2001). CNS drugs need to have sufficient lipophilicity to allow them to cross the BBB, so these influences on bioavailability need to be carefully considered in the drug discovery process (Alavijeh et al., 2005).

Drug discovery is a complex process with a combination of specific factors including drug solubility, acid dissociation constant (pKa), absorption, bioavailability, metabolism, formulation, pharmacokinetics, toxicity, and therapeutic efficacy (Alavijeh et al., 2005; Alavijeh and Palmer, 2004; Kubinyi, 2003). Drug metabolism and pharmacokinetics (DMPK) is playing an important role in drug discovery (Alavijeh and Palmer, 2004; Roberts, 2003; Riley et al., 2002; Lin et al., 2003; Edddershaw et al., 2000). Drug candidates are now selected, in part, on the basis of DMPK properties, for example, low clearance, good oral bioavailability, and an acceptable profile of metabolism. To improve the probability of success of drug leads, in vitro absorption, distribution, metabolism, and excretion (ADME) assays and in vivo DMPK studies are being performed throughout the discovery process (Alavijeh et al., 2005; Kassel, 2004).

Neuroactive drug therapies against AD have some disadvantages such as being beneficial only at higher doses, limited bioavailability, poor absorption following systemic delivery, severe peripheral side effects caused by higher uptake by normal cells, and difficulty in penetrating the highly restrictive BBB (Mufamadi et al., 2013; Roney et al., 2005; Rubin and Staddon, 1999). Smaller lipophilic molecules, peptides, and nutrients satisfy BBB penetration via endogenous transporters, but BBB restricts the entry of large molecules into the CNS (Pardridge, 2003; Kroll and Neuwelt, 1998).

Studies have shown the key structural properties for discovery of CNS drugs such as hydrogen bonds, lipophilicity, polar surface area (PSA), molecular weight (MW), and acidity (Kerns and Li, 2008; Pardridge, 1995, 1998; Liu, 2006; Doan et al., 2002; Clark, 2003). These properties are more restrictive at the BBB than at most other membrane barriers in the body. CNS drugs have fewer hydrogen bond donors, higher log P, lower PSA, and fewer rotatable bonds compared to non-CNS drugs (Doan et al., 2002).

A set of physicochemical properties that guide BBB permeability predictions has been suggested by Pardridge: the structure should have H-bonds (total) <8–10, MW <400–500, and no acids (Kroll and Neuwelt, 1998). Spraklin proposes H-bond donors <2 and H-bond acceptors <6 (Maurer et al., 2005). This proposal is in agreement with a general consensus that H-bond donors are more limiting than H-bond acceptors. According to Clark and Lobell et al. the structure should have the following: $N+O<6$, PSA <60–70 Å^2, MW <450, log $D=1$–3, and clog $P-(N+O)>0$ (Kerns and Li, 2008; Lobell et al., 2003). These rules are helpful to assess BBB permeability before synthesis, including ability to evaluate compounds being brought into a project, identifying poor in vivo brain penetration, and managing which structural modifications might best improve BBB permeation of compounds. Positively charged amines interact with the negatively charged groups of phospholipids at the BBB. Nearly 75% of CNS drugs are basic, 19% are neutral, and 6% are acids. The amine functional group has been described as essential for CNS activity (Kerns and Li, 2008).

P-glycoprotein (Pgp) efflux is the most important limitation to BBB permeation of discovery lead series. Structure–efflux relationships can be established in an in vitro Pgp assay. These relationships will indicate which portions of the molecule might be modified to attempt efflux reduction. Reducing the total number of hydrogen bonds, elimination of acidic group, increasing lipophilicity, and intramolecular hydrogen bond will increase BBB permeation. The BBB permeation of some drugs is enhanced by membrane transporters. Carrier-mediated transporters enhance the penetration of compounds with poor passive BBB permeation if those compounds happen to resemble natural substrates (Kerns and Li, 2008).

AD involves multiple pathogenic factors, thus its treatment should aim to target many factors by integrating numerous functions in a single drug molecule (Bolognesi et al., 2011; Zhang, 2005). Physicochemical properties are useful in the quest to evaluate abilities of drugs to cross biological membranes and oral absorption (El-Gendy and Adejare, 2004; Horter and Dressman, 2001). Aqueous solubility as a function of pH along with pKa determinations are important and fundamental in determining the degree of dissolution (for solid dosage forms) and subsequent permeation through cell membrane. Prior to drug administration, they are of value in drug design, selection of formulation, and development processes. Octanol/water partition coefficient has been used as a measure of lipophilicity of compounds and correlates well with biological availability (Paschke et al., 2001). A chromatographic technique referred to as immobilized artificial membrane phosphatidylcholine chromatography (Pidgeon et al., 1995) utilizing columns packed with phosphatidylcholine bound to silica support has been developed and validated as a model to predict intestinal permeability. We conducted pharmaceutical profiling studies on a novel prototype γ-secretase inhibitor (sulfonamide **1**, Fig. 5.1) to determine the potential of its oral absorption. The studies included determination of solubility, dissociation constant (pKa), octanol/water partition coefficient (log P), and the capacity factor (k'_{IAM}) on immobilized artificial membrane (IAM) chromatographic columns. The compound is very slightly soluble in water ($120 \pm 50\,\mu g/mL$) but the solubility increased considerably in basic medium ($270 \pm 60\,\mu g/mL$). The compound exhibited pKa of (10.36 ± 0.11) and log P of (3.36 ± 0.16) determined by shake-flask method and (3.31 ± 0.01) determined by high-performance liquid chromatography. The experimentally determined log P values correlated well with the calculated one of 3.44. The observed log k'_{IAM} value of (2.79 ± 0.04) indicates that the compound can reasonably be expected to have high membrane permeability and therefore good absorption profile if taken orally (El-Gendy and Adejare, 2004).

Peptides and proteins have become important targets in neuropharmaceutical drug design for the treatment of a wide variety of CNS disorders (Brasnjevic et al., 2009; Datar et al., 2004; Gentilucci, 2004; Balasubramaniam, 2002). Although they have potential, peptide and protein drugs (P/P drugs) are ineffective in the treatment of CNS disorders because of the inability to effectively deliver and hold up within the brain. Some small (mostly lipophilic) P/P drugs following intraventricular administration have been described to have successful permeability.

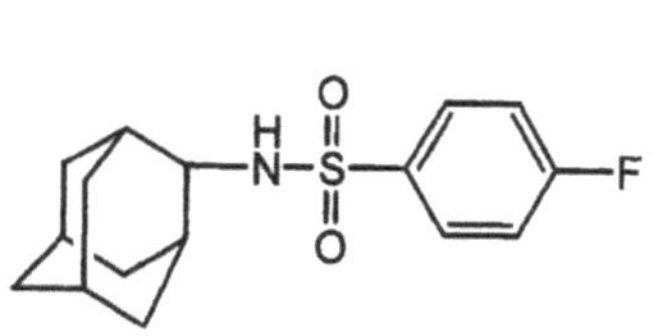

FIGURE 5.1 Structure of sulfonamide **1**.

Also the molecule must have an MW below a threshold of 400–500 Da to cross the BBB in pharmacologically significant amounts (Brasnjevic et al., 2009; Misra et al., 2003; Pavan et al., 2008). Examples of diseases responsive to treatment with P/P drugs and for which small peptide drugs have been shown to cross the BBB include depression, affective disorders, insomnia, chronic pain, and epilepsy (Brasnjevic et al., 2009; Ajay et al., 1999). Such interventions have been successful in dealing with peripheral diseases but with no damage in the CNS because the BBB restricted entry of these P/P drugs to the brain. The CNS disorders include AD, Huntington's disease, Parkinson's disease, amyotrophic lateral sclerosis, multiple sclerosis, stroke, brain and spinal cord injury, and brain cancer (Brasnjevic et al., 2009; Pardridge, 1991). BBB has reduced the application of many potentially important P/P drugs in brain diseases. Therefore the need for effective BBB drug-targeting systems is obvious and urgent to develop more brain active P/P molecules into effective therapies (Brasnjevic et al., 2009).

Neurotrophins are potential therapeutic P/P agents for neurodegenerative disorders like AD, Parkinson's disease, and amyotrophic lateral sclerosis. This is because there is strong evidence that reduced neurotrophic support is a significant factor in the pathogenesis of these neurodegenerative diseases. Administration of nerve growth factor (NGF) completely restored the number of choline acetyltransferase-immunopositive neurons to normal values, reversed deposition of extracellular amyloid aggregates, and abolished the cognitive deficits in NGF knockout mice, which acquire age-dependent pathology reminiscent of human AD (Brasnjevic et al., 2009; Hefti et al., 1985; Kromer, 1987; Capsoni et al., 2002). Although the therapeutic potential of neurotrophins is great, inconvenient pharmacokinetics and adverse side-effect profiles have limited their clinical usefulness (Thorne and Frey II, 2001; Thoenen and Sendtner, 2002). Many studies have described a useful drug delivery system for transport of NGF across the BBB to the CNS, for instance, PEGylation technology (Gozes, 2001), covalent conjugation to antitransferrin receptor antibodies (Liao et al., 2001; Zhang and Pardridge, 2001; Miller, 2002), or the adsorption on liposomes (Xie et al., 2004). These studies may open new prospects for the treatment of CNS diseases (Brasnjevic et al., 2009).

Peptides containing N-methylated amino acids have been identified as promising agents to block protein–protein interactions involving β-sheet-rich interactions, as illustrated by inhibitors for Aβ peptide (Bose et al., 2010; Hughes et al., 2000; Kokkoni et al., 2006; Austen et al., 2008; Pratim Bose et al., 2009) and amylin (Tatarek-Nossol et al., 2005; Yan et al., 2006; Yan et al., 2007) fibrillation. Prevention of Aβ and amylin aggregation has emerged as potential goals in the therapy and prevention of AD, and various β-sheet disrupting peptides have been reported to preclude the aggregation of Aβ (Chalifour et al., 2003; Chacon et al., 2004; Stephenson et al., 2008) and amylin (Scrocchi et al., 2002; Scrocchi et al., 2003; Potter et al., 2009). A detailed study of how the degree of N-methylation affects the ADME and toxicity (ADMET) properties such as solubility, membrane transport, proteolytic stability, and general cell toxicity of the investigated peptides was presented by Bose et al. They chose hexapeptides corresponding to N-methylated analogs of residues of the Aβ peptide, which have previously been shown to inhibit aggregation of Aβ fibrils in vitro. It was found that poly-N-methylated peptides are nontoxic and have enriched proteolytic stability over their nonmethylated analogs. Aqueous solubility was seen to increase with increased degree of N-methylation, but membrane transport was found to be low for all investigated hexapeptides. It was suggested that poly-N-methylated peptides, particularly shorter or equal to six residues, can be suitable candidates for drug design (Bose et al., 2010).

The AMPA receptor (AMPA-R) is a subtype of the ionotropic glutamate receptor coupled to ion channels that modulate cell excitability by gating the flow of calcium and sodium ions into the cell (Doble, 1995). It was reported that AMPA-R antagonists are effective in the therapy of neurodegenerative disorders such as ischemic stroke, epilepsy, and AD (Takano et al., 2006). After 2,3-dioxo-6-nitro-1,2,3,4-tetrahydrobenzo[*f*]quinoxaline-7-sulfonamide (**2**) was demonstrated to have potent and selective AMPA-R antagonistic activity, researchers have modified the quinoxalinedione structure (Takano et al., 2006; Sheardown et al., 1990). The numerous resulting compounds can be categorized as first-generation compounds of substituted simple quinoxalinedione structure, such as compounds **2** and **3** (Fig. 5.2) (Ohmori et al., 1994; Shimizu-Sasamata et al., 1996), and second-generation compounds with a hydrophilic substituent at the N-1 position of the quinoxalinedione resulting in compounds **4** (Kawasaki-Yatsugi et al., 1998) and **5** (Fig. 5.2) (Turski et al., 1998). Compound **3** has been shown to be a potent and selective AMPA antagonist and neuroprotective in animal models of global and focal cerebral ischemia, but its limited solubility in aqueous solutions has precluded development as a clinical agent. Also simple quinoxalinediones have been reported to cause kidney toxicity, probably as a result of their physicochemical properties, especially poor solubility (Xue et al., 1994). The second-generation compounds were designed to improve the physicochemical properties of the simple quinoxalinediones. They are more soluble and do not appear to cause kidney toxicity (Takano et al., 2006).

Takano et al. (2003, 2005) reported the development of a novel third-generation AMPA-R antagonist, the 7-imidazolyl-6-nitro-3-oxoquinoxaline-2-carboxylic acid derivative (compound **6**, Fig. 5.3), which contains a carboxylic acid as a hydrophilic group as well as an imidazole moiety. This compound is characterized by a 4-carboxyphenyl group joined through a urethane linkage onto an imidazole ring at the 7 position on the 3-oxoquinoxaline-2-carboxylic acid nucleus. It shows excellent AMPA-R antagonist activity in vitro and in vivo compared with known antagonists based on the quinoxalinedione nucleus and is also water soluble. They found that introduction of a phenyl group joined through a urethane linkage at the 4 position

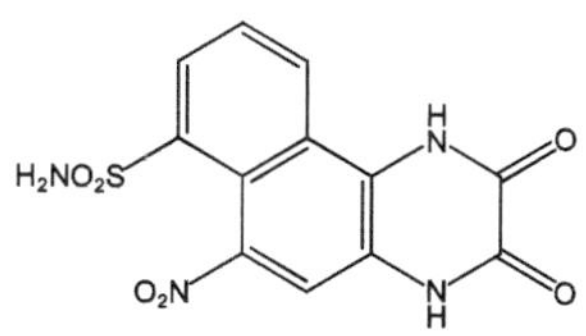

2

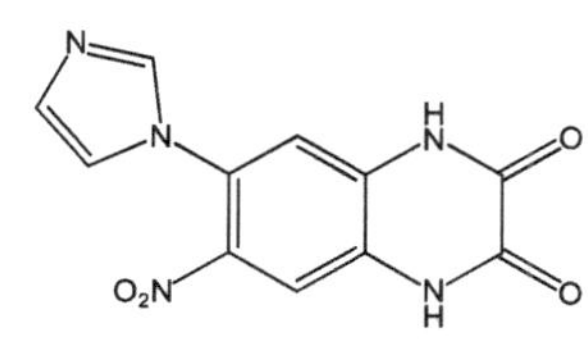

3

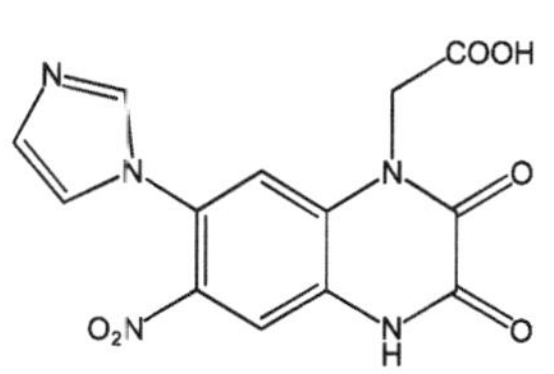

4

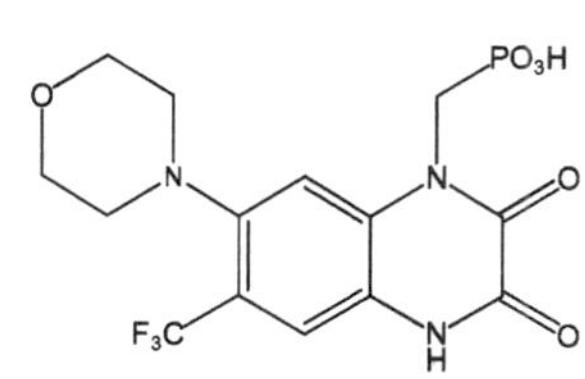

5

FIGURE 5.2 Structures of compounds **2–5**.

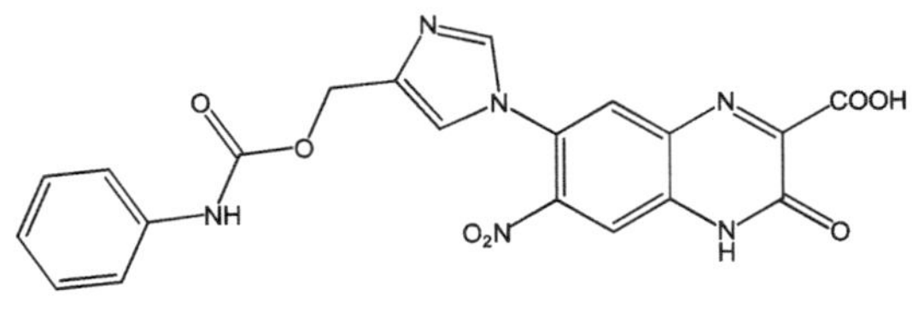

6

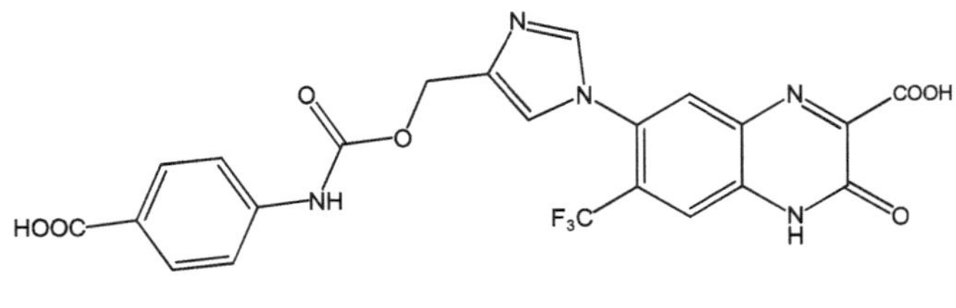

7

FIGURE 5.3 Structures of compounds **6** and **7**.

of a 7-imidazolyl group on the 6-nitro-3-oxoquinoxaline-2-carboxylic acid nucleus gives high affinity and good selectivity for the AMPA-R. However, in additional studies, they found that compound **6** has suboptimal physicochemical properties, particularly instability to fluorescent light in neutral solution (Takano et al., 2006). They reported that introduction of the trifluoromethyl group at the 6 position resulted in good biological activity, including neuroprotective effects, and good physicochemical properties. Compound **7** (Fig. 5.3), which has a 4-carboxyphenyl group joined through a urethane linkage to a 7-imidazolyl heterocycle, was found to have high potency and selectivity for the AMPA-R in vitro and to show good neuroprotective effects in vivo. Also compound **7** exhibited good physicochemical properties, including stability to light and good solubility in aqueous solutions (Takano et al., 2006).

γ-Secretase is a critical enzyme in the cellular pathway responsible for the formation of a range of β-amyloid peptides. Close et al. (2012) reported 4,4-disubstituted piperidine γ-secretase inhibitors that were optimized for in vitro cellular potency and pharmacokinetic properties in vivo. Acyl piperidine **8** (Fig. 5.4) is representative of their initial leads; it inhibits Aβ42 and Aβ40 production in SH-SY5Y cells and has promising physicochemical properties (Aleyenus, 2010; Doan, 2002). Unfortunately, it is subject to rapid clearance in vivo. When dosed orally (100 mg/kg), low drug concentrations in the brain and plasma reflected the high clearance for, and it consequently failed to lower, cerebral Aβ42 production in the APP-YAC mouse model. They did modifications to compound **8** to increase exposure by addressing metabolic liabilities and improve potency while maintaining favorable physicochemical properties. Their efforts resulted with the discovery of compound **9** (Fig. 5.4). It has an optimized medicinal chemistry profile and lowered cerebral Aβ42 production by 76% in their in vivo model (Close et al., 2012).

Pettersson et al. (2012) reported the discovery and optimization of a novel series of dihydrobenzofuran amides as γ-secretase modulators. Strategies for aligning in vitro potency with

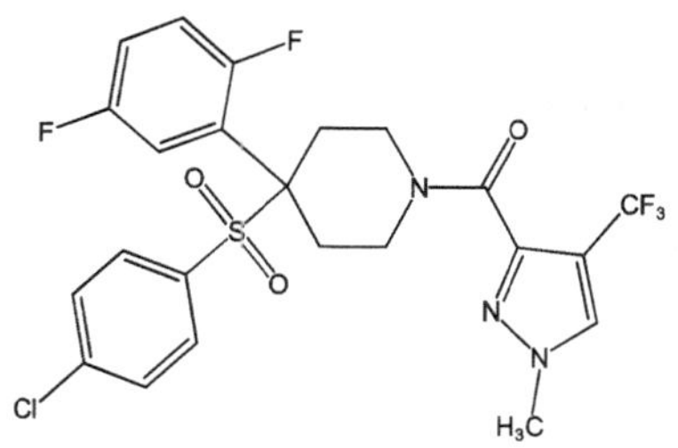

8

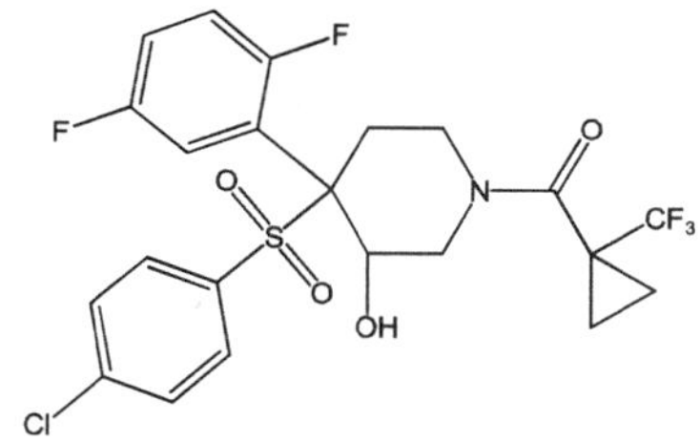

9

FIGURE 5.4 Structures of compounds **8** and **9**.

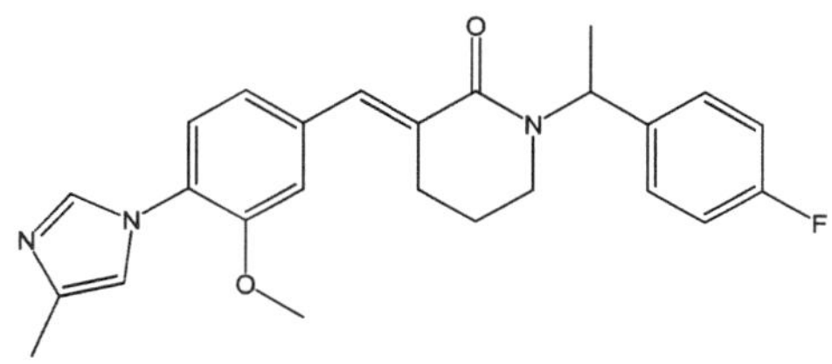

10

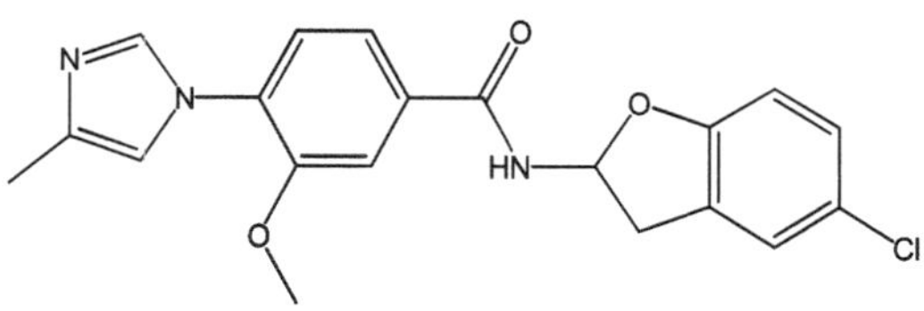

11

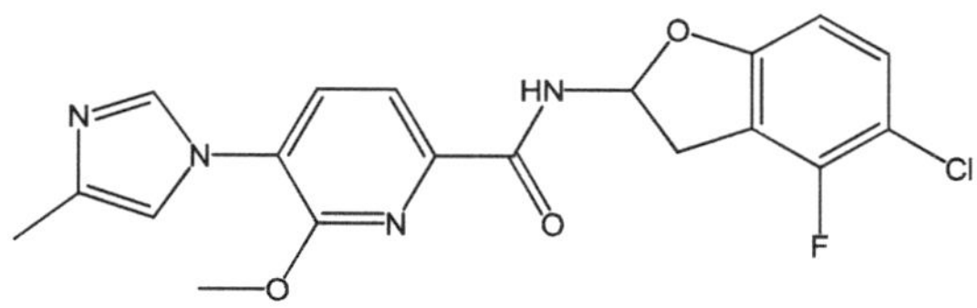

12

FIGURE 5.5 Structures of compounds **10–12**.

drug-like physicochemical properties and good microsomal stability while avoiding Pgp-mediated efflux were discussed. Using arylimidazole **10** (Fig. 5.5) as a starting point (Portelius et al., 2010), their primary objectives were to identify a series with improved CNS physicochemical properties. It defined end points for a set of four physicochemical properties that described 90% of orally active drugs that achieved phase II clinical status: (1) MW < 500 Da; (2) lipophilicity, log P or the calculate of 1-octanol-water partition coefficient, clog P < 5; (3) number of hydrogen-bond donors, OH plus NH count, <5; and (4) number of hydrogen-bond acceptors, O plus N atoms, <10 (Wager et al., 2010). The clog P values for the majority of the drugs varied from 0.4 (10th percentile) to 5.1 (90th percentile) with a median clog P value of 2.8. As expected for CNS drugs, a similar but shifted range existed for clog D, which varied from −0.5 (10th percentile) to 3.8 (90th percentile) with a median value of 1.7. In particular, they sought to reduce lipophilicity since compound **10** has a clog P of 4.8, which corresponds to a lipophilic efficiency of 2.19 and a CNS multiple parameter optimization score of 3.7 (Wager et al., 2010; Hughes et al., 2008). Thus their strategy of reducing lipophilicity was an attempt to improve the safety margin of this series, and targeting chemical space with lower clog P would increase the probability of achieving alignment of increased potency and beneficial ADME parameters such as microsomal stability. They proposed that the cinnamide and the central phenyl ring of compound **10** could be replaced with an amide bond, and heterocycles such as a pyridine or a pyrazine ring, respectively. Lead compounds **11** and **12** (Fig. 5.5) have moderate-to-good in vitro potency, and good oral bioavailability was achieved as well as robust brain Aβ42 lowering activity at 100 mg/kg oral dose (Pettersson et al., 2012).

Histamine H_3 receptor (H_3R) has received considerable interest as a potential drug target that could deliver an improved therapy for the treatment of dementia. Wilson et al. (2013) described the discovery of the benzazepine class of H_3R antagonists and the identification of lead molecule **13** (Fig. 5.6) from this series with encouraging levels of in vivo activity. By carefully controlling the physicochemical properties of the benzazepine series, the medicinal chemistry effort was able to rapidly progress the benzazepine class of H_3 antagonists through to the identification of clinical candidates with robust in vivo efficacy and excellent developability properties. To support this goal, the medicinal chemistry strategy focused on maintaining the clog P of the series around 3.0, limiting the MW (<400), and maintaining the polar surface area below 80 Å^2 to keep the series in the optimal area of chemical space for a CNS drug (Wager et al., 2011). Wilson et al. (2013) described the discovery of GSK189254 **14** and GSK239512 **15** (Fig. 5.6) that were progressed as clinical candidates to explore the potential of H_3R antagonists as novel therapies for the treatment of AD and other dementias.

Aβ peptides play an important role in the pathology of the neurodegeneration in AD. Syntheses of Aβ peptides have been difficult because of their hydrophobic character, poor aqueous solubility and high tendency for aggregation. An isopeptide precursor [iso-Aβ(1–42)] was synthesized with Fmoc chemistry and transformed at neutral pH to Aβ(1–42) by O→N acyl migration by Bozso et al. (2010). They synthesized the same precursor using Boc chemistry and studied the transformation to Aβ(1–42) by acyl migration. Several methods (circular dichroism, atomic force and transmission electron microscopy, dynamic light scattering) were used to study the peptide conformation and aggregation processes. The biological activity of

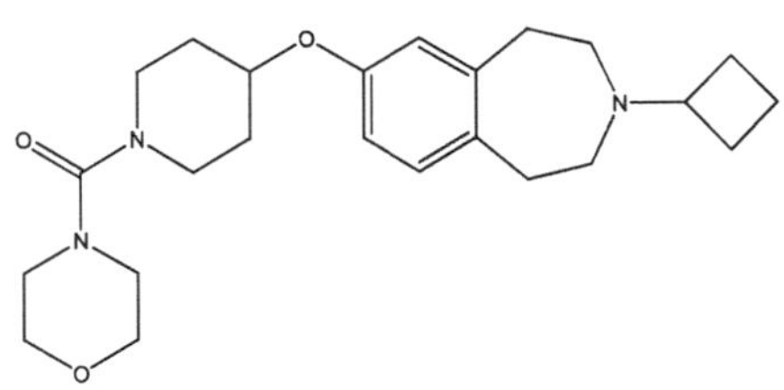

13

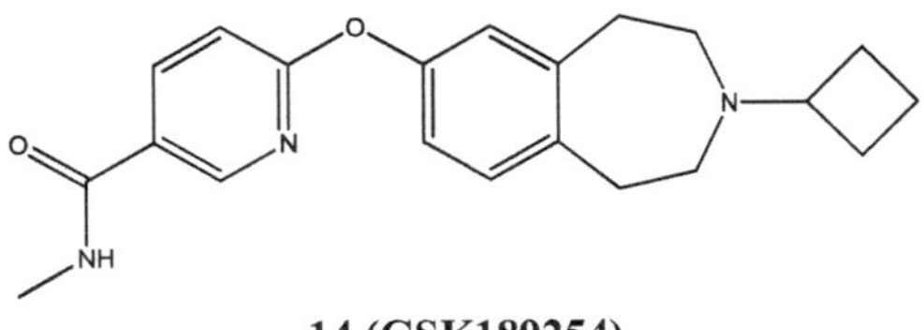

14 (GSK189254)

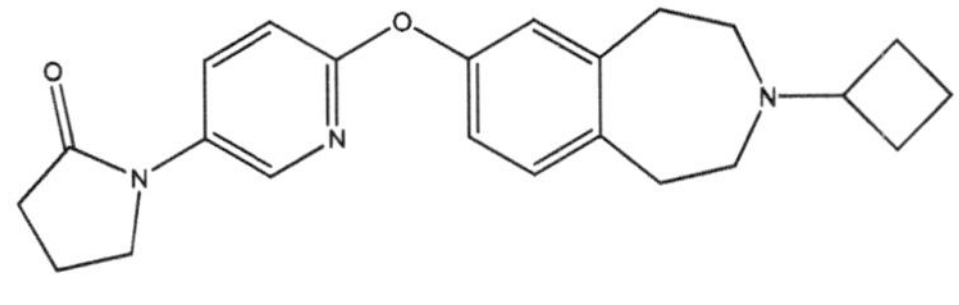

15 (GSK239512)

FIGURE 5.6 Structures of compounds **13–15**.

the synthetic Aβ(1–42) was measured by ex vivo and in vivo experiments. O→N acyl migration of the precursor isopeptide resulted in a water-soluble oligomeric mixture of neurotoxic Aβ(1–42) (Bozso et al., 2010).

The pharmacological analysis of racemic chromenotacrines (**CT**) (Fig. 5.7) in a series of experiments targeted to explore their potential use for the treatment of AD was reported by Oset-Gasque et al. (2014). It was shown that compound **16** [11-amino-12-(3,4,5-trimethoxyphenyl)-8,9,10,12-tetrahydro-7H-chromeno[2,3-b]quinolin-3-ol, Fig. 5.7] is much less hepatotoxic than THA in a range of concentrations from 1 to 300 μM, measured as cell viability in HepG2 cells. Compound **16** treatment exerts a highly protective effect against lipid peroxidation induced in H_2O_2-treated SHSY5Y cells. It behaves as a noncompetitive inhibitor ($K_i = 0.047 \pm 0.003\,\mu M$), indicating that this compound binds at the peripheral anionic site. ADMET analysis showed that this compound should have a moderate BBB permeability. These studies showed that nontoxic chromenotacrine **16** can be considered as an attractive multipotent molecule for the potential treatment of AD.

Bis(7)-tacrine (B7T, Fig. 5.8) is a novel AChEI, and its intestinal absorption is not outstanding. Passive diffusion is the main transport pathway for B7T across intestinal epithelium. It has poor intestinal permeability and low oral bioavailability (Zhang et al., 2008). The lipophilicity and solubility profiles of bis(12)-hupyridone (B12H, Fig. 5.8) and B7T were investigated over a broad pH range by Yu et al. (2008). The log P values for

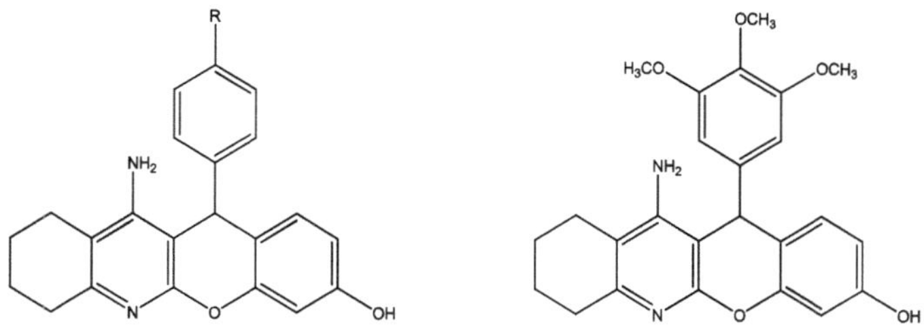

Racemic Chromenotacrines (**CT**) **16**

FIGURE 5.7 Structures of **CT** and compound **16**.

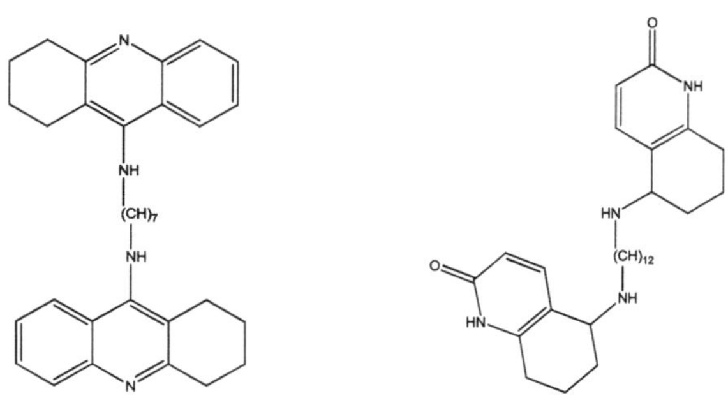

bis(7)-tacrine (B7T) bis(12)-hupyridone (B12H)

FIGURE 5.8 Structures of B7T and B12H.

B12H and B7T were found to be 5.4 and 8.2, respectively, indicating that the two dimers are highly lipophilic. The solubility of B12H was >1.41 mg/mL when the pH was <7, but <0.06 mg/mL when the pH was >8. The solubility of B7T was >0.26 mg/mL when the pH was <9, but <0.005 mg/mL when the pH was >12. The ionic strength of a solution could affect the solubilities significantly (11.16 mg/mL for B12H and 12.71 mg/mL for B7T in water; 2.07 mg/mL for B12H and 0.36 mg/mL for B7T in saline). Both dimers were found to have two pKa values: 7.5 ± 0.1 (pKa1) and 10.0 ± 0.2 (pKa2) for B12H; and 8.7 ± 0.1 (pKa1) and 10.7 ± 0.4 (pKa2) for B7T. In mice, a maximum acetylcholinesterase (AChE) inhibition occurred 15 min after the single-dose and intraperitoneal administration of either dimer. These studies showed that the two dimers may easily cross the BBB, and physiochemical characteristics of the two dimers suggest that they may be promising candidates for development of better drugs for AD (Yu et al., 2008).

Drugs should have proper ADMET properties to be approved for clinical tests. The drugs used for neurological disorder treatment should present good CNS penetration profiles and low toxic effects. BBB penetration is a crucial pharmacokinetic property in drug design because CNS-active compounds must cross it. Syntheses, biochemical evaluation, ADMET, toxicity and molecular modeling of each novel donepezil + propargylamine + 8-hydroxyquinoline (DPH) hybrids for the potential prevention and treatment of AD is described by Wang et al. (2014). **DPH** derivatives displayed moderate-to-good ADMET properties and brain penetration capacity. Compound **17** (Fig. 5.9) was less toxic than donepezil at high concentrations; while both showed similar cell viability profile at low concentrations. The antiamnesic effect of compound **17** was tested on mice. It was found to be able to significantly decrease scopolamine-induced learning deficits in healthy adult mice.

DRUG DELIVERY

Many drugs do not have adequate physicochemical characteristics which are necessary to succeed in crossing the BBB, including high lipid solubility, low MW and no charge. Numerous strategies have been developed to overcome the BBB. Combining a lipophilic moiety to the drug may cause loss of therapeutic effect making use of direct drug delivery

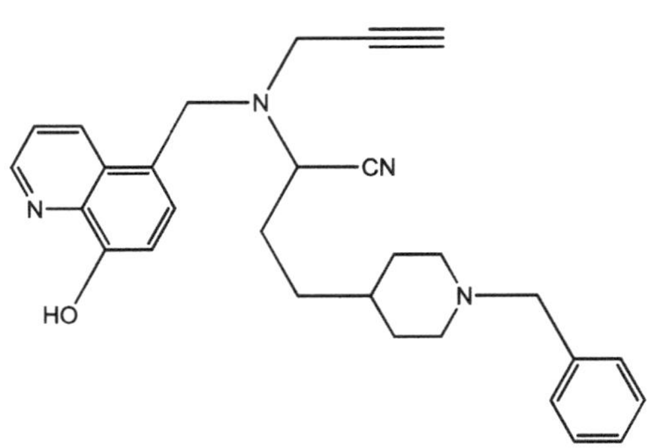

FIGURE 5.9 Structure of compound **17**.

difficult to develop. A promising strategy could be to connect drugs without any modification to colloidal carriers. Colloidal drug carriers include micelles, emulsions, liposomes, and nanoparticles (NPs). Only liposomes and NPs have been largely exploited for brain drug delivery. The reason for using colloidal carriers is usually to increase the specificity toward cells or tissues, to improve the bioavailability of drugs, and/or to protect them against enzyme inactivation. Furthermore, the colloidal systems are masking drugs' physicochemical characteristics through their encapsulation in systems, and allowing them access to cross the BBB (Garcia–Garcia et al., 2005).

NPs have been confirmed to deliver a great variety of drugs across the BBB (Kabanov, 2007; Roney et al., 2005). Drug-loaded NPs enable the brain delivery of agents that cannot independently permeate the BBB in therapeutically effective concentrations. Binding to the particles also may lead to reduction in side effects of drugs. Furthermore, because of a more effective brain delivery by NPs, the drug dose might be decreased. If any drug or larger biologically active compound or complex can be efficiently bound to the BBB-transcytosable NPs, it can be transported across the BBB, and drug released within the brain at therapeutically relevant concentrations and time profiles (Wohlfart et al., 2012). Nowadays, strategies utilizing NPs for the treatment of AD have focused on interfering with Aβ aggregation, with the idea of reducing its brain level (Matsuoka et al., 2003). A different approach with NPs is focused on treatment of symptoms, by protecting neuronal cells against oxidative damage. Because metal chelators have hepatotoxicity and neurotoxicity, their use to protect against oxidative damage is limited. The use of NPs to overcome these problems has been reported in several studies (Re et al., 2012; Krol, 2012).

Chitosan is a natural polysaccharide and a suitable nanocarrier material for delivery of anti-Alzheimer drugs because of its inherent physicochemical properties, bioactivities, and processing flexibility. The ability to become attached to varieties of molecules and the formation of the stable nanocomplex in physiological conditions make chitosan an adorable material for delivery of anti-Alzheimer drugs to the brain (Sarvaiya and Agrawal, 2015).

Melatonin (*N*-acetyl-5-methoxytryptamine) was discovered to be a direct free radical scavenger. As an antioxidant, melatonin can be used in the treatment of various cancers and neurodegenerative diseases such as Alzheimer's and Parkinson's diseases. Melatonin is easily absorbed across the mucosa, but its sensitivity to oxidation is a problem for achieving therapeutic level. In addition, its low oral bioavailability suggests the need for new routes of administration and an appropriate delivery system to be developed. The potential of lecithin/chitosan NPs as a mucoadhesive colloidal nanosystem for transmucosal delivery of melatonin was investigated by Hafner et al. The NPs were characterized by mean diameter and zeta potential ranging between 121.6 and 347.5nm, and 7.5 and 32.7mV, respectively, and increasing with lecithin-negative charge and chitosan content in the preparation. Melatonin loadings were up to 7.1%, and nearly 60–70% of melatonin was released in 4h. The permeability of melatonin was investigated using Caco-2 cells as an in vitro model of the epithelial barrier. Their results showed that NP suspension did not induce plasma membrane damage or decrease cell viability and could be safely applied to Caco-2 cells in the concentration range tested (<400 μg/mL) (Hafner et al., 2009).

Natural antioxidant compounds have been extensively studied as useful neuroprotective agents. Selective glutamatergic antagonists that also possess antioxidant capabilities represent a novel approach toward protection from excitotoxicity and oxidative stress associated with excess Aβ in AD. Sozio et al. (2013) have developed two new compounds characterized by NMDAR antagonist memantine (MEM) linked via an amide bond either to glutathione or (R)-α-lipoic acid. The new conjugates should act both as glutamate receptor antagonists and radical scavenging agents. They designed these MEM-sulfur containing antioxidants as potential new anti-AD agents. Prodrugs **18** and **19** (Fig. 5.10) showed free radical scavenging effects to both H_2O_2 and superoxide anion radical. In addition, they did not interfere with the proliferative capacity of the GL15 astroglial line. The physicochemical properties, membrane permeability, enzymatic and chemical stabilities, and antioxidant activity associated with the capacity to inhibit Aβ(1–42) aggregation make at least compound **19** a promising drug candidate in pathological events such as AD where both free radical damage and inflammatory activity in the brain are involved.

Intranasal delivery is a noninvasive method to provide effective systemic delivery of certain therapeutic compounds (Dhuria et al., 2010). If the drug could be retained and absorbed in the nasal cavity, the nasal route might also avoid the first-pass metabolism, and by this means reduce the biotransformation of the parent drug to metabolites (Wong and Zuo, 2010, 2013; Wong et al., 2012). Qian and his coworkers developed an in situ gel formulation for intranasal delivery of tacrine (THA). The pharmacokinetics and brain dispositions of the gel were compared with that from THA oral solution in rats. The gel significantly prolonged compound retention in nasal cavity compared to solution form. It was found that the gel achieved two- to threefold higher peak plasma concentration (C_{max}) and area under the curve (AUC) of THA in plasma and brain tissue compared to oral solution. It was suggested that the gel could be an effective intranasal formulation for THA because of the improved nasal residence time, enhanced bioavailability, better brain uptake of parent drug, and decreased exposure to metabolites (Qian et al., 2014).

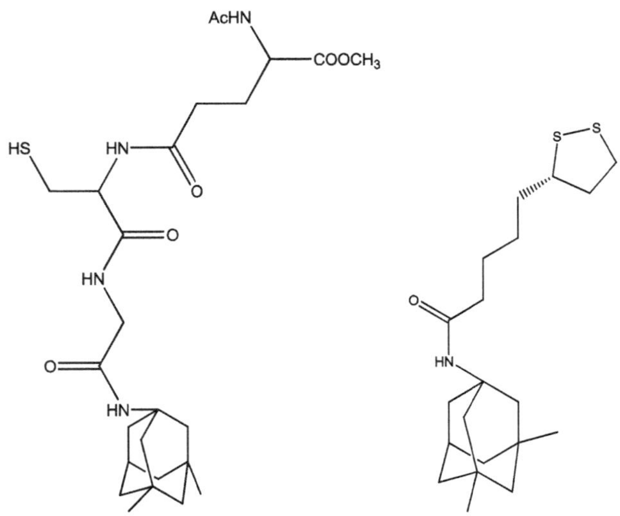

18 **19**

FIGURE 5.10 Structures of compounds **18** and **19**.

Galantamine hydrobromide (GH, Fig. 5.11) has been approved for symptomatic treatment of AD and vascular dementia because of its ability to inhibit AChE in the CNS (Li et al., 2012; Heinrich and Lee Teoh, 2004; Shytle, 2004). But because of its poor retention in the CNS and the intricacy of transporting it across the BBB, the clinical utility of the drug is impeded (De Boer and Gaillard, 2007; Ying et al., 2010). Liposomes are vesicles comprising concentric bilayer phospholipid-based membranes that can incorporate hydrophilic or hydrophobic drugs (Woodle and Lasic, 1992; Torchilin, 2005; Veerareddy and Vobalaboina, 2004). Several strategies using liposomes have been developed to improve CNS bioavailability of neuroactive drugs (Bangham et al., 1974). The effects of intranasal administration of GH-loaded flexible liposomes have been investigated for efficiency of AChE inhibition, as well as the pharmacokinetic behavior of GH in rat brain by Li and coworkers. It was found that the efficiency of AChE inhibition of GH-loaded flexible liposomes were greatly enhanced by intranasal administration compared with oral administration. They proposed that the C_{max} and $AUC_{0\to10}$ for intranasal administration of GH-loaded flexible liposomes were 3.52 and 3.36 times, respectively, higher than those of orally administered GH. Also, the T_{max} was greatly shortened for intranasal administration of GH loaded flexible liposomes. It was shown that the flexible liposome carrier is not toxic to the cultured cells by PC-12 cell viability tests and the cytotoxicity of GH to cells was clearly decreased by loading in flexible liposomes. Their results indicate that intranasal administration of GH-loaded flexible liposomes could readily transport GH into brain tissues, suggesting this approach is successful at brain–drug targeting in AD treatment (Li et al., 2012).

Mufamadi et al. (2013) also did a study to design ligand-functionalized nanoliposomes for effective intracellular delivery of galantamine into PC-12 neuronal cells to manage AD. Ligand-functionalized nanoliposomes were produced and validated for their physicochemical properties. Particle sizes of the nanoliposomes ranged from 127 to 165 nm (PdI = 0.39–0.03) with zeta potential values of −18 to −36 mV. The peptide coupling efficiency was from 40% to 78% while drug entrapment efficiency ranged from 42% to 79%. It was confirmed that galantamine and the peptide-ligand were incorporated into the inner core and surface of the nanoliposomes, respectively. Transmission electron microscopy studies revealed that native nanoliposomes, galantamine-loaded nanoliposomes, and the ligand-functionalized nanoliposomes were stable with no aggregation observed. It was found that postengineering of peptides onto the surface of galantamine-loaded nanoliposomes provide targeted delivery of galantamine directly into PC-12 neuronal cells. Native galantamine and nonfunctionalized nanoliposomes exhibited no significant accumulation into PC-12 neuronal cells after 24 h of incubation because of nonspecific drug delivery.

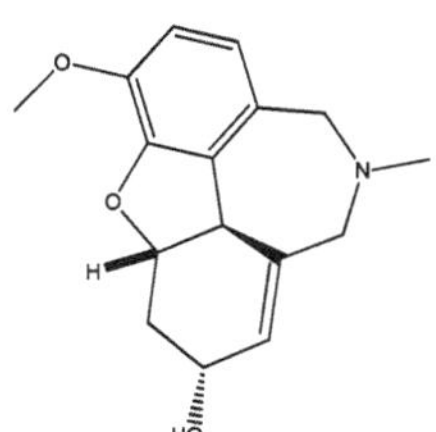

FIGURE 5.11 Galantamine.

Curcumin (Fig. 5.12) inhibits amyloid Aβ(1–42) oligomer formation and cell toxicity at micromolar concentrations in vitro (Ono et al., 2004; Kim et al., 2005; Yang et al., 2005; Kim et al., 2001; Re et al., 2010) and binds to senile plaques, reducing amyloid levels in vivo. It has a wide spectrum of therapeutic use and is thought to play a vital role against pathological conditions such as inflammation, psoriasis, various tumors, and neurodegenerative diseases like AD. But it is highly lipophilic and has very poor bioavailability. This hampers its therapeutic usefulness. Taylor et al. (2011) have been investigating a number of different ligands for their ability to bind to Aβ with high affinity to interfere with the aggregation process. Curcumin was added in the lipid phase during liposome preparation to prepare nanoliposomes incorporating curcumin. They also prepared curcumin surface-decorated liposomes by using a curcumin–lipid conjugate (lipid–S-curcumin liposomes) or by attaching a curcumin derivative on preformed liposomes by click chemistry (click-curcumin liposomes). They also incorporated the lipid ligands (phosphatidic acid, cardiolipin, or GM1) into nanoliposomes during their formation. It was found that all nanoliposomes with curcumin were able to inhibit the formation of fibrillar and/or oligomeric Aβ in vitro. The click-curcumin type was the most effective among the three forms of curcumin liposomes tested. They proposed that curcumin-based liposomes could be further developed as a novel treatment for AD.

Mulik et al. (2009) prepared poly(butyl) cyanoacrylate (PBCA) nanoparticles coated with poloxamer 188 containing curcuminoids by anionic polymerization using solvent evaporation method. The particle size and zeta potential of prepared liposomes were 178 nm and −28.33, respectively, with 77.99% encapsulation efficiency. The curcuminoids-loaded PBCA nanoparticles showed excellent chemical and physical stability. It was shown that the prepared PBCA nanoparticles are capable of controlled drug release for extended periods of time with higher release in acidic environment compared to phosphate buffer solution (PBS) (pH = 7.4) by in vitro release study, suggesting the usefulness of the prepared nanoparticles for intracellular delivery.

Donepezil (Fig. 5.13) is a reversible and noncompetitive cholinesterase inhibitor, and a far more selective inhibitor of AChE than of butyrylcholinesterase (Zhang et al., 2007).

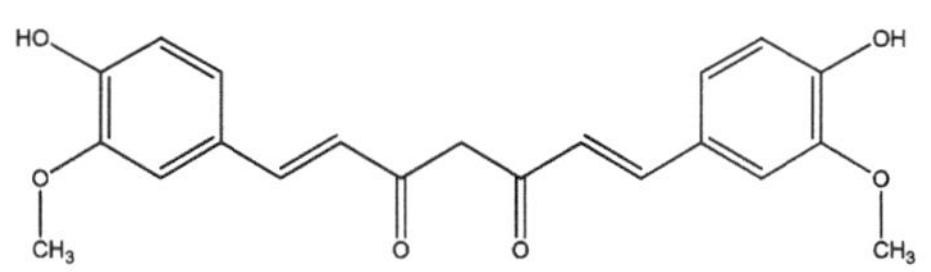

FIGURE 5.12 Curcumin.

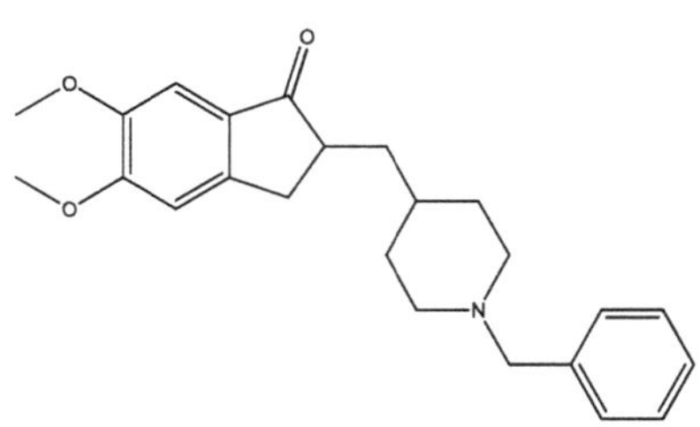

FIGURE 5.13 Donepezil.

It was shown that donepezil produces a significant improvement of cognition and global function in patients with mild-to-moderately severe AD and shows an excellent tolerability and safety profile (Rogers and Friedhoff, 1998). Donepezil is available in the market as once a day tablet or capsule (Christodoulou et al., 2006). Although oral administration is convenient for most patients, it is very difficult for AD patients not to miss scheduled self-medication. Donepezil also showed gastrointestinal side effects. Therefore it is very important to develop a long-term, nongastrointestinal delivery system of donepezil for treatment of AD. Zhang and coworkers are interested in developing a sustained-release formulation for donepezil with inexpensive, biocompatible, and convenient administration by direct subcutaneous injection. They selected poly(D,L-lactide-coglycolide) microparticles as donepezil carrier because of its excellent tissue compatibility, biodegradable property, and safety profile (Gander et al., 2001). Their purpose was to prepare donepezil microparticles (DMs), determine their physicochemical characteristics including the loading ratio, thermal profile, in vitro release, in vivo donepezil levels in rat plasma, and assess the effect of DMs as a sustained-release delivery system for treatment of AD. DMs showed a loading ratio of 13.2 ± 2.1% (w/w) and a yield of 54.8 ± 0.8% with mean particle size about 75 μm. It was shown that donepezil completely released within 28 days in water, but a slow release in PBS (pH = 7.4) by in vitro release study. They showed that subcutaneous infusion of DMs (90 mg/kg) produced a sustained release process in rats and reached steady-state concentration. That dosage was in accordance with that of free donepezil (3 mg/kg day) by oral application route, and showed the same pharmacological role. Their results implicated that a sustained release delivery strategy could substitute for oral formulation of DMs for therapy of AD but with administration of once a month as opposed to daily (Zhang et al., 2007).

CONCLUSIONS

Drug discovery is a complex process with many factors involved. Drug candidates are now selected in part on the basis of DMPK and activity properties. To improve the probability of success of drug leads, in vitro ADME assays and in vivo DMPK studies are being performed throughout the discovery process. In this review, we illustrated physicochemical properties that affect drug CNS bioavailability and access to the active site. We also evaluated the importance of various modifications, both covalent and noncovalent, of compounds, and how the physicochemical properties of these compounds relate to their activities, which can lead to useful compounds that may prevent or reverse the progression of AD.

References

Adeniji, A., 2010. Structure Activity Relationship (SAR) Studies of a Novel Gamma-Secretase Inhibitor (Dissertations & theses). University of the Sciences in Philadelphia. 166 pages; 3395655.

Ajay, Bemis, G.W., Murcko, M.A., 1999. Designing libraries with CNS activity. J. Med. Chem. 42, 4942–4951.

Alavijeh, M.S., Chishty, M., Qaiser, M.Z., Palmer, M.A., 2005. Drug metabolism and pharmacokinetics, the blood–brain barrier, and central nervous system drug discovery. NeuroRx 2, 554–571.

Alavijeh, M.S., Palmer, A.M., 2004. The pivotal role of drug metabolism and pharmacokinetics in the discovery and development of new medicines. IDrugs 7, 755–763.

Alelyunas, Y.W., Empfield, J.R., McCarthy, D., Spreen, R.C., Bui, K., Pelosi-Kilby, L., Shen, C., 2010. Experimental solubility profiling of marketed CNS drugs, exploring solubility limit of CNS discovery candidate. Bioorg. Med. Chem. Lett. 20 (24), 7312–7316.

Austen, B.M., Paleologou, K.E., Ali, S.A., Qureshi, M.M., Allsop, D., El-Agnaf, O.M., 2008. Designing peptide inhibitors for oligomerization and toxicity of Alzheimer's beta-amyloid peptide. Biochemistry 47 (7), 1984–1992.

Balasubramaniam, A., 2002. Clinical potentials of neuropeptide Y family of hormones. Am. J. Surg. 183, 430–434.

Bangham, A.D., Hill, M.W., Miller, N.G.A., 1974. Preparation and use of liposomes as models of biological membranes. Methods Membr. Biol. 1, 61–68.

Bolognesi, M.L., Bartolini, M., Tarozzi, A., Morroni, F., Lizzi, F., Milelli, A., Minarini, A., Rosini, M., Hrelia, P., Andrisano, V., Melchiorre, C., 2011. Multitargeted drugs discovery: balancing anti-amyloid and anticholinesterase capacity in a single chemical entity. Bioorg. Med. Chem. Lett. 21, 2655–2658.

Bose, P.P., Chatterjee, U., Hubatsch, I., Artursson, P., Govender, T., Kruger, H.G., Bergh, M., Johansson, J., Arvidsson, P.I., 2010. In vitro ADMET and physicochemical investigations of poly-N-methylated peptides designed to inhibit Ab aggregation. Bioorg. Med. Chem. 18, 5896–5902.

Bozso, Z., Penke, B., Simon, D., Laczko, I., Juhasz, G., Szegedi, V., Kasza, A., Soos, K., Hetenyi, A., Weber, E., Tohati, H., Csete, M., Zarandi, M., Fülöp, L., 2010. Controlled in situ preparation of Ab(1–42) oligomers from the isopeptide "iso-Ab(1–42)", physicochemical and biological characterization. Peptides 31, 248–256.

Brasnjevic, I., Steinbusch, H.W.M., Schmitz, C., Martinez-Martinez, P., 2009. Delivery of peptide and protein drugs over the blood–brain barrier. Prog. Neurobiol. 87, 212–251.

Bullock, R., Dengiz, A., 2005. Cognitive performance in patients with Alzheimer's disease receiving cholinesterase inhibitors for up to 5 years. Int. J. Clin. Pract. 59 (7), 817–822.

Cacabelos, R., Takeda, M., Winblad, B., 1999. The glutamatergic system and neurodegeneration in dementia: preventive strategies in Alzheimer's disease. Int. J. Geriatr. Psychiatry 14, 3–47.

Capsoni, S., Giannotta, S., Cattaneo, A., 2002. Nerve growth factor and galantamine ameliorate early signs of neurodegeneration in anti-nerve growth factor mice. Proc. Natl. Acad. Sci. U.S.A. 99, 12432–12437.

Chacón, M.A., Barría, M.I., Soto, C., Inestrosa, N.C., 2004. Beta-sheet breaker peptide prevents Abeta-induced spatial memory impairments with partial reduction of amyloid deposits. Mol. Psychiatry 9 (10), 953–961.

Chalifour, R.J., McLaughlin, R.W., Lavoie, L., Morissette, C., Tremblay, N., Boulé, M., Sarazin, P., Stéa, D., Lacombe, D., Tremblay, P., Gervais, F., 2003. Stereoselective interactions of peptide inhibitors with the beta-amyloid peptide. J. Biol. Chem. 278 (37), 34874–34881.

Chamberlain, S.R., Blackwell, A.D., Nathan, P.J., Hammond, G., Robbins, T.W., Hodges, J.R., Michael, A., Semple, J.M., Bullmore, E.T., Sahakian, B.J., 2011. Differential cognitive deterioration in dementia: a two year longitudinal study. J. Alzheimers Dis. 24, 125–136.

Chen, H.-S.V., Lipton, S.A., 2006. The chemical biology of clinically tolerated NMDA receptor antagonists. J. Neurochem. 97, 1611–1626.

Christodoulou, C., Melville, P., Scherl, W.F., MacAllister, W.S., Elkins, L.E., Krupp, L.B., 2006. Effects of donepezil on memory and cognition in multiple sclerosis. J. Neurol. Sci. 245, 127–136.

Clark, D.E., 2003. In silico prediction of blood–brain barrier permeation. Drug Discov. Today 8, 927–933.

Close, J., Heidebrecht Jr., R., Hendrix, J., Li, C., Munoz, B., Surdi, L., Kattar, S., Tempest, P., Moses, P., Geng, X., Hughes, B., Smotrov, N., Moxhama, C., Chapnick, J., Kariv, I., Nikov, G., Burke, J.E., Deshmukh, S., Jeliazkova-Mecheva, V., Leach, J.K., Diaz, D., Xu, L., Yang, Z., Kwei, G., Moya, L., Shah, S., Tanga, F., Kenefic, C., Savage, D., Shearman, M., Ball, R.G., McNevin, M.J., Markarewicz, A., Miller, T., 2012. Lead optimization of 4,4-biaryl piperidine amides as c-secretase inhibitors. Bioorg. Med. Chem. Lett. 22, 3203–3207.

Cull-Candy, S., Brickley, S., Farrant, M., 2001. NMDA receptor subunits: diversity, development and disease. Curr. Opin. Neurobiol. 11, 327–335.

Cummings, J.L., 2004. Alzheimer's disease. N. Engl. J. Med. 351, 56–67.

De Boer, A.G., Gaillard, P.J., 2007. Drug targeting to the brain. Ann. Rev. Pharmacol. Toxicol. 47, 323–355.

De Mattos, R.B., Bales, K.R., Parsadanian, M., O'Dell, M.A., Foss, E.M., Paul, S.M., Holtzman, D.M., 2002. Plaque-associated disruption of CSF and plasma amyloid-beta (Abeta) equilibrium in a mouse model of Alzheimer's disease. J. Neurochem. 81, 229–236.

Datar, P., Srivastava, S., Coutinho, E., Govil, G., Substance, P., 2004. structure, function, and therapeutics. Curr. Top. Med. Chem. 4, 75–103.

Dhuria, S.V., Hanson, L.R., Frey 2nd, W.H., 2010. Intranasal delivery to the central nervous system: mechanisms and experimental considerations. J. Pharm. Sci. 99, 1654–1673.

Dingledine, R., Borges, K., Bowie, D., Traynelis, S.F., 1999. The glutamate receptor ion channels. Pharmacol. Rev. 51, 7–61.

Doan, K.M.M., Humphreys, J.E., Webster, L.O., Wring, S.A., Shampine, L.J., Serabjit-Singh, C.J., et al., 2002. Passive permeability and P-glycoprotein-mediated efflux differentiate central nervous system (CNS) and non-CNS marketed drugs. J. Pharmacol. Exp. Ther. 303, 1029–1037.

Doble, A., 1995. Excitatory amino acid receptors and neurodegeneration. Therapie 50, 319–337.

Eddershaw, P.J., Beresford, A.P., Bayliss, M.K., 2000. ADME/PK as part of a rational approach to drug discovery. Drug Discov. Today 5, 409–414.

El-Gendy, A.M., Adejare, A., 2004. Membrane permeability related physicochemical properties of a novel δ-secretase inhibitor. Int. J. Pharmaceutics 280, 47–55.

Fan, M.M.Y., Raymond, L.A., 2007. N-methyl-D-aspartate (NMDA) receptor function and excitotoxicity in Huntington's disease. Prog. Neurobiol. 81, 272–293.

Farlow, M., 2002. A clinical overview of cholinesterase inhibitors in Alzheimer's disease. Int. Psychogeriatr. 14 (Suppl. 1), 93–126.

Farrall, A.J., Wardlaw, J.M., 2009. Blood–brain barrier: ageing and microvascular disease - systematic review and meta-analysis. Neurobiol. Aging 30, 337–352.

Florent-Béchard, S., Malaplate-Armand, C., Koziel, V., Kriem, B., Olivier, J.-L., Pillot, T., Oster, T., 2007. Towards a nutritional approach for prevention of Alzheimer's disease: biochemical and cellular aspects. J. Neurol. Sci. 262, 27–36.

Forsyth, D.R., Surmon, D.J., Morgan, R.A., Wilcock, G.K., 1989. Clinical experience with and side-effects of tacrine hydrochloride in Alzheimer's disease: a pilot study. Age Ageing 18, 223–229.

Forsyth, E., Ritzline, P.D., 1998. An overview of the etiology, diagnosis, and treatment of Alzheimer disease. Phys. Ther. 78, 1325–1331.

Gander, B., Meinel, M., Walter, E., Merkle, H.P., 2001. Polymers as a platform for drug delivery: reviewing our current portfolio on poly(lactide-co-glycolide) (PLGA) microspheres. Chimia 55, 212–217.

Gandy, S., 2005. The role of cerebral amyloid beta accumulation in common forms of Alzheimer disease. J. Clin. Invest. 115, 1121–1129.

Garcia-Garcia, E., Andrieux, K., Gil, S., Couvreur, P., 2005. Colloidal carriers and blood–brain barrier (BBB) translocation: a way to deliver drugs to the brain? Int. J. Pharmaceutics 298, 274–292.

Gentilucci, L., 2004. New trends in the development of opioid peptide analogues as advanced remedies for pain relief. Curr. Top. Med. Chem. 4, 19–38.

Gozes, I., 2001. Neuroprotective peptide drug delivery and development: potential new therapeutics. Trends Neurosci. 24, 700–705.

Greenblatt, H.M., Kryger, G., Lewis, T., Silman, I., Sussman, J.L., 1999. Structure of acetylcholinesterase complexed with (_)-galanthamine at 2.3 A resolution. FEBS Lett. 463, 321–326.

Hafner, A., Lovric, J., Voinovich, D., Filipovic-Grcic, J., 2009. Melatonin-loaded lecithin/chitosan nanoparticles: physicochemical characterisation and permeability through Caco-2 cell monolayers. Int. J. Pharmaceutics 381, 205–213.

Hefti, F., Hartikka, J., Eckenstein, F., Gnahn, H., Heumann, R., Schwab, M., 1985. Nerve growth factor increases choline acetyltransferase but not survival or fiber outgrowth of cultured fetal septal cholinergic neurons. Neuroscience 14, 55–68.

Heinrich, M., Lee Teoh, H., 2004. Galanthamine from snowdrop-the development of a modern drug against Alzheimer's disease from local Caucasian knowledge. J. Ethnopharmacol. 92, 147–162.

Horter, D., Dressman, J.B., 2001. Influence of physicochemical properties on dissolution of drugs in the gastrointestinal tract. Adv. Drug Deliv. Rev. 46, 75–87.

Hughes, E., Burke, R.M., Doig, A.J., 2000. Inhibition of toxicity in the beta-amyloid peptide fragment beta -(25-35) using N-methylated derivatives: a general strategy to prevent amyloid formation. J. Biol. Chem. 275, 25109–25115.

Hughes, J.D., Blagg, J., Price, D.A., Bailey, S., DeCrescenzo, G.A., Devraj, R.V., Ellsworth, E., Fobian, Y.M., Gibbs, M.E., Gilles, R.W., Greene, N., Huang, E., Krieger-Burke, T., Loesel, J., Wager, T., Whiteley, L., Zhang, Y., 2008. Bioorg. Med. Chem. Lett. 18, 4872.

Iversen, L.L., Iversen, S.D., Bloom, F.E., Roth, R.H., 2009. Introduction to Neuropsychopharmacology. Oxford University Press, Oxford, UK, p. 93.

Javitt, D.C., Zukin, S.R., 1989. Biexponential kinetics of [3H]MK-801 binding: evidence for access to closed and open N-methyl-D-aspartate receptor channels. Mol. Pharmacol. 35, 387–393.

Johnson, W.G., 2000. Late-onset neurodegenerative diseases–the role of protein insolubility. J. Anat. 196 (Pt 4), 609–616.

Kabanov, A.V., Gendelman, H.E., 2007. Nanomedicine in the diagnosis and therapy of neurodegenerative disorders. Prog. Polym. Sci. 32, 1054–1082.

Kassel, D.B., 2004. Applications of high-throughput ADME in drug discovery. Curr. Opin. Chem. Biol. 8, 339–345.

Kawasaki-Yatsugi, S., Yatsugi, S., Takahashi, M., Toya, T., Ichiki, C., Shimizu-Sasamata, M., Yamaguchi, T., Minematsu, K., 1998. A novel AMPA receptor antagonist, YM872, reduces infarct size after middle cerebral artery occlusion in rats. Brain Res. 793 (1–2), 39–46.

Kerns, E., Li, D., 2008. Blood–Brain barrier. In: Drug-Like Properties: Concepts, Structure Design and Methods: From ADME to Toxicity Optimization. Elsevier/Academic Press, San Diego, CA, USA. ISBN: 978-0-1236-9520-8, pp. 122–136 (Chapter 10).

Kim, D.S., Park, S.Y., Kim, J.K., 2001. Curcuminoids from *Curcuma longa* L. (Zingiberaceae) that protect PC12 rat pheochromocytoma and normal human umbilical vein endothelial cells from βA(1-42) insult. Neurosci. Lett. 303, 57–61.

Kim, H., Park, B.S., Lee, K.G., Choi, C.Y., Jang, S.S., Kim, Y.H., et al., 2005. Effects of naturally occurring compounds on fibril formation and oxidative stress of β-amyloid. J. Agric. Food Chem. 53, 8537–8541.

Kokkoni, N., Stott, K., Amijee, H., Mason, J.M., Doig, A.J., 2006. *N*-methylated peptide inhibitors of beta-amyloid aggregation and toxicity. Optimization of the inhibitor structure. Biochemistry 45, 9906–9918.

Krol, S., 2012. Challenges in drug delivery to the brain: nature is against us. J. Control. Release 164, 145–155.

Kroll, R.A., Neuwelt, E.A., 1998. Outwitting the blood–brain barrier for therapeutic purposes: osmotic opening and other means. Neurosurgery 42, 1083–1099.

Kromer, L.F., 1987. Nerve growth factor treatment after brain injury prevents neuronal death. Science 235, 214–216.

Kryger, G., Silman, I., Sussman, J.L., 1998. Three-dimensional structure of a complex of E2020 with acetylcholinesterase from *Torpedo californica*. J. Physiol. Paris 92, 191–194.

Kubinyi, H., 2003. Drug research: myths, hype and reality. Nat. Rev. Drug Discov. 2, 665–668.

Lam, F.C., Liu, R., Lu, P., Shapiro, A.B., Renoir, J.M., Sharom, F.J., Reiner, P.B., 2001. Beta-amyloid efflux mediated by p-glycoprotein. J. Neurochem. 76, 1121–1128.

Li, W., Zhou, Y., Zhao, N., Hao, B., Wang, X., Kong, P., 2012. Pharmacokinetic behavior and efficiency of acetylcholinesterase inhibition in rat brain after intranasal administration of galanthamine hydrobromide loaded flexible liposomes. Environ. Toxicol. Pharmacol. 34, 272–279.

Liao, G.S., Li, X.B., Zhang, C.Y., Shu, Y.Y., Tang, S.X., 2001. Pharmacological actions of nerve growth factor-transferrin conjugate on the central nervous system. J. Nat. Toxin. 10, 291–297.

Lin, J., Sahakian, D.C., de Morais, S.M., Xu, J.J., Polzer, R.J., Winter, S.M., 2003. The role of absorption, distribution, metabolism, excretion and toxicity in drug discovery. Curr. Top Med. Chem. 3, 1125–1154.

Liu, X., 2006. Factors affecting total and free drug concentration in the brain. In: AAPS Conference: Critical Issues in Discovering Quality Clinical Candidates Philadelphia, PA.

Liu, Y., Zhang, J., 2000. Recent development in NMDA receptors. Chin. Med. J. 113, 948–956.

Lobell, M., Molnar, L., Keseru, G.M., 2003. Recent advances in the prediction of blood–brain partitioning from molecular structure. J. Pharm. Sci. 92, 360–370.

Lyketsos, C.G., Carrillo, M.C., Ryan, J.M., Khachaturian, A.S., Trzepacz, P., Amatniek, J., Cedarbaum, J., Brashear, R., Miller, D.S., 2011. Neuropsychiatric symptoms in Alzheimer's disease. Alzheimers Dement. 7 (5), 532–539.

Madden, D.R., 2002. The structure and function of glutamate receptor ion channels. Nat. Rev. Neurosci. 3, 91–101.

Matsuoka, Y., Saito, M., LaFrancois, J., et al., 2003. Novel therapeutic approach for the treatment of Alzheimer's disease by peripheral administration of agents with an affinity to beta-amyloid. J. Neurosci. 23, 29–33.

Maurer, T.S., DeBartolo, D.B., Tess, D.A., Scott, D.O., 2005. Relationship between exposure and nonspecific binding of thirty-three central nervous system drugs in mice. Drug Metab. Disposition 33, 175–181.

Miller, G., 2002. Drug targeting, breaking down barriers. Science 297, 1116–1118.

Misra, A., Ganesh, S., Shahiwala, A., Shah, S.P., 2003. Drug delivery to the central nervous system: a review. J. Pharm. Pharm. Sci. 6, 252–273.

Mody, I., MacDonald, J.F., 1995. NMDA receptor-dependent excitotoxicity: the role of intracellular Ca^{2+}release. Trends Pharmacol. Sci. 16, 356–359.

Mufamadi, M.S., Choonara, Y.E., Kumar, P., Modi, G., Naidoo, D., Vuuren, S.V., Ndesendo, V.M.K., du Toit, L.C., Iyuke, S.E., Pillay, V., 2013. Ligand-functionalized nanoliposomes for targeted delivery of galantamine. Int. J. Pharmaceutics 448, 267–281.

Mulik, R., Mahadik, K., Paradkar, A., 2009. Development of curcuminoids loaded poly(butyl) cyanoacrylate nanoparticles: physicochemical characterization and stability study. Eur. J. Pharm. Sci. 37, 395–404.

Nag, S. (Ed.), 2003. The Blood–Brain Barrier: Biology and Research Protocols. Humana Press, New Jersey.

Ohmori, J., Sakamoto, S., Kubota, H., Shimizu-Sasamata, M., Okada, M., Kawasaki, S., Hidaka, K., Togami, J., Furuya, T., Murase, K., 1994. 6-(1H-imidazol-1-yl)-7-nitro-2,3(1H,4H)-quinoxalinedione hydrochloride (YM90K) and related compounds: structure-activity relationships for the AMPA-type non-NMDA receptor. J. Med. Chem. 37 (4), 467–475.

Ono, K., Hasegawa, K., Naiki, H., Yamada, M., 2004. Curcumin has potent anti-amyloidogenic effects for Alzheimer's β-amyloid fibrils in vitro. J. Neurosci. Res. 75, 742–750.

Oset-Gasque, M.J., González, M.P., Pérez-Peña, J., Nt, G.-F., Romero, A., del Pino, J., Ramos, E., Hadjipavlou-Litina, D., Soriano, E., Chioua, M., Samadi, A., Raghuvanshi, D.S., Singh, K.N., Marco-Contelles, J., 2014. Toxicological and pharmacological evaluation, antioxidant, ADMET and molecular modeling of selected racemic chromenotacrines {11-amino-12-aryl-8,9,10,12-tetrahydro-7H-chromeno[2,3-b]quinolin-3-ols} for the potential prevention and treatment of Alzheimer's disease. Eur. J. Med. Chem. 74, 491–550.

Pahnke, J., Walker, L.C., Scheffler, K., Krohn, M., 2009. Alzheimer's disease and blood–brain barrier function—Why have anti-b-amyloid therapies failed to prevent dementia progression? Neurosci. Biobehavioral Rev. 33, 1099–1108.

Pardridge, W.M., 2003. Blood–brain barrier genomics and the use of endogenous transporters to cause drug penetration into the brain. Curr. Opin. Drug Discov. Devel. 6, 683–691.

Pardridge, W.M., 1998. CNS drug design based on principles of blood–brain barrier transport. J. Neurochem. 70, 1781–1792.

Pardridge, W.M., 1991. Peptide Drug Delivery to the Brain. Raven Press, New York, NY.

Pardridge, W.M., 1995. Transport of small molecules through the blood–brain barrier: biology and methodology. Adv. Drug Deliv. Rev. 15, 5–36.

Parsons, C.G., Danysz, W., Quack, G., 1998. Glutamate in CNS disorders as a target for drug development: an update. Drug News Perspect. 11, 523–569.

Paschke, A., Manz, M., Schuurmann, G., 2001. Application of different RP-HPLC methods for the determination of the octanol/water partition coefficient of selected tetrachlorobenzyltoluenes. Chemosphere 45, 721–728.

Pavan, B., Dalpiaz, A., Ciliberti, N., Biondi, C., Manfredini, S., Vertuani, S., 2008. Progress in drug delivery to the central nervous system by the prodrug approach. Molecules 13, 1035–1065.

Pettersson, M., Johnson, D.S., Subramanyam, C., Bales, K.R., Ende, C.W., Fish, B.A., Green, M.E., Kauffman, G.W., Lira, R., Mullins, P.B., Navaratnam, T., Sakya, S.M., Stiff, C.M., Tran, T.P., Vetelino, B.C., Xie, L., Zhang, L., Pustilnik, L.R., Wood, K.M., O'Donnell, C.J., 2012. Design and synthesis of dihydrobenzofuran amides as orally bioavailable, centrally active c-secretase modulators. Bioorg. Med. Chem. Lett. 22, 2906–2911.

Pidgeon, C., Ong, S., Liu, H., Qiu, X., Pidgeon, M., Dantzig, A.H., Munroe, J., Hornback, W.J., Kasher, J.S., Glunz, L., et al., 1995. IAM chromatography: an in vitro screen for predicting drug membrane permeability. J. Med. Chem. 17, 590–594.

Portelius, E., Van Broeck, B., Andreasson, U., Gustavsson, M.K., Mercken, M., Zetterberg, H., Borghys, H., Blennow, K.J.: Alzheimers Dis. 2010, 1005, 21. In general, oral drugs tend to have a LipE between 5 and 7; see: Leeson, P.D., Springthorpe, B., Nat. Rev. Drug Disc. 2007, 6, 881.LogD at pH 7.4 calculated using ACD version 9.03.

Potter, K.J., Scrocchi, L.A., Warnock, G.L., Ao, Z., Younker, M.A., Rosenberg, L., Lipsett, M., Verchere, C.B., Fraser, P.E., 2009. Amyloid inhibitors enhance survival of cultured human islets. Biochim. Biophys. Acta 1790 (6), 566–574.

Pratim Bose, P., Chatterjee, U., Nerelius, C., Govender, T., Norström, T., Gogoll, A., Sandegren, A., Göthelid, E., Johansson, J., Arvidsson, P.I., 2009. Poly-N-methylated amyloid beta-peptide (Abeta) C-terminal fragments reduce Abeta toxicity in vitro and in *Drosophila melanogaster*. J. Med. Chem. 52 (24), 8002–8009.

Qian, S., Wong, Y.C., Zuo, Z., 2014. Development, characterization and application of in situ gel systems for intranasal delivery of tacrine. Int. J. Pharmaceutics 468, 272–282.

Raymond, L.A., 2003. Excitotoxicity in Huntington disease. Clin. Neurosci. Res. 3, 121–128.

Re, F., Airoldi, C., Zona, C., Masserini, M., La Ferla, B., Quattrocchi, N., et al., 2010. β-Amyloid aggregation inhibitors: small molecules as candidate drugs for therapy of Alzheimer's disease. Curr. Med. Chem. 17, 2990–3006.

Re, F., Gregori, M., Masserini, M., 2012. Nanotechnology for neurodegenerative disorders. Maturitas 73, 45–51.

Riley, R.J., Martin, I.J., Cooper, A.E., 2002. The influence of DMPK as an integrated partner in modern drug discovery. Curr. Drug Metab. 3, 527–550.

Riley, R.J., Parker, A.J., Trigg, S., Manners, C.N., 2001. Development of a generalized, quantitative physicochemical model of CYP3A4 inhibition for use in early drug discovery. Pharm. Res. 18, 652–655.

Roberts, S.A., 2003. Drug metabolism and pharmacokinetics in drug discovery. Curr. Opin. Drug Discov. Dev. 6, 66–80.

Rogers, S.L., Friedhoff, L.T., 1998. Long-term efficacy and safety of donepezil in the treatment of Alzheimer's disease: an interim analysis of the results of a US multicenter open label extension study. Eur. Neuropsychopharmacol. 8, 67–75.

Roney, C., Kulkarni, P., Arora, V., Antich, P., Bonte, F., Wu, A., Mallikarjuana, N.N., Manohar, S., Liang, H., Kulkarni, A.R., Sung, H.W., Sairam, M., Aminabhavi, T.M., 2005. Targeted nanoparticles for drug delivery through the blood–brain barrier for Alzheimer's disease. J. Control. Release 108, 193–214.

Rothman, S.M., Olney, J.W., 1987. Excitotoxicity and the NMDA receptor. Trends Neurosci. 10, 299–302.

Rowinska-Zyreka, M., Salernob, M., Kozlowski, H., 2015. Review neurodegenerative diseases – understanding their molecular bases and progress in the development of potential treatments. Coordination Chem. Rev. 284, 298–312.

Rubin, L.L., Staddon, J.M., 1999. The cell biology of the blood–brain barrier. Ann. Rev. Neurosci. 22, 11–28.

Sahni, J.K., Doggui, S., Ali, J., Baboota, S., Dao, L., Ramassamy, C., 2011. Neurotherapeutic applications of nanoparticles in Alzheimer's disease. J. Control. Release 152, 208–231.

Sarvaiya, J., Agrawal, Y.K., 2015. Chitosan as a suitable nanocarrier material for anti-Alzheimer drug delivery. Int. J. Biol. Macromolecules 72, 454–465.

Sattler, R., Tymianski, M., 2000. Molecular mechanisms of calcium-dependent excitotoxicity. J. Mol. Med. 78, 3–13.

Schiller, J., Schiller, Y., Clapham, D.E., 1998. NMDA receptors amplify calcium influx into dendritic spines during associative pre- and postsynaptic activation. Nat. Neurosci. 1, 114–118.

Scrocchi, L.A., Chen, Y., Waschuk, S., Wang, F., Cheung, S., Darabie, A.A., McLaurin, J., Fraser, P.E., 2002. Design of peptide-based inhibitors of human islet amyloid polypeptide fibrillogenesis. J. Mol. Biol. 318 (3), 697–706.

Scrocchi, L.A., Ha, K., Chen, Y., Wu, L., Wang, F., Fraser, P.E., 2003. Identification of minimal peptide sequences in the (8-20) domain of human islet amyloid polypeptide involved in fibrillogenesis. J. Struct. Biol. 141 (3), 218–227.

Sheardown, M.J., Nielsen, E.O., Hansen, A.J., Jacobsen, P., Honoré, T., 1990. 2,3-Dihydroxy-6-nitro-7-sulfamoyl-benzo(F)quinoxaline: a neuroprotectant for cerebral ischemia. Science 247 (4942), 571–574.

Shimizu-Sasamata, M., Kawasaki-Yatsugi, S., Okada, M., Sakamoto, S., Yatsugi, S., Togami, J., Hatanaka, K., Ohmori, J., Koshiya, K., Usuda, S., Murase, K., 1996. YM90K: pharmacological characterization as a selective and potent alpha-amino-3-hydroxy-5-methylisoxazole-4-propionate/kainate receptor antagonist. J. Pharmacol. Exp. Ther. 276 (1), 84–89.

Shytle, R.D., Mori, T., Vendrame, M., Sun, N., Zeng, J., Ehrhart, J., Silver, A.A., Sanberg, P.R., Tan, J., 2004. Cholinergic modulation of microglial activation by alpha7 nicotinic receptors. J. Neurochem. 89, 337–343.

Sozio, P., Cerasa, L.S., Laserra, S., Cacciatore, I., Cornacchia, C., DiFilippo, E.S., Fulle, S., Fontana, A., DiCrescenzo, A., Grilli, M., Marchi, M., Stefano, A.D., 2013. Memantine-sulfur containing antioxidant conjugates as potential prodrugs to improve the treatment of Alzheimer's disease. Eur. J. Pharm. Sci. 49, 187–198.

Stephenson, K.A., Reid, L.C., Zubieta, J., Babich, J.W., Kung, M.P., Kung, H.F., Valliant, J.F., 2008. Synthesis and screening of a library of Re/Tc-based amyloid probes derived from beta-breaker peptides. Bioconjug. Chem. 19 (5), 1087–1094.

Takano, Y., Shiga, F., Asano, J., Ando, N., Uchiki, H., Anraku, T., 2003. Synthesis and AMPA receptor antagonistic activity of a novel class of quinoxalinecarboxylic acid with a substituted phenyl group at the C-7 position. Bioorg. Med. Chem. Lett. 13 (20), 3521–3525.

Takano, Y., Shiga, F., Asano, J., Ando, N., Uchiki, H., Fukuchi, K., Anraku, T., 2005. Design, synthesis, and AMPA receptor antagonistic activity of a novel 6-nitro-3-oxoquinoxaline-2-carboxylic acid with a substituted phenyl group at the 7 position. Bioorg. Med. Chem. 13 (20), 5841–5863.

Takano, Y., Shiga, F., Asano, J., Hori, W., Fukuchi, K., Anraku, T., Uno, T., 2006. Design and synthesis of novel 7-heterocycle-6-trifluoromethyl-3-oxoquinoxaline-2-carboxylic acids bearing a substituted phenyl group as superior AMPA receptor antagonists with good physicochemical properties. Bioorg. Med. Chem. 14, 776–792.

Tatarek-Nossol, M., Yan, L.M., Schmauder, A., Tenidis, K., Westermark, G., Kapurniotu, A., 2005. Inhibition of hIAPP amyloid-fibril formation and apoptotic cell death by a designed hIAPP amyloid- core-containing hexapeptide. Chem. Biol. 12 (7), 797–809.

Taylor, M., Moore, S., Mourtas, S., Niarakis, A., Re, F., Zona, C., Ferla, B.L., Nicotra, F., Masserini, M., Antimisiaris, S.G., Gregori, M., Allsop, D., 2011. Effect of curcumin-associated and lipid ligand-functionalized nanoliposomes on aggregation of the Alzheimer's Aβ peptide. Nanomed. Nanotech. Biol. Med. 7, 541–550.

Thoenen, H., Sendtner, M., 2002. Neurotrophins: from enthusiastic expectations through sobering experiences to rational therapeutic approaches. Nat. Neurosci. 5 (Suppl.), 1046–1050.

Thorne, R.G., Frey II, W.H., 2001. Delivery of neurotrophic factors to the central nervous system: pharmacokinetic considerations. Clin. Pharmacokinet. 40, 907–946.

Tolnay, M., Probst, A., 1999. REVIEW: tau protein pathology in Alzheimer's disease and related disorders. Europathol Appl. Eurobiol. 25, 171–187.

Torchilin, V.P., 2005. Recent advances with liposomes as pharmaceutical carriers. Nat. Rev. Drug Discov. 4 (2), 145–160.

Turski, L., Huth, A., Sheardown, M., McDonald, F., Neuhaus, R., Schneider, H.H., Dirnagl, U., Wiegand, F., Jacobsen, P., Ottow, E., 1998. ZK200775: a phosphonate quinoxalinedione AMPA antagonist for neuroprotection in stroke and trauma. Proc. Natl. Acad. Sci. U.S.A. 95 (18), 10960–10965.

Veerareddy, P.R., Vobalaboina, V., 2004. Lipid-based formulations of amphotericin B. Drugs Today 40, 133–145.

Wager, T.T., Chandrasekaran, R.Y., Hou, X., Troutman, M.D., Verhoest, P.R., Villalobos, A., 2010. Will, Y: defining desirable central nervous system drug space through the alignment of molecular properties, in vitro ADME, and safety attributes. ACS Chem. Neurosci. 1 (6), 420–434.

Wager, T.T., Villalobos, A., Verhoest, P.R., Hou, X., Shaffer, C.L., 2011. Strategies to optimize the brain availability of central nervous system drug candidates. Expert Opin. Drug Discov. 6 (4), 371–381.

Walker, L.C., LeVine 3rd, H., 2000. The cerebral proteopathies. Neurobiol. Aging 21, 559–561.

Walsh, D.M., Klyubin, I., Fadeeva, J.V., Rowan, M.J., Selkoe, D.J., 2002. Amyloidbeta oligomers: their production, toxicity and therapeutic inhibition. Biochem. Soc. Trans. 30, 552–557.

Wang, L., Esteban, G., Ojima, M., Bautista-Aguilera, O.M., Inokuchi, T., Moraleda, I., Iriepa, I., Samadi, A., Youdim, M.B.H., Romero, A., Soriano, E., Herrero, R., Fernández, A.P.F., Martínez-Murillo, R., Marco-Contelles, J., Unzeta, M., 2014. Donepezil+propargylamine+ 8-hydroxyquinoline hybrids as new multifunctional metal-chelators, ChE and MAO inhibitors for the potential treatment of Alzheimer's disease. Eur. J. Med. Chem. 80, 543–561.

Watkins, P.B., Zimmerman, H.J., Knapp, M.J., Gracon, S.I., Lewis, K.W., 1994. Hepatotoxic effects of tacrine administration in patients with Alzheimer's disease. J. Am. Med. Assoc. 271, 992–998.

Wilson, D.M., Apps, J., Bailey, N., Bamford, M.J., Beresford, I.J., Brackenborough, K., Briggs, M.A., Brough, S., Calver, A.R., Crook, B., Davis, R.K., Davis, R.P., Davis, S., Dean, D.K., Harris, L., Heslop, T., Holland, V., Jeffrey, P., Panchal, T.A., Parr, C.A., Quashie, N., Schogger, J., Sehmi, S.S., Stean, T.O., Steadman, J.G.A., Trail, B., Wald, J., Worby, A., Takle, A.K., Witherington, J., Medhurst, A.D., 2013. Identification of clinical candidates from the benzazepine class of histamine H3 receptor antagonists. Bioorg. Med. Chem. Lett. 23, 6890–7689.

Wohlfart, S., Gelperina, S., Kreuter, J., 2012. Transport of drugs across the blood–brain barrier by nanoparticles. J. Control. Release 161, 264–273.

Wong, Y., Zuo, Z., 2013. Brain disposition and catalepsy after intranasal delivery of loxapine: role of metabolism in PK/PD of intranasal CNS drugs. Pharm. Res. 30, 2368–2384.

Wong, Y.C., Qian, S., Zuo, Z., 2012. Regioselective biotransformation of CNS drugs and its clinical impact on adverse drug reactions. Expert Opin. Drug Metab. Toxicol. 8, 833–854.

Wong, Y.C., Zuo, Z., 2010. Intranasal delivery – modification of drug metabolism and brain disposition. Pharm. Res. 27, 1208–1223.

Woodle, M.C., Lasic, D.D., 1992. Sterically stabilized liposomes. Biochim. Biophys. Acta 1113, 171–199.

Xie, Y., Ye, L.Y., Cui, W., Xu, K., Zhang, X.B., Lou, J.N., Hou, X.P., 2004. Study on nevre growth factor liposomes on crossing blood–brain barrier in vitro and in vivo. Yao Xue Xue Bao 39, 944–948.

Xue, D., Huang, Z.-G., Barnes, K., Lesiuk, H.J., Smith, K.E., Buchan, A.M., 1994. Delayed treatment with AMPA, but not NMDA, antagonists reduces neocortical infarction. J. Cereb. Blood Flow Metab. 14 (2), 251–261.

Yan, L.M., Tatarek-Nossol, M., Velkova, A., Kazantzis, A., Kapurniotu, A., 2006. Design of a mimic of nonamyloidogenic and bioactive human islet amyloid polypeptide (IAPP) as nanomolar affinity inhibitor of IAPP cytotoxic fibrillogenesis. Proc. Natl. Acad. Sci. U.S.A. 103 (7), 2046–2051.

Yan, L.M., Velkova, A., Tatarek-Nossol, M., Andreetto, E., Kapurniotu, A., 2007. IAPP mimic blocks Abeta cytotoxic self-assembly: cross-suppression of amyloid toxicity of Abeta and IAPP suggests a molecular link between Alzheimer's disease and type II diabetes. Angew. Chem. Int. Ed. Engl. 46 (8), 1246–1252.

Yang, F., Lim, G.P., Begum, A.N., Ubeda, O.J., Simmons, M.R., Ambegaokar, S.S., et al., 2005. Curcumin inhibits formation of amyloid β oligomers and fibrils, binds plaques, and reduces amyloid in vivo. J. Biol. Chem. 280, 5892–5901.

Ying, X., Wen, H., Lu, W., Du, J., Guo, J., Tian, W., Men, Y., Zhang, Y., Li, R.J., Yang, T.Y., Shang, D.W., Lou, J.N., Zhang, L.R., Zhang, Q., 2010. Dual-targeting daunorubicin liposomes improve the therapeutic efficacy of brain glioma in animals. J. Control. Release 141, 183–192.

Yu, H., Li, W.M., Kan, K.K.W., Ho, J.M.K., Carlier, P.R., Pang, Y.P., Gu, Z.M., Zhong, Z., Chan, K., Wang, Y.T., Han, Y.F., 2008. The physicochemical properties and the *in vivo* AChE inhibition of two potential anti-Alzheimer agents, bis(12)-hupyridone and bis(7)-tacrine. J. Pharm. Biomed. Anal. 46, 75–81.

Yuste, R., Majewska, A., Cash, S.S., Denk, W., 1999. Mechanisms of calcium influx into hippocampal spines: heterogeneity among spines, coincidence detection by NMDA receptors, and optical quantal analysis. J. Neurosci. 196, 1976–1987.

Zhang, H.Y., 2005. One-compound-multiple-targets strategy to combat Alzheimer's disease. FEBS Lett. 579, 5260–5264.

Zhang, L., Yu, H., Li, W.M., Cheung, M.C., Pang, Y.P., Gu, Z.M., Chan, K., Wang, Y.T., Zuo, Z., Han, Y.F., 2008. Preclinical characterization of intestinal absorption and metabolism of promising anti-Alzheimer's dimer bis(7)-tacrine. Int. J. Pharmaceutics 357, 85–94.

Zhang, P., Chen, L., Gu, W., Xu, Z., Gao, Y., Li, Y., 2007. In vitro and in vivo evaluation of donepezil-sustained release microparticles for the treatment of Alzheimer's disease. Biomaterials 28, 1882–1888.

Zhang, Y., Pardridge, W.M., 2001. Conjugation of brain-derived neurotrophic factor to a blood–brain barrier drug targeting system enables neuroprotection in regional brain ischemia following intravenous injection of the neurotrophin. Brain Res. 889, 49–56.

CHAPTER

6

Receptor Targets in Alzheimer's Disease Drug Discovery

J. Wallach, T. Colestock, A. Adejare

OUTLINE

INTRODUCTION

Hundreds of drugs have been evaluated in clinical trials of Alzheimer's disease (AD). Unfortunately, the majority of these have failed to show significant efficacy and have therefore been abandoned. These drugs target an array of CNS receptors and may provide symptomatic and/or

Drug Discovery Approaches for the Treatment of Neurodegenerative Disorders
http://dx.doi.org/10.1016/B978-0-12-802810-0.00006-4

disease-modifying effects. Existing treatment strategies in AD are limited and are used to provide symptomatic relief. In the United States, these include the Food and Drug Administration (FDA)-approved acetylcholinesterase inhibitors (AChEIs) donepezil, galantamine, and rivastigmine, and the *N*-methyl-D-aspartate (NMDA) receptor (NMDAR) antagonist memantine (Namenda). Clinical improvements from current therapies remain modest at best. The average life expectancy is 8 years after diagnosis, illustrating the need for better therapies. Although a number of drug candidates are in various phases along the clinical development pipeline, from preclinical to phase III trials, current prognosis looks poor based on the historical low success rate. Therefore, systematic examination of possible therapeutic targets including receptors is highly warranted.

Drug discovery in AD continues to be a significant challenge and novel approaches are needed. Early diagnosis and interventions, inclusion of biomarkers and neuroimaging in diagnosis, clinical trials and patient monitoring, and investigation of novel strategies are all likely to help advance the effort. For example, the potential for polypharmacological intervention is great, and may be achieved through single agent drugs with multiple targets or drug combinations.

Although an AD "cure" is a crucial goal of these efforts, even modest improvements in clinical outcomes can be very important. For example, it has been estimated by the Alzheimer's Association in their 2015 report that by 2050, the number of people ages 65 years and older diagnosed with AD may almost triple from the current 5.1 million (2015) to 13.8 million (Alzheimer's, 2015). This increase may cause an unbearable economic and social burden. The association has reported that the development of a therapy that could delay onset or progression of the disease by 5 years would limit these huge economic and social burdens. Although certainly a benefit, such achievements do not necessarily require a complete understanding of AD etiology. Thus, it is important to investigate therapeutic strategies that fit these criteria.

This chapter will review some of the receptors that have been targeted or are currently under investigation for modulation in AD. The goal is to present a brief overview of some of the recent developments in this area. We hope the reader takes away an appreciation of the complexity and difficulty common in this field while knowing that some successes, even if modest, have been found. The chapter focuses on protein-based receptor sites. The receptors have been organized by functional characterization into four classes: G protein-coupled receptors (GPCRs), enzymatic, ionotropic, and hormonal. Targets were chosen based on promising physiological rationale, existence of drug candidates, or evaluation in clinical trials. Finally, we introduce some alternate approaches including a discussion on advances in the use of polypharmacology in the treatment of AD.

G PROTEIN-COUPLED RECEPTORS

A number of GPCRs have been investigated as targets in AD treatment. These include histaminergic, GABAergic, serotonergic, adrenergic, cholinergic, and cannabinoid receptors as well as others. Several of these are reviewed next.

Histaminergic Receptors

The histaminergic family of receptors currently comprises four druggable targets: H_1, H_2, H_3, and H_4. These sites are being investigated because of their involvement with immune system regulation and neurotransmitter modulation (Naddafi and Mirshafiey, 2013). Initially used for seasonal allergies, it was soon realized that H_1 antagonists had potential for treatment of CNS disorders including sleep issues and neurodegenerative diseases (NDDs). For example, a clinical trial with the H_1 antagonist latrepirdine in AD and Huntington's disease found improvements in patients (Sabbagh and Shill, 2010). However, further investigations were terminated after a phase III clinical trial did not show efficacy over placebo in patients with moderate-to-severe AD receiving 20 mg doses three times daily (clinicaltrials.gov trial ID: NCT00912288).

H_2 receptor antagonism is a strategy for treating peptic ulcers. Because a large elderly population was receiving H_2R antagonists for this indication, and studies suggested H_2R antagonism might prevent onset of AD diagnosis, H_2R antagonists were investigated in patients with AD (Anthony et al., 2000). A double-blind, placebo-controlled trial found no significant effects for the H_2R antagonist nazitidine, given at 75 mg, twice daily (Carlson et al., 2002). The failure of nazitidine in this case may have been caused by dosage, but more importantly that treatment was started after patients were diagnosed with AD. A prospective population-based cohort study was more recently conducted using a higher (300 mg) dose of nazitidine, as well as other H_2R antagonists including cimetidine, ranitidine, and famotidine, on 65-year-old patients who did not exhibit early-onset AD symptoms. However, the study found no correlation between the usage of these H_2R antagonists and AD (Gray et al., 2011).

One of the functions of H_3 is as a presynaptic autoreceptor regulating synaptic release of neurotransmitters. H_3R antagonism in preclinical models caused an increase in both histamine and acetylcholine (ACh) levels in the prefrontal cortex of rats, and to a lesser extent the monoamines dopamine and norepinephrine—all theoretical beneficial strategies to treat AD-like symptoms (Brioni et al., 2011). The H_3 antagonist GSK-239512 was well tolerated and demonstrated positive effects on attention and memory (40 and 80 μg oral) through phase II clinical trials in patients with mild-to-moderate AD, but further details on clinical investigation since this 2012 study have not been found (Grove et al., 2014). In addition, MK-0249, an inverse agonist at H_3R, failed to show symptomatic relief (5 mg oral) over placebo in a phase II clinical study (Egan et al., 2013). The H_4R is the most recent histaminergic receptor in terms of discovery. It is expressed throughout the body and is believed to have numerous different functions (Leurs et al., 2009). Whether the H_4R will find a role in AD drug therapy remains to be found.

Serotonergic Receptors

All but one of the known serotonin receptor types are GPCRs. Numerous serotonergic (5-HT), receptors exist in humans, where they are implicated in a host of functions.

The 5-HT_{1A} antagonist lecozotan appeared promising in preclinical animal models for its ability to enhance cognitive function (Schechter et al., 2005). A phase II double-blind clinical trial using patients with mild-to-moderate AD was conducted to assess its efficacy at different doses (2, 5, and 10 mg) co-administered with donepezil, an FDA-approved AChEI for AD patients, and compared to donepezil alone (clinicaltrials.gov trial ID: NCT00151398). The trial was completed in 2008 but the results were not found.

5-HT_4 is expressed throughout the periphery as well as the CNS. Full agonists of 5-HT_4 receptors, such as prucalopride (Resolor), are frequently used to treat gastrointestinal (GI) blockage. Interestingly, prucalopride administration increased levels of ACh and histamine and positively influenced hippocampal oscillatory actions in rat brains (Johnson et al., 2012). Further research established that partial agonism at 5-HT_4 diminished GI effects while preserving the desired CNS efficacy in vivo (Ahmad and Nirogi, 2011). It was believed that these effects would be desirable in the treatment of AD and related neurodegenerative diseases. Partial agonists of 5-HT_4 include the compound PRX-03140, which has shown promising activity in vitro and in animal models of AD (Shen et al., 2011). A phase II clinical trial with PRX-03140 in AD patients was terminated in 2009 for undisclosed reasons (clinicaltrials.gov trial ID: NCT00693004).

5-HT_6 receptor antagonism has similar outcomes to 5-HT_4 partial agonists, with preclinical candidates displaying improved cognitive functions and attenuation of negative behavioral symptoms such as depression in vivo (Upton et al., 2008). The 5-HT_6 receptor antagonist SB-742457 underwent two phase II clinical trials in 2008 and 2009 for patients with mild-to-moderate AD (clinicaltrials.gov trial ID: NCT00224497, clinicaltrials.gov trial ID: NCT00348192). Results of either trial were not found, but, interestingly, Axovant Sciences purchased the rights to SB-742457 (now called RVT-101) and announced an upcoming phase III clinical trial for AD.

Adrenergic Receptors

A number of adrenergic receptor subtypes exist. Epinephrine and norepinephrine are major monoamine neurotransmitters of the peripheral and central nervous systems.

The α_1 selective adrenergic receptor antagonist prazosin (Minipress) has been indicated for the treatment of cardiac hypertension for many years. A double-blind, placebo-controlled parallel study was conducted to determine if prazosin reduced disruptive agitation in AD patients (clinicaltrials.gov trial ID: NCT01126099). Results demonstrated that 2 mg administered in the morning, followed by 4 mg in the afternoon, significantly reduced agitation and aggression relative to placebo (Wang et al., 2009).

Ergoloid (Hydergine) is a combination drug consisting of three ergoloid mesylates developed by Albert Hofmann at Sandoz. Although the exact mechanism of action is unknown, these compounds act on numerous neurotransmitter systems including adrenergic sites and related monoamine transmitters such as serotonin and dopamine (Wadworth and Chrisp, 1992). Hydergine has been used in the treatment of AD and related dementias in Europe and the United States for decades. A large meta-analysis of clinical use of Hydergine in dementias found that "overall, ergoloid mesylates were more effective than placebo." Unfortunately, the study concluded that the effect in patients with potential AD were modest at best (Schneider and Olin, 1994).

Nicergoline is a semi-synthetic ergoline, which acts as an α_{1A} adrenergic receptor antagonist as well as at other receptors. It has numerous pharmacological effects relevant to AD. These include the enhancement of cholinergic and catecholaminergic neurotransmitter functions, improvement of age-related cognitive deficits, modulation of protein kinase C (PKC)-mediated α-secretase processing of amyloid precursor protein, neuroprotection, and interaction with endogenous nerve growth factor-mediated processes (Winblad et al., 2001). Nicergoline has several uses including treatment of cerebral metabolic-vascular disorders, vascular migraines, and dementias. In a European multicenter double-blind, placebo-controlled trial, it was well tolerated (30 mg twice a day) and exerted a positive effect on the cognitive symptoms of mild-to-moderate AD measured via multiple outcomes including the Alzheimer's Disease Assessment Scale-cognitive subscale (ADAS-cog) (Winblad et al., 2001). Meta-analysis of various studies has also shown some potential in dementia (Fioravanti and Flicker, 2001). These results justify further investigation of nicergoline as well as related ergoloid derivatives.

Cannabinoid Receptors

Cannabinoid receptors include CB_1 and CB_2. CB_1 is often stated to be the most highly expressed GPCR in the CNS and plays essential roles in numerous processes including learning, memory, sensory processing, and pain perception (Mackie, 2006). CB_1 and CB_2 cannabinoid receptor agonists show promise in neurodegenerative diseases including AD (Campbell and Gowran, 2007; Scotter et al., 2010). For example, the CB_1 agonist tetrahydrocannabinol (THC), in addition to decreasing presynaptic glutaminergic signaling and AChEI activity, impairs Aβ aggregation (Eubanks et al., 2006). A great deal of promising preclinical research has been performed supporting the endocannabinoid system as relevant territory in the search for AD modification and symptomatic therapies (Scotter et al., 2010; Ramírez et al., 2005; Aso and Ferrer, 2014; Caoa et al., 2014). Anecdotal reports on the efficacy of cannabis, the cannabinoid-rich flowers of the *Cannabis* genus, in a large number of therapeutic areas exist and find strong support in preclinical research. Still, controlled clinical trials are drastically needed. Medicinal cannabis and cannabis products are frequently used, with reported benefits, in related NDDs including multiple sclerosis, amyotrophic lateral sclerosis (ALS) as well as epilepsy (Chong et al., 2006; Consroe et al., 1997; Maa and Figi, 2014; Carter and Rosen, 2001).

A few clinical trials evaluating Δ^9-THC (dronabinol) and its derivative nabilone in AD patients have been undertaken. In a trial of 15 AD patients treated with dronabinol for 6 weeks, a decrease in altered behaviors was observed as well as an increase in body weight in those previously refusing food. Side effects were those common to cannabis and included euphoria, somnolence, and tiredness, but did not warrant abandonment of the therapy (Volicer et al., 1997). Similar benefits (reduction in night-time agitation and behavioral disturbances) were reported in two pilot studies involving dementia patients (Walther et al., 2006, 2011). Nabilone provided prompt and dramatic improvements in agitation and aggressiveness in advanced AD patients refractory to antipsychotic and anxiolytic treatment (Passmore, 2008). Unfortunately, these studies were small and did not evaluate cognitive or neurodegenerative disease markers. Still, the promising results reported warrant further investigations with larger controlled trials, particularly given the potential for novel selective cannabinoid receptor ligands, which may have reduced psychoactive effects (Aso and Ferrer, 2014).

$GABA_B$ Receptors

GABA (γ-aminobutyric acid) is the major inhibitory neurotransmitter in the CNS. Two main subtypes of GABA receptors are recognized: $GABA_A$, an ionotropic receptor discussed later, and $GABA_B$, a GPCR. The process of forming and storing memories, long-term potentiation (LTP), has been indirectly associated with $GABA_B$ signaling. Agonism of $GABA_B$ can impede memory formation, while antagonism can restore synaptic plasticity (Kerr and Ong, 1995). $GABA_B$ antagonism may thus have potential use in enhancing memory and cognitive function. A phase

II, double-blind, placebo-controlled study with SG742 in patients with mild-to-moderate AD was conducted (clinicaltrials.gov trial ID: NCT00093951). Results of the trial were not found, but SG742 was previously reported as well tolerated at a dose of 600 mg oral administration, three times a day, in a study investigating mild cognitive impairment (Froestl et al., 2004).

Muscarinic Cholinergic Receptors

Two main classes of cholinergic receptors are recognized: the ionotropic nicotinic receptors discussed later and the muscarinic GPCRs. Cholinergic deficits are well recognized in AD and AChEIs are one of the major existing symptomatic treatment options in AD. Agonism of muscarinic ACh GPCRs may offer an alternative to the enzymatic inhibition of AChEIs. However, until recently, compounds were nonselective for the five subtypes M_1–M_5 (Daval et al., 2012). Developing M_1-selective compounds prevented adverse side effects and displayed cognitive enhancement in animal models (Fisher, 2008). Numerous M_1-selective compounds have been synthesized and are undergoing preclinical investigations (Nickols and Conn, 2014). More work is needed to determine what role the other subtypes may play in AD.

KINASES/ENZYMES

Acetylcholinesterase

AChEIs were the first class of pharmacological agents approved for AD treatment in the United States (McGleenon et al., 1999). AChE catalyzes the breakdown of ACh into physiologically inert choline and acetate. The mechanism of efficacy for these inhibitors is believed to be a restoration of ACh function through elevation of its level, thus ameliorating deficiency resulting from degeneration of ACh neurons (Craig et al., 2011). FDA-approved AChEIs include donepezil, galantamine, and rivastigmine. These agents have shown modest symptomatic benefits in AD patients and a few studies have suggested disease modification including slowing of AD progression (Munoz-Torrero, 2008). The AChEIs are widely prescribed and commercially successful.

Protein Kinases

The tau protein is necessary for both cytoskeletal structure and pathway signaling in neurons, and is regulated by kinase phosphorylation (Kimura et al., 2014). Excessive, or hyperphosphorylation, of tau protein is implicated in neurological disorders including AD; thus preventing the hyperphosphorylated state by kinase inhibition has become a therapeutic approach. Bryostatins, compounds isolated from the marine species *Bugula neritina*, were earlier assessed as chemotherapeutics, but it was discovered that they enhance cognitive function (Sun and Alkon, 2006). Bryostatin-1 acts as a partial agonist to bolster PKC activity, which has been shown to diminish with age, serving a multifaceted beneficial role in both reducing Aβ levels and preventing hyperphosphorylated tau protein (Lucke-Wold et al., 2015). A phase II clinical trial is currently recruiting patients to assess 10, 20, and 40 μg doses I.V. in patients with moderate severe-to-severe AD (clinicaltrials.gov trial ID: NCT02431468).

Originally developed as a treatment for solid tumors, AZD-0530 (saracatinib) is an inhibitor of the protein tyrosine kinase Fyn, which was later found to be involved in Aβ signal transduction and tau phosphorylation (Nygaard et al., 2015). A phase II multicenter clinical trial is currently recruiting patients to assess 100 and 125 mg oral doses in patients with mild-to-moderate AD (clinicaltrials.gov trial ID: NCT02167256). Masitinib (AB-1010) also inhibits Fyn, but to a greater extent than tyrosine kinases c-Kit and Lyn. This activity reduces proinflammatory mediators released from immunological mast cells, which tend to be overactive in pathological conditions such as AD (Piette et al., 2011). Masitinib has been evaluated clinically for rheumatoid arthritis and different forms of cancer, and is sold in the United States under the name Kinavet-CA1 to treat canine tumors. A phase III double-blind multicenter clinical trial is currently recruiting patients to assess efficacy of 3 versus 4.5 mg/kg/day orally in patients with mild-to-moderate AD (clinicaltrials.gov trial ID: NCT01872598).

Glycogen synthase kinase-3β (GSK3β) inhibition has been found to reduce Aβ and phospho-tau levels in AD models (Beurel et al., 2015). GSK3β inhibition may also indirectly increase synaptic levels of AChE (Jing et al., 2013). Lithium, a potent GSK3β inhibitor approved to treat bipolar disorder, has been investigated alone, co-administered with the FDA-approved anti-epileptic divalproex (Depakote), and completed a phase II clinical trial evaluating phospho-tau reduction (clinicaltrials.gov trial ID: NCT00088387). Another phase II trial is currently recruiting patients to measure symptomatic relief of psychosis and agitation in AD patients who are being given up to 600 mg orally per day (clinicaltrials.gov trial ID: NCT02129348).

Phosphodiesterase Enzymes

Cyclic nucleotides, such as cyclic adenosine monophosphate (cAMP), are crucial molecules required for cell signal transduction and secondary messenger pathways, and are regulated by the phosphodiesterase (PDE) superfamily (Bollen and Prickaerts, 2012). Thus, neuronal dysfunction seen in neurological disorders may be a function of aberrant PDE activity. Inhibition of PDE4 has demonstrated cognitive enhancement in mammalian models of aging, and may involve elevation of levels of cAMP, which decreases neuronal release of inflammatory cytokines and aids long-term potentiation (Gallant et al., 2010). Major clinical drawbacks to using PDE4 inhibitors are nausea and vomiting. However, milder inhibitors have been discovered (García-Osta et al., 2012). A phase II trial with PDE4 inhibitor MK-0952 in patients with mild-to-moderate AD in 2007 was completed, but results from the study could not be located (clinicaltrials.gov trial ID: NCT00362024). The PDE5 inhibitor etazolate (EHT0202) was coadministered with an AChEI and assessed in patients with the same indication in 2009 (clinicaltrials.gov trial ID: NCT00880412). It was well tolerated at 40 and 80 mg oral doses, but was not assessed for efficacy in disease progression (Vellas et al., 2011). EHT0202 also modulates $GABA_A$ chloride channels as discussed later (Rissman et al., 2007).

HMG-CoA Reductase

Research in transgenic mice models strongly suggested that a high total serum cholesterol level, as a result of diet, altered amyloid protein processing leading to decreased levels of soluble amyloid sAPPα and increased levels of pathological Aβ (Refolo et al., 2000). Studies have since demonstrated that treatment with statins not only lower cholesterol levels, but bring about cognitive enhancement with decreased levels of amyloid plaques (Kurata et al., 2012). Statins, or HMG-CoA reductase inhibitors, have been used clinically to treat high cholesterol levels for many years. Several clinical trials have been conducted to assess their efficacy in patients with AD, but results are not readily available. One of the most well-known statins, atorvastatin (Lipitor), did show a significant improvement on the ADAS-cog testing versus placebo when taken 80 mg orally per day (Sparks et al., 2005).

Histone Deacetylase

Epigenetic modification of histones, the macromolecules that form the core of nuclear chromatin, is an emerging field of research and has strongly demonstrated a role in memory formation (Stilling and Fischer, 2011). There appears to be a fine balance between the levels of histone acetylation and pathological features of AD, and histone deacetylase (HDAC) inhibition has led to improved cognitive function in rodent models of AD (Fischer, 2014). FMR0334 (formerly EVP0334), an HDAC inhibitor, displayed cognitive improvements of mice in various tasks (Patzke et al., 2008). FMR0334 completed phase I clinical trial and is being continued in a phase II study for patients with genetic predisposition to frontotemporal dementia (clinicaltrials.gov trial ID: NCT02149160).

Monoamine Oxidase

Monoamine oxidases (MAOs) catalyze the breakdown of monoamine neurotransmitters including dopamine, serotonin, and epinephrine in the CNS (Cai, 2014). Inhibition of MAO-B, the predominant isoform in the human brain, is a therapeutic strategy for treating Parkinson's disease, and the drug rasagiline is clinically approved to relieve symptoms (Chen et al., 2007). It was investigated clinically as an adjuvant therapy with donepezil in AD and a phase II clinical trial was completed in 2007, but no further data were found (clinicaltrials.gov trial ID: NCT00104273).

IONOTROPIC CHANNELS

Ionotropic receptors play essential roles throughout the body. In the CNS, ion channels are essential to regulating membrane potential, propagation of action potentials, neurotransmitter release, and intercellular communication. Not surprisingly, dysfunction of ion channel signaling can lead to cognitive impairment. Drugs that target ionotropic receptor sites are used in treatment of numerous disease states including AD and other neurodegenerative diseases. With respect to neurodegeneration, ionotropic dysfunction can lead to neuronal cell toxicity (discussed later) and a number of compounds that target ion channels have been investigated as neuroprotective agents (Schurr, 2004). These compounds can have both symptomatic and disease-modifying benefits. Memantine, which inhibits the NMDA ion channel, is a successful example of a channel blocker used in AD for symptomatic and mild disease-modifying effects (discussed further later) (Lipton and Chen, 2004). Some of the relevant ion channels include glutamatergic, cholinergic, and GABAergic channels.

IONOTROPIC GLUTAMATE RECEPTORS

Three classes of ionotropic glutamate receptors are recognized based on synthetic agonist selectivity. These are AMPA, NMDA, and KA receptors for agonists α-amino-3-hydroxy-5-methyl-4-isoxazolepropionic acid (AMPA), NMDA acid, and kainic acid (KA), respectively. Glutamate receptors are implicated in CNS cell degeneration associated with neurodegenerative diseases including AD, frontotemporal dementia, ALS, and many related disorders (Meldrum and Garthwaite, 1990; Doble, 1999; Albin and Greenamyre, 1992). Excessive glutamatergic signaling has been shown to mediate excitotoxicity in vitro and in vivo and ionotropic glutamate receptors are important therapeutic drug targets (Lodge et al., 2002). Several reviews on the molecular basis of glutamatergic excitotoxicity have been published (Dong et al., 2009; Arundine and Tymianski, 2003).

AMPA Receptors

The AMPA receptor is a ligand-gated ionotropic glutamate receptor. A number of AMPA receptor subtypes exist based on subunit composition ($GluR_{1-4}$) of the functional tetramer. AMPA receptors are expressed throughout the CNS and play essential roles in neuronal communication, sensory processing, as well as learning, memory, and synaptic plasticity (Shepherd and Huganir, 2007). Dysfunction of AMPA channels and resultant changes in LTP and neuronal communication have been implicated in the pathophysiology underlying AD (Shepherd and Huganir, 2007).

The important role of AMPA in synaptic plasticity and learning support AMPA as a target for cognitive enhancement (nootropic effects) and a whole class of drugs, called the ampakines, have grown out of this theory (Lynch and Gall, 2006). Ampakines are positive allosteric modulators of the AMPA receptor. Many ampakines show interesting and promising nootropic effects such as memory enhancement in animals (Zheng et al., 2011; Granger et al., 1996) including aged humans (Lynch, 2004; Lynch et al., 1997; Ingvar et al., 1997; Wezenberg et al., 2007). Memory-enhancing effects are, however, not universal, for example, while the ampakine farampator (500mg) improved short-term memory, it appeared to impair episodic memory (Wezenberg et al., 2007).

As a result of the cognitive and memory-enhancing effects, AMPA modulation is a target in a number of neurological disorders including AD, schizophrenia, and Parkinson's disease (O'Neill et al., 2004; Black, 2005). While efficacy has been predicted, the effects of ampakines on cognitive deficits characteristic of neurodegenerative diseases are not clear and to date only a limited number of ampakines have been evaluated in controlled clinical studies of AD. Ampakine CX516 was evaluated in patients with mild-to-moderate cognitive impairment in a randomized, double-blind, placebo-controlled phase II trial (Johnson and Simmon, 2002). A phase II trial in AD was completed (clinicaltrials.gov trial ID: NCT00001662). Unfortunately, details of the outcomes of these studies could not be located. However, a chemically distinct AMPA modulator, LY415395, did not improve cognition in a trial of AD because no statistically significant difference was seen between patients treated with drug or placebo using the ADAS-cog (Chappell et al., 2007).

N-Methyl-D-Aspartate Receptors

Overstimulation of NMDAR mediates excitotoxicity in vitro and in vivo, which can lead to apoptotic or necrotic cell death. Pathological dysfunction of NMDAR signaling can lead to excitotoxic signaling even with physiologically normal levels of channel activation. NMDAR antagonists show neuroprotection in a large number of in vitro models including glutamate excitotoxicity (Drian et al., 1999), traumatic brain injury (Raghavendra Rao et al., 2001), and hippocampal ischemia (Pringle et al., 1997). A portion of the pathology underlying a number of CNS disorders is hypothesized to involve glutamate-mediated excitotoxicity, and NMDAR-mediated excitotoxicity is implicated in the pathology of AD and a number of related neurodegenerative disorders.

The neuroprotective action of NMDAR antagonism has been validated in numerous animal models of neurodegenerative diseases. For example, NMDAR antagonists have shown efficacy in vivo in multiple transgenic mouse models of AD (Rammes et al., 2008), including 3xTg-AD mice (Martinez-Coria et al., 2010) and APP/PS1 Tg mice (Scholtzova et al., 2008), and in traumatic brain injury models (Raghavendra Rao et al., 2001; Faden et al., 1989; Hayes et al., 1988). Naturally aged rat may better model features of neurodegenerative processes and aging and it is possible this model may be superior to classic transgenic models for predicting drug action in certain neurodegenerative diseases such as AD (Lecanu and Papadopoulos, 2013).

At present, memantine (Namenda) is the only FDA-approved NMDAR antagonist indicated for moderate-to-severe AD. In addition to memantine, a few other neuroprotective agents have been found to have NMDAR antagonist actions including riluzole in ALS (Debono et al., 1993). Memantine, an uncompetitive NMDAR antagonist, has consistently shown modest but statistically significant improvements in AD and related dementias. Clinically significant outcomes reported include cognition improvements as well as improvements on functional and global endpoints on a number of AD scales. Benefits have been observed in numerous clinical trials, meta-analyses, and large-scale responder analyses (Hellweg et al., 2012; Ditzler, 1991; Herrmann et al., 2011; Winblad et al., 2007; Winblad and Poritis, 1999; Görtelmeyer and Erbler, 1992; Reisberg et al., 2003; Rossom and Dysken, 2004). More so, evidence of disease-modifying effects in the form of slowing disease progression has been reported in several studies (Hellweg et al., 2012; Beister et al., 2004; Uitti et al., 1996).

Despite promising results with several uncompetitive NMDAR antagonists, numerous clinical failures, caused by tolerability issues, have discouraged many efforts (Muir, 2006). The issue is also partially confounded by the limitation of using current animal models in testing for the undesired psychoactive side effects of these compounds combined with the great financial cost of clinical trials. Memantine's tolerability is rather unique and Lipton and colleagues first hypothesized that it is because of uncompetitive use-dependent inhibition as well as rapid off-rate from the channel (Rammes et al., 2008; Chen et al., 1992; Lipton, 2006). It is believed that potent high-affinity antagonists have slow on-/off-rates and exhibit the phenomenon known as channel trapping in which they remain in the channel for long periods, sometimes even after channel deactivation. It is believed that this long off-rate leads to absence of physiologically required NMDAR signaling and the classic NMDAR antagonist side effects (Hardingham and Bading, 2003; Papadia and Hardingham, 2007). In this way, NMDAR signaling is an example of the Goldilocks principle where the degree of channel signaling must be within a specific window: too much leads to excitotoxicity whereas too little leads to no effects. Understanding the relationship between NMDAR antagonism and tolerability is extremely important to improve success in this drug class.

Limited successes with NMDAR antagonists continue to appear. This observation is illustrated by a recently published phase II, randomized, double-blind, placebo-controlled study in AD, which reported promising results with AVP-923 (Nuedexta), a two-drug therapy containing an uncompetitive moderate affinity NMDAR channel blocker dextromethorphan with the cytochrome P450 (CYP2D6) inhibitor quinidine. AVP-923 was well tolerated, reduced AD-associated agitation, and decreased "caregiver burden" (Cummings et al., 2015). It was approved for pseudobulbar affect, a syndrome of uncontrolled episodes of laughing and/or crying, associated with numerous NDDs including AD (Tan and Dubovsky, 2011). A phase IV trial investigating use of AVP-923 in AD-specific pseudobulbar affect is ongoing (clinicaltrials.gov trial ID: NCT01832350).

A number of NMDAR subtypes exist, made up of varying combinations of subunits, and it has been speculated that subtype-specific NMDAR antagonists may have improved tolerability profiles (Carter et al., 1997). One subtype that has been investigated is NR2B containing NMDAR populations (Williams, 1993). The NR2B selective antagonists ifenprodil and eliprodil have shown neuroprotection in a number of in vitro and in vivo models (Carter et al., 1997). More so, NR2B antagonists appear to have better tolerability in animal studies and humans than classic competitive and uncompetitive NMDAR antagonists like PCP and MK-801 (Carter et al., 1997). These results led to clinical investigations of these compounds. Eliprodil was well tolerated in a phase I study of healthy volunteers (Carter et al., 1997). However, a phase III trial in ischemic stroke was halted because of lack of efficacy (De Keyser et al., 1999).

EVT 101 and EVT 103 are second-generation NR2B selective antagonists. EVT 101 was investigated in several phase I clinical trials including one investigating the potential role of NR2B receptors in cognitive function in healthy adults (clinicaltrials.gov trial ID: NCT00526968). Indications include AD, neuropathic pain, and treatment-resistant depression.

Kainate Receptors

The final type of ionotropic glutamatergic receptors are KA receptors. KA is a potent glutaminergic neurotoxin (Nadler and Cuthbertson, 1980). KA competitive antagonists have anticonvulsant activities (Collins et al., 1984; Chapman et al., 1985). Whereas AMPA and NMDAR play roles in fast synaptic communication and processing, KA receptors have a modulatory function where they fine-tune the delicate balance between neuronal excitation and inhibition (Swanson, 2009). As such, drugs targeting the KA receptor may have potential in NDDs including AD.

CHOLINERGIC RECEPTORS

Acetylcholine plays an important role in the mammalian CNS and is implicated in the regulation of numerous CNS functions including arousal, reward, learning, and memory (Gotti et al., 2006). ACh receptors may be classified into two types: ionotropic, represented by the nicotinic receptors, and GPCR, represented by the muscarinic receptors (described earlier). These distinctions are based on differential binding of the ligands nicotine and muscarine.

Alterations in nicotinic receptors subtype expressions have been observed in AD patients (Gotti et al., 2006; Sugaya et al., 1990). This observation led to the investigation and FDA approval of AChEIs as symptomatic therapy in AD (McGleenon et al., 1999). These compounds are believed to act largely by preventing ACh breakdown, thus elevating synaptic concentrations of ACh, compensating for reduced cholinergic signaling from AD-associated neuronal (and glial) cell death or degeneration.

Nicotinic receptors are homo- or heteropentamers made up from a combination of several distinct subunits. As such, a large number of nicotinic receptor subtypes have been identified, several of which are believed to be relevant to AD including $\alpha_4\beta_2$ and α_7 (Gotti et al., 2006; Levin, 2002). Clinical trials with a number of ligands targeting nicotinic receptors including AZD1446 (TC-6683) ($\alpha_4\beta_2$) (clinicaltrials.gov trial ID: NCT01039701) have been performed or are ongoing. A number of studies unfortunately have been discontinued because of poor recruitment status (Misra and Medhi, 2013). In addition, nicotine has many useful effects on mood, arousal, and cognition (Stolerman, 1991). A phase II study looking at nicotine in mild cognitive decline is currently recruiting (clinicaltrials.gov trial ID: NCT01778946).

$GABA_A$ RECEPTORS

$GABA_A$ is the ionotropic Cl^- channel gated by the major inhibitory neurotransmitter γ-aminobutyric acid. $GABA_A$ receptors are expressed widely throughout the CNS where they represent one of the major inhibitory receptors (Wisden and Seeburg, 1992). $GABA_A$ therefore plays essential functions in regulating neuronal membrane potential, action potential, intercellular communication, network synchronization, and neurotransmitter release (Buzsáki and Chrobak, 1995). Functional $GABA_A$ protein is a pentamer with several subtypes recognized. These subtypes arise from $GABA_A$ subunit composition (α, β, γ, δ) of the functional pentamer (Wisden and Seeburg, 1992; Chang et al., 1996) and give rise to differences in pharmacological effects (discussed further later) (Rowlett et al., 2005; Maubach, 2003; Chambers et al., 2004).

Research in rats has shown differential distributions of $GABA_A$ subtypes throughout the CNS (Fritschy and Mohler, 1995). Likewise, differences in expression have been reported with developmental stages and age (Laurie et al., 1992). GABAergic neurons are largely spared in AD, in contrast to their cholinergic and glutamatergic counterparts, making them a potential useful target. However, this observation should not be taken to mean $GABA_A$ receptors are not involved in AD pathology as age- and disease-related changes in $GABA_A$ receptor subtypes and their regional distributions have been reported and may play roles in disease pathophysiology and/or drug response (Rissman et al., 2007).

In addition to competitive binding site for GABA on the $GABA_A$ receptor, a number of allosteric binding sites on $GABA_A$ channels exist, which may provide unique pharmacological actions on the channel and could be investigated as drug targets (Sieghart, 2006).

An example of a $GABA_A$ modulator is etazolate (EHT0202). In addition to its effects on $GABA_A$, it has additional pharmacological effects relevant to AD including PDE5 inhibition. Desirable pharmacological effects are believed to include $GABA_A$ receptor mediated α-secretase stimulation, which leads to reduced Aβ plaque formation (Desire et al., 2009). Etazolate has shown neuroprotective and cognitive enhancing effects in a number of in vitro and in vivo AD and age-related models (Desire et al., 2009). It was well tolerated in a phase I trial (Desire et al., 2009), as well as in a randomized, placebo-controlled, double-blind phase IIA study in 159 randomized patients with mild-to-moderate AD as an adjunct to AChE treatment (Vellas et al., 2011). In the latter, except for ratings on the Alzheimer's Disease

Cooperative Study-Activities of Daily Living scale, no differences were observed between groups. However, this study was not designed to show drug efficacy (Vellas et al., 2011). Follow-up research with etazolate or related $GABA_A$ modulators is needed.

The most well-studied and clinically used $GABA_A$ allosteric modulators are the benzodiazepines. Benzodiazepines were discovered, through a series of serendipitous events, by Leo Sternbach at Hoffman-La Roche in the 1950s (Sternbach, 1979). Since this discovery, an impressive number of benzodiazepines have entered the global pharmacopeia with diverse clinical uses. The widespread adoption of benzodiazepines has to do with their extensive applicability as anxiolytics, antispasmolytics, tranquilizers, sedatives/sleep aids, mood enhancers, and anticonvulsants (Bianchi, 2010), combined with a generally excellent therapeutic index.

In general, benzodiazepines act via binding to the allosteric benzodiazepine binding site on $GABA_A$ channels and as modulators of channel function by enhancing the inhibitory Cl^- current via increasing channel opening frequency (Bianchi, 2010; Twyman et al., 1989; Paul et al., 1981). A large body of research suggesting enhanced inhibitory GABA neurotransmission may actually limit glutamatergic excitotoxicity and exert neuroprotective effects (Egashira et al., 2007). Benzodiazepines have shown neuroprotective effects in many in vitro and in vivo models (Schwartz-Bloom et al., 1998, 2000). They are commonly prescribed in elderly patients to relieve agitation and anxiety (de Gage et al., 2014; Kirby et al., 1999). Although unfortunate, it is not too surprising, given common benzodiazepines side effects, that a number of studies show a relationship between use of these drug and serious issues in the elderly including cognitive impairment, increased risk of motor vehicle accidents, and hip fractures (Kirby et al., 1999; Wagner et al., 2004).

Even more concerning, epidemiological studies have shown correlations between benzodiazepine use and dementia, with a correlation between length of use and disease risk (de Gage et al., 2014; Paterniti et al., 2002). While epidemiological studies establish correlation they should not be used as sole support for a causative relationship as any number of noncausative factors may explain the correlations. For example, early disease manifestation could lead to the display of symptoms commonly treated with benzodiazepines. Another possibility is that common side effects from use of the benzodiazepines (and related GABAergics) are consistent with many symptoms seen in dementias including memory impairment, drowsiness, motor impairment, intoxication, and loss of inhibition. Thus, benzodiazepine use in elderly patients may lead to behaviors consistent with dementia leading to misdiagnosis. For example, hip fractures and car accidents would likely lead to concerns from family, care takers, and medical professionals and thus medical consultation. Reliance on symptomatic diagnosis as opposed to biomarkers could lead to inaccurate dementia diagnosis. This perspective is partially supported by several studies involving short-term benzodiazepine use (Foy et al., 1995). Significant cognitive improvements including memory were found in at least one controlled study in which benzodiazepine treatment was gradually discontinued from elderly nursing home residents (as compared to continually treated controlled) (Salzman et al., 1992). Furthermore, current but not past benzodiazepine use in elderly patients was associated with cognitive impairments (Hanlon et al., 1998).

An interesting possibility to limit side effects of benzodiazepines is the use of subtype selective inverse agonists, which may provide symptomatic relief in AD. Inverse $GABA_A$ agonists (eg, methyl-6,7-dimethoxy-4-ethyl-beta-carboline-3-carboxylate) attenuate $GABA_A$ receptor function and show improvements in learning and memory in animal models (Maubach, 2003). However, the early non-subtype selective ligands also induced anxiety and convulsions

(Maubach, 2003). Follow-up research found that selective α5 $GABA_A$ inverse agonists could have potential in AD and related disorders because α5 $GABA_A$ subtypes are found preferentially in the hippocampus and inverse agonists enhanced memory in animal models including the Morris water maze (spatial learning) while being devoid of adverse effects associated with the nonselective inverse agonists (Maubach, 2003; Chambers et al., 2004; Koh et al., 2013). With recent advances made by several laboratories in our understanding of $GABA_A$ subtype pharmacology, allosteric modulators with tailored subtype-specific profiles for anxiolytic, neuroprotective, and procognitive actions devoid of undesirable effects like drowsiness, motor impairment, intoxication and memory impairments seem possible.

5-HT_3 RECEPTORS

5-HT_3 is the only ionotropic serotonin receptor currently recognized. Functional 5-HT_3 receptors are a pentamer made up from a number of subunits, giving rise to several subtypes (5-HT_{3a-3e}), which can have distinct pharmacological activities (Niesler et al., 2007). Current approved use of 5-HT_3 antagonists is as an antiemetic in chemotherapy. 5-HT_3 is highly expressed throughout the CNS and is involved in excitatory neurotransmission and regulation of ACh. Furthermore, evidence suggests 5-HT_3 activation may lead to inhibition of LTP and memory impairment (Rogawski and Wenk, 2003). Thus 5-HT_3 antagonists may have procognitive actions. Consistent with this hypothesis, a number of 5-HT_3 antagonists show cognitive enhancing effects in animal models. For example, WAY-100579 and ondansetron enhanced learning in lesioned rats and similar effects were reported with the related WAY-100289 (Hodges et al., 1996). A study of ondansetron in patients with age-associated memory impairments showed dose-dependent improvements in several memory tests (Crook and Lakin, 1991). Unfortunately, ondansetron failed to slow cognitive decline in AD patients in a multicenter, double-blind, placebo-controlled clinical trial (Dysken et al., 2002).

The significance of 5-HT_3 in AD therapy remains unknown. Normal concentrations of 5-HT_3 receptor sites were observed in a study of AD patients (Barnes et al., 1990). Interestingly, NMDAR antagonist memantine and NMDAR NR2B antagonist ifenprodil have been found to act as 5-HT_3 channel blockers at low μM concentrations (Rammes et al., 2001; Barann et al., 1998). While it is unclear how 5-HT_3 antagonism contributes to the therapeutic activity of NMDAR antagonism in AD, the potential for polypharmacological activity between NMDAR, 5-HT_3, and other ion channels as well as other receptors is worthy of further investigation.

CATION CHANNELS

Dysfunction in calcium and zinc homeostasis has been implicated in AD pathophysiology (Corona et al., 2011; Yu et al., 2009). As discussed under the NMDAR section, excessive levels of Ca^{2+} can cause excitotoxic cascade ending in cellular damage or death. A number of distinct calcium channels exist in the CNS and these regulate a host of physiological functions including Ca^{2+} gradients, signaling processes, synaptic neurotransmitter release, and biomolecule activation/inactivation (Yu et al., 2009). The widely used anticonvulsant and mood stabilizer valproic acid has a number of pharmacological actions that are relevant to

AD including blockage of ionotropic cation (sodium, potassium, and calcium) channels, GABAergic actions, HDAC inhibition, and inhibition of tau hyperphosphorylation (Hu et al., 2011; Chateauvieux et al., 2010). However, valproic acid failed to show cognitive or functional status improvements in a phase III trial of AD, although, consistent with its action as a mood stabilizer, agitation and psychosis incidents were reduced (Mangialasche et al., 2010).

HORMONE RECEPTORS

Hormones are essential biological signaling molecules, which can be distinguished from neurotransmitters in their release and signaling properties. They can be subdivided based on chemical compositions (peptide, steroid, and amino acid derived). Hormonal imbalances are associated with a host of disease states including diabetes, gigantism, dwarfism, thyroid disorders, low testosterone, as well as numerous reproductive and psychological disorders.

Alterations in hormone systems may have complex effects on AD risk and pathology, which are highly dependent on age, sex, past exposure to hormone therapies, hormone type, and genetic factors (Resnick and Henderson, 2002; Shahrokhi et al., 2012). For example, age-associated loss of sex hormones in male and females is a risk factor in developing AD (Vest and Pike, 2013; Pike et al., 2009). While this loss could be coincidental, evidence suggests there may be a real relationship. Female patients treated with sex hormones for 10 years showed a slight reduction in risk of developing AD (Resnick and Henderson, 2002). Though not conclusive, this observation strengthens the belief in the link between AD and hormonal changes as well as illustrates a major current issue in AD therapy: time dependence of intervention. To decrease risk of AD with sex hormone replacement therapy may require early intervention, which may extend a decade or more prior to diagnosis. Without advances in existing diagnosis techniques, identification of high-risk patients remains a challenge.

Steroid Hormones

Investigations into the use of sex hormones, such as estrogen-based strategies to treat AD and slow disease onset or progression, have been performed or are ongoing, although in some cases no benefit was found (Pike et al., 2009; Henderson et al., 2000). Pharmacological support for the role of hormones in AD pathology and as a promising drug target for AD comes from the fact that many steroid hormones have potent antiinflammatory mechanisms of action and inflammation has been implicated in AD pathophysiology (McGeer and Rogers, 1992; McGeer and McGeer, 2007). Many steroid hormones including estrogen and androgens also exhibit neuroprotective activities in vivo including models of neurodegenerative diseases (Pike et al., 2009; Vongher and Frye, 1999). Antioxidant effects observed with many hormones are proposed to underlie a part of this neuroprotection (Shahrokhi et al., 2012). Testosterone has shown beneficial effects including improvement in spatial memory and quality of life in men with AD (Cherrier et al., 2005; Lu et al., 2006).

Selective Estrogen-Receptor Modulator

Raloxifene is a selective estrogen-receptor modulator currently approved for preventing and treating osteoporosis in postmenopausal women. During a large trial of raloxifene in osteoporosis, a cognitive outcome substudy was included (Yaffe et al., 2014). Following 3 years of treatment, the 120-mg (but not 60-mg) dose correlated with a reduced risk for minimal cognitive impairment and AD. A 1-year phase II placebo-controlled trial of raloxifene in 72 AD patients has been completed and some differences between groups were seen though they do not appear to be statistically significant (clinicaltrials.gov trial ID: NCT00368459).

Another hormone that has been evaluated in AD is the gonadotropin-releasing hormone analog leuprolide acetate. Leuprolide acetate's mechanism of action is believed to involve the suppression of gonadotrope-induced secretion of luteinizing hormone (LH) (Wilson et al., 2007). A large body of experimental evidence supports a role of LH in AD (Meethal et al., 2005; Casadesus et al., 2004; Webber et al., 2007). A study using transgenic mice developed to overproduce LH showed cognitive impairment (Webber et al., 2007). LH also modulates Aβ processing in vitro and in vivo (Webber et al., 2007). Up to twofold elevated LH levels were found in AD patients compared to age-matched controls (Short et al., 2001).

The limited number of clinical trials with leuprolide acetate have been promising. In women with mild-to-moderate AD, it was well tolerated over a 48-week period. In addition, it was reported to have a "stabilizing effect on cognitive and global functioning" in the study (LaPlante et al., 2006). Likewise, a phase III study of 109 women with mild-to-moderate AD showed a stabilizing effect with co-treatment of leuprolide acetate and an AChEI (Bowen et al., 2015). A pooled analysis of two studies with VP4896, a proprietary implantable form of leuprolide acetate, showed a non-significant improvement on the ADAS-cog and a significant effect ($p = .048$) in which 50.9% of treated patients remained unchanged or improved on the Alzheimer's Disease Cooperative Study-Clinical Global Impression of Change at 48 weeks compared to 34.5% of the placebo group (Susman, 2006). These results are particularly promising and warrant further investigation of leuprolide acetate as well as alternate hormone-based therapies.

Nerve Growth Factor

Dysfunction in nerve growth factor (NGF) has been implicated in activation of the amyloidogenic pathway and neurodegeneration in AD (Cattaneo et al., 2008). Targeted administration of NGF to cholinergic neurons of the basal forebrain prevented cell death, enhanced synaptic cholinergic activity and promoted cognitive improvement in animals (Cattaneo et al., 2008). Intracerebroventricular-infused NGF has been evaluated in a small number of AD patients. Despite improvements in cognition and physiological measurements of CNS functions, adverse effects including weight loss and pain were reported in these patients (Olson et al., 1992; Eriksdotter Jönhagen et al., 1998). Alternate routes of NGF delivery including intranasal and topical are under investigation as means to limit side effects (Mangialasche et al., 2010). Likewise, use of NGF gene therapy and encapsulated-NGF-producing cell-based biodelivery are being investigated clinically (Mangialasche et al., 2010). NGF gene therapy was well tolerated in a phase I trial, supporting follow-up investigation to determine efficacy (Tuszynski et al., 2005).

POLYPHARMACOLOGY

The importance of polypharmacology in the treatment of complex disease states is becoming increasingly recognized (Kroeze and Roth, 2012; Anighoro et al., 2014). It involves at least two strategies: single agent with multiple pharmacological mechanisms, or combinations of drugs to act via multiple mechanisms. Memantine is an NMDAR antagonist that has several pharmacological mechanisms including 5-HT_3 and nicotinic α7ACh channel antagonism, which may contribute to its efficacy and tolerability. An example of multidrug polypharmacology involves use of memantine with the AChEI/nicotinic receptor allosteric modulator (potentiator) galantamine, which has become commonplace in contemporary AD therapy (Lopes et al., 2013). Another example is donecopride (RS67333), which was developed as a dual binding site inhibitor. The chemical structure of an AChEI was modified until partial agonist activity at 5-HT_4 was achieved (Rochais et al., 2015). The polypharmacological benefits include ACh elevation, and altered amyloid protein processing leading to generation of the more favorable soluble amyloid protein sAPPα (Lecoutey et al., 2014). Ladostigil (TV-3326) was designed from the structure of the MAO-B inhibitor rasagiline and modified to achieve AChEI activity (Youdim, 2013). A phase II clinical study concluded in 2013 investigating the effectiveness of 160 mg/day of the hemitartrate salt given orally, for patients with mild-to-moderate AD (clinicaltrials.gov trial ID: NCT01354691). A phase IIB trial is currently active studying the effects of 10 mg/day oral for participants with mild cognitive impairment (clinicaltrials.gov trial ID: NCT01429623). Another novel multitarget drug investigated for AD is memoquin, an AChE/β-secretase inhibitor, which also exhibits antioxidant activity. Memoquin has shown desirable cognitive enhancing effects in in vivo animal models (Capurro et al., 2013).

CONCLUSIONS

Despite an abundance of diverse targets investigated, successful development of drugs for AD has been very limited. Limitations in our understanding of disease pathology, inaccurate in vitro and in vivo models coupled with biases toward present monotherapy are likely central factors. Despite the difficulty, even modestly active compounds could have dramatic economic, social, and therapeutic impacts and are therefore desperately needed. In addition, there is drastic need for fresh perspectives, improved diagnostics, disease prevention strategies, a biological systems approach, and polypharmacology, some of which were reviewed in this chapter.

References

Ahmad, I., Nirogi, R., 2011. 5-HT_4 receptor agonists for the treatment of Alzheimer's disease. Neurosci. Med. 2, 87.

Albin, R.L., Greenamyre, J.T., 1992. Alternative excitotoxic hypotheses. Neurology 42, 733.

Alzheimer's, A., 2015. 2015 Alzheimer's disease facts and figures. Alzheimers Dement. J. Alzheimers Assoc. 11, 332.

Anighoro, A., Bajorath, J., Rastelli, G., 2014. Polypharmacology: challenges and opportunities in drug discovery: miniperspective. J. Med. Chem. 57, 7874–7887.

Anthony, J., Breitner, J., Zandi, P., Meyer, M., Jurasova, I., Norton, M., Stone, S., C.C.M.S. Group, 2000. Reduced prevalence of AD in users of NSAIDs and H2 receptor antagonists: the Cache County Study. Neurology 54, 2066–2071.

Arundine, M., Tymianski, M., 2003. Molecular mechanisms of calcium-dependent neurodegeneration in excitotoxicity. Cell Calcium 34, 325–337.

Aso, E., Ferrer, I., 2014. Cannabinoids for treatment of Alzheimer's disease: moving toward the clinic. Front. Pharmacol. 5.

Barann, M., Bönisch, H., Urban, B.W., Göthert, M., 1998. Inhibition of 5-HT3 receptor cation channels by ifenprodil in excised patches of N1E-115 cells. Naunyn Schmiedebergs Arch. Pharmacol. 358, 145–152.

Barnes, N.M., Costall, B., Naylor, R.J., Williams, T.J., Wischik, C.M., 1990. Normal densities of 5-HT_3 receptor recognition sites in Alzheimer's disease. Neuroreport.

Beister, A., Kraus, P., Kuhn, W., Dose, M., Weindl, A., Gerlach, M., 2004. The *N*-methyl-D-aspartate Antagonist Memantine Retards Progression of Huntington's Disease. Springer.

Beurel, E., Grieco, S.F., Jope, R.S., 2015. Glycogen synthase kinase-3 (GSK3): regulation, actions, and diseases. Pharmacol. Ther. 148, 114–131.

Bianchi, M.T., 2010. Context dependent benzodiazepine modulation of $GABA_A$ receptor opening frequency. Curr. Neuropharmacol. 8, 10.

Black, M.D., 2005. Therapeutic potential of positive AMPA modulators and their relationship to AMPA receptor subunits. A review of preclinical data. Psychopharmacology 179, 154–163.

Bollen, E., Prickaerts, J., 2012. Phosphodiesterases in neurodegenerative disorders. IUBMB Life 64, 965–970.

Bowen, R.L., Perry, G., Xiong, C., Smith, M.A., Atwood, C.S., 2015. A clinical study of lupron depot in the treatment of women with Alzheimer's disease: preservation of cognitive function in patients taking an acetylcholinesterase inhibitor and treated with high dose lupron over 48 weeks. J. Alzheimers Dis. 44, 549–560.

Brioni, J.D., Esbenshade, T.A., Garrison, T.R., Bitner, S.R., Cowart, M.D., 2011. Discovery of histamine H3 antagonists for the treatment of cognitive disorders and Alzheimer's disease. J. Pharmacol. Exp. Ther. 336, 38–46.

Buzsáki, G., Chrobak, J.J., 1995. Temporal structure in spatially organized neuronal ensembles: a role for interneuronal networks. Curr. Opin. Neurobiol. 5, 504–510.

Carter, C., et al., 1997. In: Herrling, P. (Ed.), Ifenprodil and Liprodil: Neuroprotective NMDA Receptor Antagonists and Calcium Channel Blockers, 6. Academic Press, pp. 57–87.

Cai, Z., 2014. Monoamine oxidase inhibitors: promising therapeutic agents for Alzheimer's disease (Review). Mol. Med. Rep. 9, 1533–1541.

Campbell, V., Gowran, A., 2007. Alzheimer's disease; taking the edge off with cannabinoids? Br. J. Pharmacol. 152, 655–662.

Cao, C., Li, Y., Liu, H., Bai, G., Mayl, J., Lin, X., Sutherland, K., Nabar, N., Cai, J., 2014. The potential therapeutic effects of THC on Alzheimer's disease. Neurodegeneration 24, 25.

Capurro, V., Busquet, P., Lopes, J.P., Bertorelli, R., Tarozzo, G., Bolognesi, M.L., Piomelli, D., Reggiani, A., Cavalli, A., 2013. Pharmacological characterization of memoquin, a multi-target compound for the treatment of Alzheimer's disease. PLoS One 8, e56870.

Carlson, M.C., Tschanz, J.T., Norton, M.C., Welsh-Bohmer, K., Martin, B.K., Breitner, J.C., 2002. H2 histamine receptor blockade in the treatment of Alzheimer disease: a randomized, double-blind, placebo-controlled trial of nizatidine. Alzheimer Dis. Assoc. Disord. 16, 24–30.

Carter, G.T., Rosen, B.S., 2001. Marijuana in the management of amyotrophic lateral sclerosis. Am. J. Hosp. Palliat. Care 18, 264–270.

Casadesus, G., Zhu, X., Atwood, C.S., Webber, K.M., Perry, G., Bowen, R.L., Smith, M.A., 2004. Beyond estrogen: targeting gonadotropin hormones in the treatment of Alzheimer's disease. Curr. Drug Targets CNS Neurol. Disord. 3, 281–285.

Cattaneo, A., Capsoni, S., Paoletti, F., 2008. Towards non invasive nerve growth factor therapies for Alzheimer's disease. J. Alzheimers Dis. 15, 255–283.

Chambers, M.S., Atack, J.R., Carling, R.W., Collinson, N., Cook, S.M., Dawson, G.R., Ferris, P., Hobbs, S.C., O'Connor, D., Marshall, G., 2004. An orally bioavailable, functionally selective inverse agonist at the benzodiazepine site of GABAA $\alpha 5$ receptors with cognition enhancing properties. J. Med. Chem. 47, 5829–5832.

Chang, Y., Wang, R., Barot, S., Weiss, D.S., 1996. Stoichiometry of a recombinant GABAA receptor. J. Neurosci. 16, 5415–5424.

Chapman, A., Hart, G., Meldrum, B., Turski, L., Watkins, J., 1985. Anticonvulsant activity of two novel piperazine derivatives with potent kainate antagonist activity. Neurosci. Lett. 55, 325–330.

Chappell, A., Gonzales, C., Williams, J., Witte, M., Mohs, R., Sperling, R., 2007. AMPA potentiator treatment of cognitive deficits in Alzheimer disease. Neurology 68, 1008–1012.

Chateauvieux, S., Morceau, F., Dicato, M., Diederich, M., 2010. Molecular and therapeutic potential and toxicity of valproic acid. BioMed Res. Int. 2010.

Chen, H., Pellegrini, J., Aggarwal, S., Lei, S.Z., Warach, S., Jensen, F.E., Lipton, S., 1992. Open-channel block of *N*-methyl-D-aspartate (NMDA) responses by memantine: therapeutic advantage against NMDA receptor-mediated neurotoxicity. J. Neurosci. 12, 4427–4436.

Chen, J.J., Swope, D.M., Dashtipour, K., 2007. Comprehensive review of rasagiline, a second-generation monoamine oxidase inhibitor, for the treatment of Parkinson's disease. Clin. Ther. 29, 1825–1849.

Cherrier, M., Matsumoto, A., Amory, J., Asthana, S., Bremner, W., Peskind, E., Raskind, M., Craft, S., 2005. Testosterone improves spatial memory in men with Alzheimer disease and mild cognitive impairment. Neurology 64, 2063–2068.

Chong, M., Wolff, K., Wise, K., Tanton, C., Winstock, A., Silber, E., 2006. Cannabis use in patients with multiple sclerosis. Mult. Scler. 12, 646–651.

Collins, J., Dixon, A., Badman, G., De Sarro, G., Chapman, A., Hart, G., Meldrum, B., 1984. Kainic acid derivatives with anticonvulsant activity. Neurosci. Lett. 51, 371–376.

Consroe, P., Musty, R., Rein, J., Tillery, W., Pertwee, R., 1997. The perceived effects of smoked cannabis on patients with multiple sclerosis. Eur. Neurol. 38, 44–48.

Corona, C., Pensalfini, A., Frazzini, V., Sensi, S., 2011. New therapeutic targets in Alzheimer's disease: brain deregulation of calcium and zinc. Cell Death Dis. 2, e176.

Craig, L.A., Hong, N.S., McDonald, R.J., 2011. Revisiting the cholinergic hypothesis in the development of Alzheimer's disease. Neurosci. Biobehav. Rev. 35, 1397–1409.

Crook, T., Lakin, M., 1991. Effects of Ondansetron in Age-Associated Memory Impairment. The Role of Ondansetron, a Novel., p. 5.

Cummings, J., Lyketsos, C., Tariot, P., Peskind, E., Nguyen, U., Knowles, N., Shin, P., Siffert, J., 2015. Dextromethorphan/Quinidine (AVP-923) efficacy and safety for treatment of agitation in persons with Alzheimer's disease: results from a phase 2 study (NCT01584440). Neurology 84, S16. 007.

Daval, S.B., Valant, C.l., Bonnet, D., Kellenberger, E., Hibert, M., Galzi, J.-L., Ilien, B., 2012. Fluorescent derivatives of AC-42 to probe bitopic orthosteric/allosteric binding mechanisms on muscarinic M1 receptors. J. Med. Chem. 55, 2125–2143.

de Gage, S.B., Moride, Y., Ducruet, T., Kurth, T., Verdoux, H., Tournier, M., Pariente, A., Bégaud, B., 2014. Benzodiazepine use and risk of Alzheimer's disease: case-control study. BMJ 349, g5205.

De Keyser, J., Sulter, G., Luiten, P.G., 1999. Clinical trials with neuroprotective drugs in acute ischaemic stroke: are we doing the right thing? Trends Neurosci. 22, 535–540.

Debono, M.-W., Le Guern, J., Canton, T., Doble, A., Pradier, L., 1993. Inhibition by riluzole of electrophysiological responses mediated by rat kainate and NMDA receptors expressed in *Xenopus* oocytes. Eur. J. Pharmacol. 235, 283–289.

Desire, L., Marcade, M., Peillon, H., Drouin, D., Sol, O., Pando, M., 2009. Clinical trials of EHT 0202, a neuroprotective and procognitive alpha-secretase stimulator for Alzheimer's disease. Alzheimers Dement. 5, P255–P256.

Ditzler, K., 1991. Efficacy and tolerability of memantine in patients with dementia syndrome. A double-blind, placebo controlled trial. Arzneimittelforschung 41, 773–780.

Doble, A., 1999. The role of excitotoxicity in neurodegenerative disease: implications for therapy. Pharmacol. Ther. 81, 163–221.

Dong, X.X., Wang, Y., Qin, Z.H., 2009. Molecular mechanisms of excitotoxicity and their relevance to pathogenesis of neurodegenerative diseases. Acta Pharmacol. Sin. 30, 379–387.

Drian, M., Kamenka, J., Privat, A., 1999. In vitro neuroprotection against glutamate toxicity provided by novel non-competitive *N*-methyl-D-aspartate antagonists. J. Neurosci. Res. 57, 927–934.

Dysken, M., Kuskowski, M., Love, S., Group, O.S., 2002. Ondansetron in the treatment of cognitive decline in Alzheimer dementia. Am. J. Geriatr. Psychiatry 10, 212–215.

Egan, M.F., Zhao, X., Gottwald, R., Harper-Mozley, L., Zhang, Y., Snavely, D., Lines, C., Michelson, D., 2013. Randomized crossover study of the histamine H3 inverse agonist MK-0249 for the treatment of cognitive impairment in patients with schizophrenia. Schizophr. Res. 146, 224–230.

Egashira, N., Hayakawa, K., Osajima, M., Mishima, K., Iwasaki, K., Oishi, R., Fujiwara, M., 2007. Involvement of $GABA_A$ receptors in the neuroprotective effect of theanine on focal cerebral ischemia in mice. J. Pharmacol. Sci. 105, 211–214.

Eriksdotter Jönhagen, M., Nordberg, A., Amberla, K., Bäckman, L., Ebendal, T., Meyerson, B., Olson, L., Seiger, Shigeta, M., Theodorsson, E., 1998. Intracerebroventricular infusion of nerve growth factor in three patients with Alzheimer's disease. Dement. Geriatr. Cogn. Disord. 9, 246–257.

Eubanks, L.M., Rogers, C.J., Beuscher IV, A.E., Koob, G.F., Olson, A.J., Dickerson, T.J., Janda, K.D., 2006. A molecular link between the active component of marijuana and Alzheimer's disease pathology. Mol. Pharm. 3, 773–777.

Faden, A.I., Demediuk, P., Panter, S.S., Vink, R., 1989. The role of excitatory amino acids and NMDA receptors in traumatic brain injury. Science 244, 798–800.

Fioravanti, M., Flicker, L., 2001. Nicergoline for dementia and other age associated forms of cognitive impairment. Cochrane Database Syst. Rev. 4.

Fischer, A., 2014. Targeting histone-modifications in Alzheimer's disease. What is the evidence that this is a promising therapeutic avenue? Neuropharmacology 80, 95–102.

Fisher, A., 2008. Cholinergic treatments with emphasis on m1 muscarinic agonists as potential disease-modifying agents for Alzheimer's disease. Neurotherapeutics 5, 433–442.

Foy, A., O'Connell, D., Henry, D., Kelly, J., Cocking, S., Halliday, J., 1995. Benzodiazepine use as a cause of cognitive impairment in elderly hospital inpatients. J. Gerontol. A Biol. Sci.Med. Sci. 50, M99–M106.

Fritschy, J.M., Mohler, H., 1995. GABAA-receptor heterogeneity in the adult rat brain: differential regional and cellular distribution of seven major subunits. J. Comp. Neurol. 359, 154–194.

Froestl, W., Gallagher, M., Jenkins, H., Madrid, A., Melcher, T., Teichman, S., Mondadori, C.G., Pearlman, R., 2004. SGS742: the first $GABA_B$ receptor antagonist in clinical trials. Biochem. Pharmacol. 68, 1479–1487.

Gallant, M., Aspiotis, R., Day, S., Dias, R., Dubé, D., Dubé, L., Friesen, R.W., Girard, M., Guay, D., Hamel, P., 2010. Discovery of MK-0952, a selective PDE4 inhibitor for the treatment of long-term memory loss and mild cognitive impairment. Bioorg. Med. Chem. Lett. 20, 6387–6393.

García-Osta, A., Cuadrado-Tejedor, M., García-Barroso, C., Oyarzábal, J., Franco, R., 2012. Phosphodiesterases as therapeutic targets for Alzheimer's disease. ACS Chem. Neurosci. 3, 832–844.

Görtelmeyer, R., Erbler, H., 1992. Memantine in the treatment of mild to moderate dementia syndrome. A double-blind placebo-controlled study. Arzneimittelforschung 42, 904–913.

Gotti, C., Zoli, M., Clementi, F., 2006. Brain nicotinic acetylcholine receptors: native subtypes and their relevance. Trends Pharmacol. Sci. 27, 482–491.

Granger, R., Deadwyler, S., Davis, M., Moskovitz, B., Kessler, M., Rogers, G., Lynch, G., 1996. Facilitation of glutamate receptors reverses an age-associated memory impairment in rats. Synapse 22, 332–337.

Gray, S.L., Walker, R., Dublin, S., Haneuse, S., Crane, P.K., Breitner, J., Bowen, J., McCormick, W., Larson, E.B., 2011. Histamine-2 receptor antagonist use and incident dementia in an older cohort. J. Am. Geriatr. Soc. 59, 251–257.

Grove, R.A., Harrington, C.M., Mahler, A., Beresford, I., Maruff, P., Lowy, M.T., Nicholls, A.P., Boardley, R.L., Berges, A.C., Nathan, P.J., 2014. A randomized, double-blind, placebo-controlled, 16-week study of the H3 receptor antagonist, GSK239512 as a monotherapy in subjects with mild-to-moderate Alzheimer's disease. Curr. Alzheimer Res. 11, 47–58.

Hanlon, J.T., Horner, R.D., Schmader, K.E., Fillenbaum, G.G., Lewis, I.K., Wall, W.E., Landerman, L.R., Pieper, C.F., Blazer, D.G., Cohen, H.J., 1998. Benzodiazepine use and cognitive function among community-dwelling elderly. Clin. Pharmacol. Ther. 64, 684–692.

Hardingham, G.E., Bading, H., 2003. The Yin and Yang of NMDA receptor signalling. Trends Neurosci. 26, 81–89.

Hayes, R., Jenkins, L., Lyeth, B., Balster, R., Robinson, S., Clifton, G., Stubbins, J., Young, H., 1988. Pretreatment with phencyclidine, an *N*-methyl-D-aspartate antagonist, attenuates long-term behavioral deficits in the rat produced by traumatic brain injury. J. Neurotrauma 5, 259–274.

Hellweg, R., Wirth, Y., Janetzky, W., Hartmann, S., 2012. Efficacy of memantine in delaying clinical worsening in Alzheimer's disease (AD): responder analyses of nine clinical trials with patients with moderate to severe AD. Int. J. Geriatr. Psychiatry 27, 651–656.

Henderson, V.W., Paganini-Hill, A., Miller, B., Elble, R., Reyes, P., Shoupe, D., McCleary, C., Klein, R., Hake, A., Farlow, M., 2000. Estrogen for Alzheimer's disease in women randomized, double-blind, placebo-controlled trial. Neurology 54, 295.

Herrmann, N., Li, A., Lanctôt, K., 2011. Memantine in dementia: a review of the current evidence. Expert Opin. Pharmacother. 12, 787–800.

Hodges, H., Sowinski, P., Turner, J., Fletcher, A., 1996. Comparison of the effects of the 5-HT3 receptor antagonists WAY-100579 and ondansetron on spatial learning in the water maze in rats with excitotoxic lesions of the forebrain cholinergic projection system. Psychopharmacology 125, 146–161.

Hu, J.-P., Xie, J.-W., Wang, C.-Y., Wang, T., Wang, X., Wang, S.-L., Teng, W.-P., Wang, Z.-Y., 2011. Valproate reduces tau phosphorylation via cyclin-dependent kinase 5 and glycogen synthase kinase 3 signaling pathways. Brain Res. Bull. 85, 194–200.

Ingvar, M., Ambros-Ingerson, J., Davis, M., Granger, R., Kessler, M., Rogers, G.A., Schehr, R.S., Lynch, G., 1997. Enhancement by an ampakine of memory encoding in humans. Exp. Neurol. 146, 553–559.

Jing, P., Zhang, J.-Y., Ouyang, Q., Wu, J., Zhang, X.-J., 2013. Lithium treatment induces proteasomal degradation of over-expressed acetylcholinesterase (AChE-S) and inhibit GSK3β. Chem. Biol. Interact. 203, 309–313.

Johnson, S.A., Simmon, V.F., 2002. Randomized, double-blind, placebo-controlled international clinical trial of the Ampakine CX516 in elderly participants with mild cognitive impairment. J. Mol. Neurosci. 19, 197–200.

Johnson, D.E., Drummond, E., Grimwood, S., Sawant-Basak, A., Miller, E., Tseng, E., McDowell, L.L., Vanase-Frawley, M.A., Fisher, K.E., Rubitski, D.M., 2012. The 5-hydroxytryptamine4 receptor agonists prucalopride and PRX-03140 increase acetylcholine and histamine levels in the rat prefrontal cortex and the power of stimulated hippocampal θ oscillations. J. Pharmacol. Exp. Ther. 341, 681–691.

Kerr, D., Ong, J., 1995. GABA B receptors. Pharmacol. Ther. 67, 187–246.

Kimura, T., Ishiguro, K., Hisanaga, S., 2014. Physiological and pathological phosphorylation of tau by Cdk5. Front. Mol. Neurosci.

Kirby, M., Denihan, A., Bruce, I., Radic, A., Coakley, D., Lawlor, B.A., 1999. Benzodiazepine use among the elderly in the community. Int. J. Geriatr. Psychiatry 14, 280–284.

Koh, M.T., Rosenzweig-Lipson, S., Gallagher, M., 2013. Selective $GABA_A$ α5 positive allosteric modulators improve cognitive function in aged rats with memory impairment. Neuropharmacology 64, 145–152.

Kroeze, W., Roth, B., 2012. Polypharmacological Drugs: Magic Shotguns for Psychiatric Diseases. Polypharmacology in Drug Discovery. , pp. 133–148.

Kurata, T., Kawai, H., Miyazaki, K., Kozuki, M., Morimoto, N., Ohta, Y., Ikeda, Y., Abe, K., 2012. Statins have therapeutic potential for the treatment of Alzheimer's disease, likely via protection of the neurovascular unit in the AD brain. J. Neurol. Sci. 322, 59–63.

LaPlante, B.J., Powers, C.F., Gault, J.L., Reynolds, B.D., Gregory, C.W., 2006. P4-353: stabilization of cognitive decline in Alzheimer's disease following treatment with leuprolide acetate. Alzheimers Dement. 2, S620–S621.

Laurie, D., Wisden, W., Seeburg, P., 1992. The distribution of thirteen GABAA receptor subunit mRNAs in the rat brain. III. Embryonic and postnatal development. J. Neurosci. 12, 4151–4172.

Lecanu, L., Papadopoulos, V., 2013. Modeling Alzheimer's disease with non-transgenic rat models. Alzheimer Res. Ther. 5, 17.

Lecoutey, C., Hedou, D., Freret, T., Giannoni, P., Gaven, F., Since, M., Bouet, V., Ballandonne, C., Corvaisier, S., Fréon, A.M., 2014. Design of donecopride, a dual serotonin subtype 4 receptor agonist/acetylcholinesterase inhibitor with potential interest for Alzheimer's disease treatment. Proc. Natl. Acad. Sci. U.S.A. 111, E3825–E3830.

Leurs, R., Chazot, P.L., Shenton, F.C., Lim, H.D., de Esch, I.J., 2009. Molecular and biochemical pharmacology of the histamine H4 receptor. Br. J. Pharmacol. 157, 14–23.

Levin, E.D., 2002. Nicotinic receptor subtypes and cognitive function. J. Neurobiol. 53, 633–640.

Lipton, S., Chen, H.-S., 2004. Paradigm shift in neuroprotective drug development: clinically tolerated NMDA receptor inhibition by memantine. Cell Death Differ. 11, 18–20.

Lipton, S.A., 2006. Paradigm shift in neuroprotection by NMDA receptor blockade: memantine and beyond. Nat. Rev. Drug Discov. 5, 160–170.

Lodge, D., Danysz, W., Parsons, C.G., 2002. Ionotropic Glutamate Receptors as Therapeutic Targets. F.P Graham Publishing Co.

Lopes, J.P., Tarozzo, G., Reggiani, A., Piomelli, D., Cavalli, A., 2013. Galantamine potentiates the neuroprotective effect of memantine against NMDA-induced excitotoxicity. Brain Behav. 3, 67–74.

Lu, P.H., Masterman, D.A., Mulnard, R., Cotman, C., Miller, B., Yaffe, K., Reback, E., Porter, V., Swerdloff, R., Cummings, J.L., 2006. Effects of testosterone on cognition and mood in male patients with mild Alzheimer disease and healthy elderly men. Arch. Neurol. 63, 177–185.

Lucke-Wold, B.P., Turner, R.C., Logsdon, A.F., Simpkins, J.W., Alkon, D.L., Smith, K.E., Chen, Y.-W., Tan, Z., Huber, J.D., Rosen, C.L., 2015. Common mechanisms of Alzheimer's disease and ischemic stroke: the role of protein kinase C in the progression of age-related neurodegeneration. J. Alzheimers Dis. 43, 711–724.

Lynch, G., Gall, C.M., 2006. Ampakines and the threefold path to cognitive enhancement. Trends Neurosci. 29, 554–562.

Lynch, G., Granger, R., Ambros-Ingerson, J., Davis, C.M., Kessler, M., Schehr, R., 1997. Evidence that a positive modulator of AMPA-type glutamate receptors improves delayed recall in aged humans. Exp. Neurol. 145, 89–92.

Lynch, G., 2004. AMPA receptor modulators as cognitive enhancers. Curr. Opin. Pharmacol. 4, 4–11.

Maa, E., Figi, P., 2014. The case for medical marijuana in epilepsy. Epilepsia 55, 783–786.

Mackie, K., 2006. Cannabinoid receptors as therapeutic targets. Annu. Rev. Pharmacol. Toxicol. 46, 101–122.

Mangialasche, F., Solomon, A., Winblad, B., Mecocci, P., Kivipelto, M., 2010. Alzheimer's disease: clinical trials and drug development. Lancet Neurol. 9, 702–716.

Martinez-Coria, H., Green, K.N., Billings, L.M., Kitazawa, M., Albrecht, M., Rammes, G., Parsons, C.G., Gupta, S., Banerjee, P., LaFerla, F.M., 2010. Memantine improves cognition and reduces Alzheimer's-like neuropathology in transgenic mice. Am. J. Pathol. 176, 870–880.

Maubach, K., 2003. $GABA_A$ receptor subtype selective cognition enhancers. Curr. Drug Targets CNS Neurol. Disord. 2, 233–239.

McGeer, P.L., McGeer, E.G., 2007. NSAIDs and Alzheimer disease: epidemiological, animal model and clinical studies. Neurobiol. Aging 28, 639–647.

McGeer, P.L., Rogers, J., 1992. Anti-inflammatory agents as a therapeutic approach to Alzheimer's disease. Neurology 42, 447–449.

McGleenon, B., Dynan, K., Passmore, A., 1999. Acetylcholinesterase inhibitors in Alzheimer's disease. Br. J. Clin. Pharmacol. 48, 471–480.

Meethal, S.V., Smith, M.A., Bowen, R.L., Atwood, C.S., 2005. The gonadotropin connection in Alzheimer's disease. Endocrine 26, 317–325.

Meldrum, B.S., Garthwaite, J., 1990. Excitatory amino acid neurotoxicity and neurodegenerative disease. Trends Pharmacol. Sci. 11, 379–387.

Misra, S., Medhi, B., 2013. Drug development status for Alzheimer's disease: present scenario. Neurol. Sci. 34, 831–839.

Muir, K.W., 2006. Glutamate-based therapeutic approaches: clinical trials with NMDA antagonists. Curr. Opin. Pharmacol. 6, 53–60.

Munoz-Torrero, D., 2008. Acetylcholinesterase inhibitors as disease-modifying therapies for Alzheimer's disease. Curr. Med. Chem. 15, 2433–2455.

Naddafi, F., Mirshafiey, A., 2013. The neglected role of histamine in Alzheimer's disease. Am. J. Alzheimers Dis. Other Demen. 1533317513488925.

Nadler, J.V., Cuthbertson, G.J., 1980. Kainic acid neurotoxicity toward hippocampal formation: dependence on specific excitatory pathways. Brain Res. 195, 47–56.

Nickols, H.H., Conn, P.J., 2014. Development of allosteric modulators of GPCRs for treatment of CNS disorders. Neurobiol. Dis. 61, 55–71.

Niesler, B., Walstab, J., Combrink, S., Möller, D., Kapeller, J., Rietdorf, J., Bönisch, H., Göthert, M., Rappold, G., Brüss, M., 2007. Characterization of the novel human serotonin receptor subunits 5-HT3C, 5-HT3D, and 5-HT3E. Mol. Pharmacol. 72, 8–17.

Nygaard, H.B., Wagner, A.F., Bowen, G.S., Good, S.P., MacAvoy, M.G., Strittmatter, K.A., Kaufman, A.C., Rosenberg, B.J., Sekine-Konno, T., Varma, P., 2015. A phase Ib multiple ascending dose study of the safety, tolerability, and central nervous system availability of AZD0530 (saracatinib) in Alzheimer's disease. Alzheimers Res. Ther. 7, 35.

Olson, L., Nordberg, A., Von Holst, H., Bäckman, L., Ebendal, T., Alafuzoff, I., Amberla, K., Hartvig, P., Herlitz, A., Lilja, A., 1992. Nerve growth factor affects 11C-nicotine binding, blood flow, EEG, and verbal episodic memory in an Alzheimer patient (case report). J. Neural Transm. Park. Dis. Dement. Sect. 4, 79–95.

O'Neill, M.J., Bleakman, D., Zimmerman, D.M., Nisenbaum, E.S., 2004. AMPA receptor potentiators for the treatment of CNS disorders. Curr. Drug Targets CNS Neurol. Disord. 3, 181–194.

Papadia, S., Hardingham, G.E., 2007. The dichotomy of NMDA receptor signaling. Neuroscientist 13, 572–579.

Passmore, M.J., 2008. The cannabinoid receptor agonist nabilone for the treatment of dementia-related agitation. Int. J. Geriatr. Psychiatry 23, 116.

Paterniti, S., Dufouil, C., Alpérovitch, A., 2002. Long-term benzodiazepine use and cognitive decline in the elderly: the epidemiology of vascular aging study. J. Clin. Psychopharmacol. 22, 285–293.

Patzke, H., Albayya, F., Besterman, J., 2008. Development of the novel histone deacetylase inhibitor EVP-0334 for CNS indications. In: Society for Neuroscience Conference.

Paul, S.M., Marangos, P.J., Skolnick, P., 1981. The benzodiazepine-GABA-chloride ionophore receptor complex: common site of minor tranquilizer action. Biol. Psychiatry 16, 213–229.

Piette, F., Belmin, J., Vincent, H., Schmidt, N., Pariel, S., Verny, M., Marquis, C., Mely, J., Hugonot-Diener, L., Kinet, J.-P., 2011. Masitinib as an adjunct therapy for mild-to-moderate Alzheimer's disease: a randomised, placebo-controlled phase 2 trial. Alzheimers Res. Ther. 3, 16.

Pike, C.J., Carroll, J.C., Rosario, E.R., Barron, A.M., 2009. Protective actions of sex steroid hormones in Alzheimer's disease. Front. Neuroendocrinol. 30, 239–258.

Pringle, A., Iannotti, F., Wilde, G., Chad, J., Seeley, P., Sundstrom, L., 1997. Neuroprotection by both NMDA and non-NMDA receptor antagonists in in vitro ischemia. Brain Res. 755, 36–46.

Raghavendra Rao, V.L., Dogan, A., Todd, K.G., Bowen, K.K., Dempsey, R.J., 2001. Neuroprotection by memantine, a non-competitive NMDA receptor antagonist after traumatic brain injury in rats. Brain Res. 911, 96–100.

Ramírez, B.G., Blázquez, C., del Pulgar, T.G., Guzmán, M., de Ceballos, M.L., 2005. Prevention of Alzheimer's disease pathology by cannabinoids: neuroprotection mediated by blockade of microglial activation. J. Neurosci. 25, 1904–1913.

Rammes, G., Rupprecht, R., Ferrari, U., Zieglgänsberger, W., Parsons, C., 2001. The *N*-methyl-D-aspartate receptor channel blockers memantine, MRZ 2/579 and other amino-alkyl-cyclohexanes antagonise 5-HT(3) receptor currents in cultured HEK-293 and N1E-115 cell systems in a non-competitive manner. Neurosci. Lett. 306, 81–84.

Rammes, G., Danysz, W., Parsons, C., 2008. Pharmacodynamics of memantine: an update. Curr. Neuropharmacol. 6, 55.

Refolo, L.M., Pappolla, M.A., Malester, B., LaFrancois, J., Bryant-Thomas, T., Wang, R., Tint, G.S., Sambamurti, K., Duff, K., 2000. Hypercholesterolemia accelerates the Alzheimer's amyloid pathology in a transgenic mouse model. Neurobiol. Dis. 7, 321–331.

Reisberg, B., Doody, R., Stöffler, A., Schmitt, F., Ferris, S., Möbius, H.J., 2003. Memantine in moderate-to-severe Alzheimer's disease. N. Engl. J. Med. 348, 1333–1341.

Resnick, S.M., Henderson, V.W., 2002. Hormone therapy and risk of Alzheimer disease: a critical time. JAMA 288, 2170–2172.

Rissman, R.A., De Blas, A.L., Armstrong, D.M., 2007. $GABA_A$ receptors in aging and Alzheimer's disease. J. Neurochem. 103, 1285–1292.

Rochais, C., Lecoutey, C., Gaven, F., Giannoni, P., Hamidouche, K., Hedou, D., Dubost, E., Genest, D., Yahiaoui, S., Freret, T., 2015. Novel multitarget-directed ligands (MTDLs) with acetylcholinesterase (AChE) inhibitory and serotonergic subtype 4 receptor (5-HT4R) agonist activities as potential agents against Alzheimer's disease: the design of donecopride. J. Med. Chem. 58, 3172–3187.

Rogawski, M.A., Wenk, G.L., 2003. The neuropharmacological basis for the use of memantine in the treatment of Alzheimer's disease. CNS Drug Rev. 9, 275–308.

Rossom, R., Dysken, M., 2004. Efficacy and tolerability of memantine in the treatment of dementia. Am. J. Geriatr. Pharmacother. 2, 303–312.

Rowlett, J.K., Platt, D.M., Lelas, S., Atack, J.R., Dawson, G.R., 2005. Different GABAA receptor subtypes mediate the anxiolytic, abuse-related, and motor effects of benzodiazepine-like drugs in primates. Proc. Natl. Acad. Sci. U.S.A. 102, 915–920.

Sabbagh, M.N., Shill, H.A., 2010. Latrepirdine, a potential novel treatment for Alzheimer's disease and Huntington's chorea. Curr. Opin. Investig. Drugs 11, 80.

Salzman, C., Fisher, J., Nobel, K., Glassman, R., Wolfson, A., Kelley, M., 1992. Cognitive improvement following benzodiazepine discontinuation in elderly nursing home residents. Int. J. Geriatr. Psychiatry 7, 89–93.

Schechter, L.E., Smith, D., Rosenzweig-Lipson, S., Sukoff, S., Dawson, L., Marquis, K., Jones, D., Piesla, M., Andree, T., Nawoschik, S., 2005. Lecozotan (SRA-333): a selective serotonin 1A receptor antagonist that enhances the stimulated release of glutamate and acetylcholine in the hippocampus and possesses cognitive-enhancing properties. J. Pharmacol. Exp. Ther. 314, 1274–1289.

Schneider, L.S., Olin, J.T., 1994. Overview of clinical trials of hydergine in dementia. Arch. Neurol. 51, 787–798.

Scholtzova, H., Wadghiri, Y.Z., Douadi, M., Sigurdsson, E.M., Li, Y.S., Quartermain, D., Banerjee, P., Wisniewski, T., 2008. Memantine leads to behavioral improvement and amyloid reduction in Alzheimer's disease model transgenic mice shown as by micromagnetic resonance imaging. J. Neurosci. Res. 86, 2784–2791.

Schurr, A., 2004. Neuroprotection against ischemic/hypoxic brain damage: blockers of ionotropic glutamate receptor and voltage sensitive calcium channels. Curr. Drug Targets 5, 603–618.

Schwartz-Bloom, R.D., McDonough, K.J., Chase, P.J., Chadwick, L.E., Inglefield, J.R., Levin, E.D., 1998. Long-term neuroprotection by benzodiazepine: full versus partial agonists after transient cerebral ischemia in the gerbil. J. Cereb. Blood Flow Metab. 18, 548–558.

Schwartz-Bloom, R., Miller, K., Evenson, D., Crain, B., Nadler, J., 2000. Benzodiazepines protect hippocampal neurons from degeneration after transient cerebral ischemia: an ultrastructural study. Neuroscience 98, 471–484.

Scotter, E.L., Abood, M.E., Glass, M., 2010. The endocannabinoid system as a target for the treatment of neurodegenerative disease. Br. J. Pharmacol. 160, 480–498.

Shahrokhi, N., Haddad, M.K., Joukar, S., Shabani, M., Keshavarzi, Z., Shahozehi, B., 2012. Neuroprotective antioxidant effect of sex steroid hormones in traumatic brain injury. Pak. J. Pharm. Sci. 25, 219–225.

Shen, F., Smith, J.A., Chang, R., Bourdet, D.L., Tsuruda, P.R., Obedencio, G.P., Beattie, D.T., 2011. 5-HT(4) receptor agonist mediated enhancement of cognitive function in vivo and amyloid precursor protein processing in vitro: a pharmacodynamic and pharmacokinetic assessment. Neuropharmacology 61, 69–79.

Shepherd, J.D., Huganir, R.L., 2007. The cell biology of synaptic plasticity: AMPA receptor trafficking. Annu. Rev. Cell Dev. Biol. 23, 613–643.

Short, R.A., O'Brien, P.C., Graff-Radford, N.R., Bowen, R.L., 2001. Elevated gonadotropin levels in patients with Alzheimer disease. In: Mayo Clinic Proceedings. Elsevier.

Sieghart, W., 2006. Structure, pharmacology, and function of $GABA_A$ receptor subtypes. Adv. Pharmacol. 54, 231–263.

Sparks, D.L., Sabbagh, M.N., Connor, D.J., Lopez, J., Launer, L.J., Browne, P., Wasser, D., Johnson-Traver, S., Lochhead, J., Ziolwolski, C., 2005. Atorvastatin for the treatment of mild to moderate Alzheimer disease: preliminary results. Arch. Neurol. 62, 753–757.

Sternbach, L.H., 1979. The benzodiazepine story. J. Med. Chem. 22, 1–7.

Stilling, R.M., Fischer, A., 2011. The role of histone acetylation in age-associated memory impairment and Alzheimer's disease. Neurobiol. Learn. Mem. 96, 19–26.

Stolerman, I.P., 1991. Behavioural pharmacology of nicotine: multiple mechanisms. Br. J. Addict. 86, 533–536.

Sugaya, K., Giacobini, E., Chiappinelli, V., 1990. Nicotinic acetylcholine receptor subtypes in human frontal cortex: changes in Alzheimer's disease. J. Neurosci. Res. 27, 349–359.

Sun, M.K., Alkon, D.L., 2006. Bryostatin-1: pharmacology and therapeutic potential as a CNS drug. CNS Drug Rev. 12, 1–8.

Susman, E., 2006. Alzheimer disease modifying agents are promising in preliminary clinical trials. Neurol. Today 6, 18.

Swanson, G.T., 2009. Targeting AMPA and kainate receptors in neurological disease: therapies on the horizon? Neuropsychopharmacology 34, 249.

Tan, A., Dubovsky, S.L., 2011. Dextromethorphan/quinidine for pseudobulbar affect. Curr. Psychiatry 10, 60.

Tuszynski, M.H., Thal, L., Pay, M., Salmon, D.P., Bakay, R., Patel, P., Blesch, A., Vahlsing, H.L., Ho, G., Tong, G., 2005. A phase 1 clinical trial of nerve growth factor gene therapy for Alzheimer disease. Nat. Med. 11, 551–555.

Twyman, R.E., Rogers, C.J., Macdonald, R.L., 1989. Differential regulation of γ-aminobutyric acid receptor channels by diazepam and phenobarbital. Ann. Neurol. 25, 213–220.

Uitti, R., Rajput, A., Ahlskog, J., Offord, K., Schroeder, D., Ho, M., Prasad, M., Rajput, A., Basran, P., 1996. Amantadine treatment is an independent predictor of improved survival in Parkinson's disease. Neurology 46, 1551–1556.

Upton, N., Chuang, T.T., Hunter, A.J., Virley, D.J., 2008. 5-HT6 receptor antagonists as novel cognitive enhancing agents for Alzheimer's disease. Neurotherapeutics 5, 458–469.

Vellas, B., Sol, O., Snyder, P.J., Ousset, P.-J., Haddad, R., Maurin, M., Lemarié, J.-C., Désiré, L., Pando, M.P., 2011. EHT0202 in Alzheimer's disease: a 3-month, randomized, placebo-controlled, double-blind study. Curr. Alzheimer Res. 8, 203–212.

Vest, R.S., Pike, C.J., 2013. Gender, sex steroid hormones, and Alzheimer's disease. Horm. Behav. 63, 301–307.

Volicer, L., Stelly, M., Morris, J., McLaughlin, J., Volicer, B.J., 1997. Effects of dronabinol on anorexia and disturbed behavior in patients with Alzheimer's disease. Int. J. Geriatr. Psychiatry 12, 913–919.

Vongher, J.M., Frye, C.A., 1999. Progesterone in conjunction with estradiol has neuroprotective effects in an animal model of neurodegeneration. Pharmacol. Biochem. Behav. 64, 777–785.

Wadworth, A.N., Chrisp, P., 1992. Co-dergocrine mesylate. Drugs Aging 2, 153–173.

Wagner, A.K., Zhang, F., Soumerai, S.B., Walker, A.M., Gurwitz, J.H., Glynn, R.J., Ross-Degnan, D., 2004. Benzodiazepine use and hip fractures in the elderly: who is at greatest risk? Arch. Intern. Med. 164, 1567–1572.

Walther, S., Mahlberg, R., Eichmann, U., Kunz, D., 2006. Delta-9-tetrahydrocannabinol for nighttime agitation in severe dementia. Psychopharmacology 185, 524–528.

Walther, S., Schüpbach, B., Seifritz, E., Homan, P., Strik, W., 2011. Randomized, controlled crossover trial of dronabinol, 2.5 mg, for agitation in 2 patients with dementia. J. Clin. Psychopharmacol. 31, 256–258.

Wang, L.Y., Shofer, J.B., Rohde, K., Hart, K.L., Hoff, D.J., McFall, Y.H., Raskind, M.A., Peskind, E.R., 2009. Prazosin for the treatment of behavioral symptoms in patients with Alzheimer disease with agitation and aggression. Am. J. Geriatr. Psychiatry 17, 744–751.

Webber, K.M., Perry, G., Smith, M.A., Casadesus, G., 2007. The contribution of luteinizing hormone to Alzheimer disease pathogenesis. Clin. Med. Res. 5, 177–183.

Wezenberg, E., Verkes, R.J., Ruigt, G.S., Hulstijn, W., Sabbe, B.G., 2007. Acute effects of the ampakine farampator on memory and information processing in healthy elderly volunteers. Neuropsychopharmacology 32, 1272–1283.

Williams, K., 1993. Ifenprodil discriminates subtypes of the *N*-methyl-D-aspartate receptor: selectivity and mechanisms at recombinant heteromeric receptors. Mol. Pharmacol. 44, 851–859.

Wilson, A.C., Meethal, S.V., Bowen, R.L., Atwood, C.S., 2007. Leuprolide acetate: a drug of diverse clinical applications. Expert Opin. Investig. Drugs 16 (11).

Winblad, B., Poritis, N., 1999. Memantine in severe dementia: results of the 9M-best study (benefit and efficacy in severely demented patients during treatment with memantine). Int. J. Geriatr. Psychiatry 14, 135–146.

Winblad, B., Bonura, M.L., Rossini, B.M., Battaglia, A., 2001. Nicergoline in the treatment of mild-to-moderate Alzheimer's disease. Clin. Drug Investig. 21, 621–632.

Winblad, B., Jones, R.W., Wirth, Y., Stöffler, A., Möbius, H.J., 2007. Memantine in moderate to severe Alzheimer's disease: a meta-analysis of randomised clinical trials. Dement. Geriatr. Cogn. Disord. 24, 20–27.

Wisden, W., Seeburg, P.H., 1992. $GABA_A$ receptor channels: from subunits to functional entities. Curr. Opin. Neurobiol. 2, 263–269.

Yaffe, K., Krueger, K., Cummings, S.R., Blackwell, T., Henderson, V.W., Sarkar, S., Ensrud, K., Grady, D., 2014. Effect of raloxifene on prevention of dementia and cognitive impairment in older women: the Multiple Outcomes of Raloxifene Evaluation (MORE) randomized trial. Am. J. Psychiatry.

Youdim, M.B., 2013. Multi target neuroprotective and neurorestorative anti-Parkinson and anti-Alzheimer drugs ladostigil and m30 derived from rasagiline. Exp. Neurobiol. 22, 1–10.

Yu, J.-T., Chang, R.C.-C., Tan, L., 2009. Calcium dysregulation in Alzheimer's disease: from mechanisms to therapeutic opportunities. Prog. Neurobiol. 89, 240–255.

Zheng, Y., Balabhadrapatruni, S., Masumura, C., Darlington, C.L., Smith, P.F., 2011. Effects of the putative cognitive-enhancing ampakine, CX717, on attention and object recognition memory. Curr. Alzheimer Res. 8, 876–882.

CHAPTER

7

Amyloid β Hypothesis in the Development of Therapeutic Agents for Alzheimer's Disease

A.O. Adeniji, P.W. Adams, V.V. Mody

OUTLINE

INTRODUCTION

Alzheimer's disease (AD) is a progressive, age-related neurodegenerative disease that affects discrete brain areas leading to impairments of memory, cognition, and movement. AD affects one out of every nine individuals older than 65 years and the incidence doubles every 5 years afterward (Alzheimer's, 2014). It remains the most common type of

Drug Discovery Approaches for the Treatment of Neurodegenerative Disorders
http://dx.doi.org/10.1016/B978-0-12-802810-0.00007-6

dementia and accounts for 60–80% of all cases. AD is defined by intracranial amyloidosis manifested by extracellular amyloid plaques, which is primarily composed of amyloid β (Aβ) peptide, and intracellular polymerized tau tangles in brain areas associated with cognition and memory consolidation. Neuronal cell death in these brain areas leads to memory loss, poor judgment, changes in personality, and other clinical symptoms seen in AD.

Current therapeutic agents for the treatment of AD include the cholinesterase inhibitors donepezil, rivastigmine, and galantamine as well as the noncompetitive *N*-methyl-D-aspartate (NMDA) receptor antagonist memantine. While donepezil and rivastigmine are approved for treating all stages of AD, galantamine and memantine are only approved for the treatment of mild-to-moderate AD and moderate-to-severe AD, respectively. These drugs are able to improve the symptoms of the disease; however, they do not modify the underlying pathology of the disease and are unable to slow or stop the neurodegeneration that defines the disease.

The search for disease-modifying treatment for AD was aided by the extensive research efforts aimed at understanding the molecular underpinnings of the disease. Most of the drug discovery efforts in AD over the last two decades have been based on the "Aβ hypothesis." This hypothesis posits that the overproduction and accumulation of the Aβ peptide, the main component of the amyloid plaque, is the key event that triggers the other neuropathological changes such as neurofibrillary tangles, loss of synapse between neurons, and vascular damage that are associated with AD (Hardy and Allsop, 1991; Hardy and Higgins, 1992; Hardy and Selkoe, 2002). Aβ peptide is a 4 kDa, 38–43 amino acid peptide that is obtained from the proteolytic cleavage of the amyloid precursor protein (APP). APP is a type 1 transmembrane protein with a large extracellular domain and a short cytoplasmic tail. APP is proteolytically processed via two mutually exclusive pathways involving either α- or β-secretase in combination with γ-secretase (Fig. 7.1). Shedding of APP ectodomain by either α- or β-secretase is essential for optimal γ-secretase activity.

The first pathway involves the sequential activity of α- and γ-secretases. α-Secretase cleaves APP within the Aβ peptide region to liberate an extracellular amino terminal fragment known as soluble APPα protein (sAPPα), and a transmembrane stub known as the APP-C-terminal fragment alpha (APP-CTFα, C83). C83 is subsequently processed by γ-secretase to liberate the p3 protein and the APP intracellular domain (AICD) (Haass et al., 1993). This is the dominant pathway for APP processing under normal conditions and is referred to as the nonamyloidogenic pathway because it precludes the formation of the Aβ peptide. The other pathway involves β-secretase cleavage of APP to produce soluble APPβ protein (sAPPβ) and APP-C terminal fragment beta (APP-CTFβ, C99). C99 is subsequently processed by γ-secretase to produce the Aβ peptide and AICD. Aβ40 and Aβ42 with 40 and 42 amino residues, respectively (Fig. 7.2), are the most common forms of Aβ peptide produced. Shorter forms are also produced but these are usually present in very small amounts. Under normal conditions, Aβ40 is the most abundant variant in the cerebrospinal fluid (CSF) and it accounts for ~90% of the total Aβ peptide produced while Aβ42 accounts for less than 10%. However, Aβ42 is more pathogenic and prone to aggregation because of the presence of two additional hydrophobic amino acid residues:

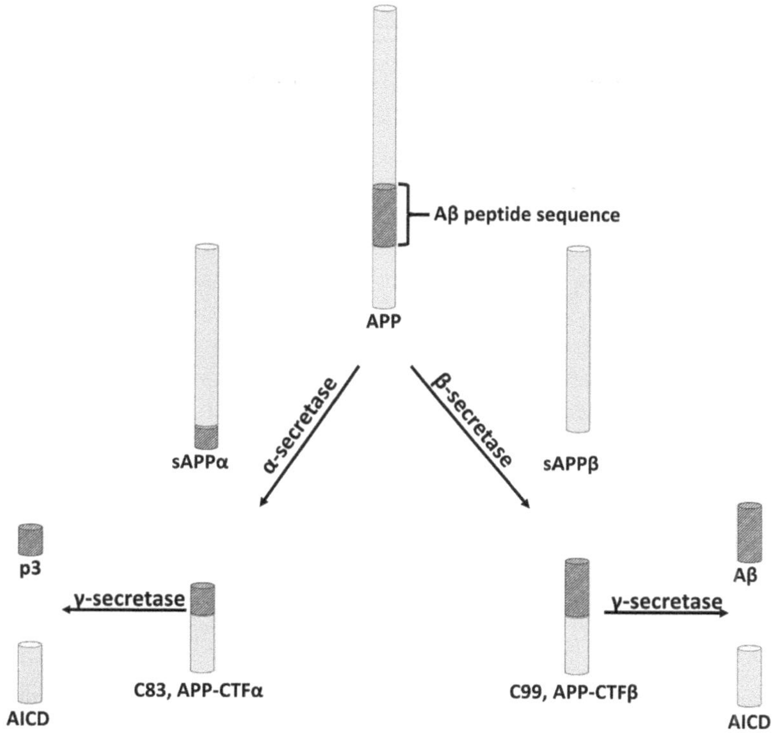

FIGURE 7.1 Amyloid precursor protein (APP) processing by α-, β-, and γ-secretases. α- and β-secretases are involved in the nonamyloidogenic pathway whereas β- and γ-secretases catalyze the formation of the Aβ peptide. *AICD*, APP intracellular domain; *APP-CTFα*, APP-C-terminal fragment alpha; *APP-CTFβ*, APP-C terminal fragment beta; *sAPPα*, soluble APPα protein; *sAPPβ*, soluble APPβ protein.

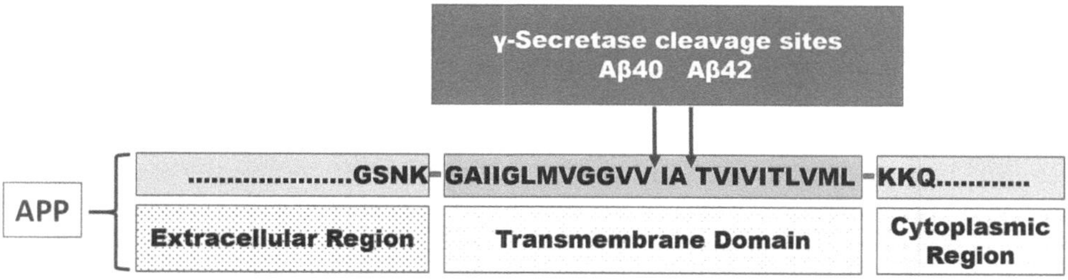

FIGURE 7.2 Amyloid precursor protein (APP) domains and γ-secretase cleavage sites leading to Aβ40/Aβ42 production.

isoleucine and alanine (Fig. 7.2). Aberrant APP processing leads to increased Aβ peptide production, particularly an increase in Aβ42, and is believed to trigger AD pathogenesis characterized by Aβ aggregation and subsequent plaque formation. This chapter focuses on the current understanding of the Aβ hypothesis and drug discovery efforts that have been based on this hypothesis.

EVOLUTION OF THE AMYLOID HYPOTHESIS

The presence of amyloid plaques in the cerebral cortex of an autopsied patient with symptoms of dementia was first described by Dr. Alois Alzheimer in 1906. For many decades after the astounding suggestion by Dr. Alzheimer that a mental defect could be related to physical changes in the brain, research was aimed at confirming that AD patients showed a consistent pattern of brain pathology and understanding how these pathological structures formed. The presence of extracellular amyloid plaques and intracellular neurofibrillary tangles in the brain have been widely accepted as common pathological findings in Alzheimer's patients since the 1960s (Tanzi and Bertram, 2005). However, it was not until the 1980s that the substances forming these structures were analyzed and described. During this time, the sequence of a 4 kDa protein isolated from amyloid deposits in meningeal microvasculature and cerebral cortex from Alzheimer's patients was reported (Glenner and Wong, 1984a,b; Masters et al., 1985). In 1987, the cDNA of a gene located on chromosome 21 and encoding a 695 residue protein was isolated and sequenced, with the results suggesting that this gene encoded the precursor protein to the previously identified 4 kDa protein (Kang et al., 1987). This gene product is now known as "amyloid precursor protein," the transmembrane glycoprotein from which Aβ peptides are produced.

Genetic Evidence: Risk Alleles for Familial and Sporadic AD

In addition to the observation that postmortem analyses of human AD brains consistently show the distinctive amyloid plaques, remarkable evidence in support of the Aβ hypothesis is provided by studies showing associations between genetic polymorphisms and different forms of AD. AD can be characterized into two broad classes based on the age of presentation: early-onset AD (EOAD) and late-onset AD (LOAD). In EOAD, symptoms tend to develop prior to age 65 and can develop as early as the third decade of life. EOAD is less common (<4% of all AD cases worldwide) but can have greater symptom severity. In LOAD, which accounts for >96% of all AD cases and approximately 50–60% of all cases of dementia in elderly patients, symptoms tend to develop after age 65.

EOAD is associated with an autosomal dominant inheritance pattern within families. For this reason, the early-onset form of the disease is also known as familial AD (FAD). Individuals with EOAD or FAD often have mutations in the genes encoding the amyloid precursor protein (*APP*), presenilin-1 (*PSEN1*), and presenilin-2 (*PSEN2*), which are located on chromosomes 21, 14, and 1, respectively. Notably, these genes code for proteins that are required for the production of Aβ peptide and transgenic animals expressing these mutations display several of the pathological hallmarks of AD (Games et al., 1995).

APP

The significance of APP processing in the neuropathological changes that drive AD emerged when mutations in the *APP gene* were reported to be associated with cases of EOAD (Goate et al., 1991; Chartier-Harlin et al., 1991; Mullan et al., 1992). The identified missense APP mutations occur near the cleavage sites for the secretase enzymes and appear to increase the risk of EOAD by disrupting normal APP processing and altering production of Aβ40 and Aβ42 peptides. Specifically, APP mutations that produce increased risk of EOAD have been associated with an increased production of Aβ peptide (particularly the more fibrillogenic Aβ42), an increased Aβ42/Aβ40 ratio, and increased Aβ aggregation. The observation that individuals with trisomy 21 (Down's syndrome), in which the *APP gene* is triplicated, often develop EOAD is also consistent with the emerging hypothesis that increased Aβ production promotes development of AD (Glenner and Wong, 1984a; Masters et al., 1985).

Presenilins

In the mid-1990s, mutations in the genes encoding presenilin-1 and -2 were implicated as additional genetic causes of certain forms of early-onset familial AD (Levy-Lahad et al., 1995; Rogaev et al., 1995; Sherrington et al., 1995). Mutations in these polytopic proteins are often responsible for some of the most aggressive forms of AD. Presenilins-1 and -2 compose one of the four integral components of the active γ-secretase complex, and the mutations described alter γ-secretase processing of APP in favor of Aβ42 relative to Aβ40. Altered APP processing caused by these mutations ultimately produce a similar biochemical effect to that seen in the previously described APP mutations: an increased Aβ42/Aβ40 ratio (reviewed in Tanzi and Bertram, 2005).

APOE4

The more common LOAD often occurs in the absence of immediate family members who suffer from the disease and has thus been referred to as sporadic AD (sAD). However, increasing evidence reported over the past decade has identified risk alleles promoting development of sAD (reviewed in Karch and Goate, 2015). Among the numerous genetic polymorphisms that have been associated with increased risk of sAD, the strongest risk allele identified to date is *APOEε4*. The *APOEε4* gene encodes the ε4 allele of apolipoprotein E (ApoE). ApoE is a lipoprotein that has roles in the transport and metabolism of lipids, including cholesterol and phospholipids. The specific mechanism by which the ε4 allele promotes the development of sAD is neither fully understood nor established. However, reducing the function of ApoE in brain, by treatment with inhibitory antibodies, by induction of low-density lipoprotein receptor-mediated removal of ApoE, or by knocking down ApoE expression, has been associated with reduction of Aβ plaque load in transgenic mouse models of AD (Kim et al., 2009, 2011, 2012; Liao et al., 2014). Likewise, overexpression of human *APOEε4* in transgenic mice increases the level of Aβ42 peptide in hippocampal interstitial fluid and greater retention of Aβ in the CNS (Hudry et al., 2013). Other transgenic mouse models of AD have also been used to demonstrate that the ApoE4-associated increase in brain Aβ peptide levels is caused by reduced clearance of Aβ peptide and not increased synthesis (Castellano et al., 2011).

Despite the differences in cause, age of onset, and rate of progression, familial and sporadic AD share common pathological characteristics. In addition to intracellular neurofibrillary tangles and extracellular amyloid plaques, other pathological changes observed in the AD brain include loss of synapses, neurotransmitter deficiencies, and inflammation. Amyloid plaques may also deposit in blood vessels of the cerebral compartment, giving rise to amyloid angiopathy. In advanced cases, gross anatomical changes occur in the brain, including loss of cortical mass and ventricular enlargement.

The common pathological characteristics suggest a convergence point in the pathological sequence of both forms of AD. The Aβ hypothesis suggests that changes in Aβ peptide production may represent this convergence point. Research over the past decades has focused on understanding the mechanisms by which Aβ peptide contributes to development of one or more of these pathological changes in the brain and whether they have a role in the progression of cognitive and behavioral defects that are observed in AD patients.

Evidence of Aβ Peptide's Role in Neurotoxicity

The invariant plaques seen in AD brains are formed by an amyloid core that is primarily composed of filamentous aggregates of Aβ peptide, dystrophic neurons, and microglia and is surrounded by astrocytes extending dendritic projections into the core (Selkoe, 2001). Aβ peptide, especially Aβ42, is relatively hydrophobic and tends to aggregate and form oligomers and fibrils. It is these fibers that tend to accumulate into the insoluble amyloid plaques of AD (Selkoe, 2001). These insoluble fibers were long considered to be the toxic moiety in AD. However, more recent evidence suggests that soluble forms of Aβ oligomers may actually constitute the pathogenic factor in AD (Walsh et al., 2002a,b; Gandy, 2005; Haass and Selkoe, 2007).

While large aggregates of insoluble fibrils have been associated with dystrophic neurons, smaller, soluble oligomers have also been shown to interfere with synaptic transmission (Walsh et al., 2002a,b). Soluble Aβ oligomers accumulate in cortical and hippocampal neurons of transgenic mouse models of AD before the appearance of cognitive impairments (as early as 1 week after birth). In the same animals, extracellular amyloid deposits do not begin to accumulate until approximately 6–10 months of age (Wirths et al., 2002; Leon et al., 2010; Iulita et al., 2014). Multiple studies have demonstrated that intraneural Aβ42 accumulation precedes the formation of extracellular amyloid plaques in human brain neurons (Walsh et al., 2000; Gouras et al., 2000; Takahashi et al., 2002; Fernandez-Vizarra et al., 2004) and that these intraneural accumulations are associated with pathological changes in synapses and/or neuronal death (D'Andrea et al., 2001; Takahashi et al., 2004).

Mechanisms for the observed Aβ-induced synaptic dysfunction have also been widely examined. In vivo studies in transgenic mice (Lesne et al., 2006) and in rats (Walsh et al., 2002a,b; Shankar et al., 2008) have suggested that low-number soluble oligomers of Aβ peptide (ie, as large as dodecamers) cause memory impairment (assessed by water maze navigation). This effect is blocked by treatment with antibodies to Aβ oligomers, and the effect is not observed with insoluble Aβ structures. Interactions of Aβ oligomers with the synaptic membrane have been associated with increased Ca^{2+} conductance across the synaptic membrane (Lauren et al., 2009; Um et al., 2012; Varga et al., 2014; Peters et al., 2015), which could explain synaptic dysfunction or neuronal death, possibly via an excitotoxic mechanism.

A variety of studies have worked to identify Aβ peptide binding proteins, leading to a long list of binding partners that have been speculated to mediate Aβ-induced memory deficits as well as other effects. These include molecular players such as α7-nicotinic acetylcholine receptors, metabotropic glutamate receptors, glutamate transporters, ephrin type-B receptors, cellular prion protein, and NMDA receptors. A number of these binding partners for Aβ peptide have roles in mediating the neuronal response to glutamate, and alterations in glutamate signaling and responsiveness have been proposed as possible mechanisms by which Aβ induces neurotoxicity or inhibits synaptic plasticity (Varga et al., 2014; Tu et al., 2014; Hamilton et al., 2015). The number and diversity of different binding partners for Aβ peptide has been speculated to be caused by its intrinsically disordered structure (Hubin et al., 2014). This intrinsically disordered structure of monomeric Aβ peptides may also explain the dynamic nature of the Aβ peptide oligomerization.

Studies have been complicated by the varying lengths of Aβ peptides that can be produced by APP processing, because of the heterogeneous cleavage pattern of γ-secretase. While the major Aβ peptides produced are Aβ40 and Aβ42, low levels of shorter Aβ peptides also are produced. Multiple studies have demonstrated that the degree of neurotoxicity of Aβ-soluble oligomers varies with the size of the oligomer, the specific Aβ peptide composition, the post-translational modification state, and the conformational structure (reviewed in Hubin et al., 2014). For example, neurotoxicity increases in oligomers with greater surface hydrophobicity. Aβ42-rich small molecular weight oligomers, which have a high level of solvent-exposed hydrophobic residues, were more likely to alter Ca^{2+} conductance and disrupt cell membranes (Williams et al., 2011; Ladiwala et al., 2012).

Because of the ability of Aβ40 and Aβ42 to directly interact during oligomerization, slight changes to the Aβ42/Aβ40 ratio can have significant effects on oligomerization kinetics and induction of synaptic toxicity (Kuperstein et al., 2010; Bate and Williams, 2010). These observations suggest that rather than a single toxic species of Aβ peptide, the composition of the Aβ pool and how it influences the dynamic equilibrium of Aβ oligomers may be an important determinant of neurotoxicity. In this regard, it is important to note that the insoluble amyloid fibrils appear to influence this pool. Data from several studies suggest that fibrils may influence the overall pool of Aβ oligomers by serving as a reservoir for neurotoxic oligomers, which can dissociate from the fibril and diffuse to induce synaptic dysfunction and eventual memory impairment (Wogulis et al., 2005; Martins et al., 2008; Koffie et al., 2009; Spires-Jones et al., 2009; Xue et al., 2010; Jan et al., 2011). However, it has also been reported that insoluble fibrils increase soluble Aβ oligomers not by releasing them but rather by promoting oligomerization of Aβ monomers in the localized region (Cohen et al., 2013). Substances that reduce the dynamic equilibrium of oligomerization, such as metals or metal chelators and chaperones, may have a role in modulating amyloid-induced neurotoxicity (Fonte et al., 2002; Syme et al., 2004; Evans et al., 2006; Rezaei-Ghaleh et al., 2011; Zhang et al., 2013; Yang et al., 2015).

The Interplay of Aβ and Tau Protein

Another hallmark lesion of AD is intracellular neurofibrillary tangles, which are formed by hyperphosphorylated forms of tau protein. An early study in a transgenic mouse model of AD demonstrated that injection of synthetic Aβ42 fibrils into the brains of mice resulted in a fivefold increase in neurofibrillary tangle formation near the injection site (Gotz et al., 2001), suggesting that Aβ peptides induce tangle formation. Another study showed that deletion of one or both copies of the gene encoding tau protein had protective effects against neuronal excitotoxicity and memory impairment that was previously observed in the parental mouse model of AD (Roberson et al., 2007). Studies in primary neurons isolated from mice revealed that neuronal degeneration resulting from treatment of cells with Aβ42 fibrils occurred in neurons from wild-type mice but not in neurons from tau knockout mice. Reexpression of tau in the tau-deficient neurons restored the Aβ-induced neuronal death (Rapoport et al., 2002). Numerous studies have suggested that tau has a role in mediating other Aβ-induced effects in neurons, including promoting microtubule disassembly and microtubule degeneration, interrupting mitochondrial transport, and impairing long-term potentiation (King et al., 2006;

Vossel et al., 2010; Shipton et al., 2011; Zempel et al., 2013). The effects on microtubule stability and transport represent significant threats to synaptic function. A number of studies have provided evidence that Aβ oligomers induce tau phosphorylation (Zempel et al., 2010; Lloret et al., 2011; Oliveira et al., 2015), an event that could impact tau's function as a microtubule regulator and precede formation of neurofibrillary tangles. Collectively, these observations suggest that Aβ-induced neurotoxicity occurs at least in part via a tau-dependent mechanism.

Despite these data, the relationship between Aβ and tau remains incompletely understood and is still debated. First, it is important to note that Aβ oligomers also induce a number of effects in neurons that are independent of tau (discussed in Bloom, 2014). Additionally, one study suggests that, at least in some AD patients, the location and chronology for formation of Aβ oligomers and hyperphosphorylated tau do not support the hypothesis that these events are functionally linked (Fornicola et al., 2014). To further complicate matters, tau also appears to mediate the paradoxical effect of inhibiting amyloid plaque load and reducing the Aβ42/Aβ40 ratio (Leroy et al., 2012).

DISEASE-MODIFYING THERAPEUTIC APPROACHES

Based on the Aβ hypothesis, compounds that lower intracranial levels of Aβ peptide, either by inhibiting its production or increasing its clearance, and those that prevent Aβ aggregation represent disease-modifying therapeutic agents, which should alter the course of the disease. The following approaches represent areas that are being pursued:

1. Inhibition of Aβ peptide aggregation.
2. Activation of α-secretase.
3. Inhibition of β-secretase.
4. Inhibition and modulation of γ-secretase.
5. Aβ peptide clearance using immunotherapy.

Inhibitors of Aβ Aggregation

Based on the Aβ hypothesis, a logical approach to prevent or delay the onset of AD is to inhibit Aβ aggregation into toxic oligomers, fibrils, and plaques and/or induce disintegration of the Aβ deposit in the brain (Nie et al., 2011). Peptide-based inhibitors of Aβ aggregation inhibitors have been reported and there is evidence that these peptides may inhibit aggregation and induce disassembly of Aβ peptide aggregates (Sigurdsson et al., 2000; Permanne et al., 2002). However, peptide-based inhibitors often do not have the requisite physicochemical and pharmacokinetic properties to be effective in vivo.

Developing small molecule inhibitors of Aβ aggregation is particularly challenging because of the need for specific interactions between inhibitors and the significantly larger Aβ peptide. This need is in contrast to the peptide-based inhibitors that are able to interact with a greater region of the Aβ peptide. Additionally, these small molecule inhibitors may occupy approximately one-third of the Aβ protein and cause multiple nonspecific interactions, which can interfere with the potential therapeutic effect (Nie et al., 2011; Jones and Thornton, 1996; Lo Conte et al., 1999; Teichmann, 2002; Smith et al., 2006; Cheng et al., 2007; Keskin et al., 2008). Fortunately, the roles of various regions of Aβ peptide in aggregation and regulation of the process have now been identified (Maji et al., 2009). For example, the N-terminus, C-terminus, and

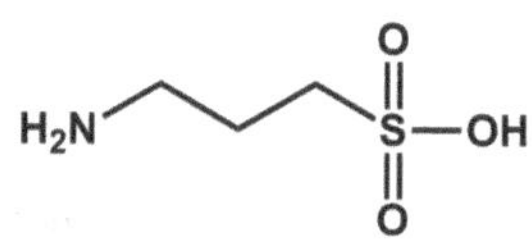

FIGURE 7.3 Structure of the Aβ aggregation inhibitor tramiprosate.

the hydrophobic regions are all responsible for aggregation of Aβ (Nie et al., 2011; Permanne et al., 2002; McLaurin et al., 2002, 2006; Gardberg et al., 2007; Wasmer et al., 2008; Fradinger et al., 2008). This phenomenon offers an opportunity to design and use small molecules that target these regions to inhibit the aggregation process.

Tramiprosate (Alzhemed, Fig. 7.3) is one of the first small molecules reported to inhibit Aβ aggregation (Nie et al., 2011). It is a synthetic glycosaminoglycan (GAG) mimetic designed to interfere with the HHQK ($A\beta_{13-16}$) subregion at the N-terminus and prevent Aβ aggregation. GAGs bind to Aβ peptides and accelerate their aggregation. Tramiprosate binds to soluble Aβ peptide and blocks its interaction with GAGs thereby inhibiting their aggregation. Tramiprosate was found to inhibit Aβ aggregation in phase II clinical trials but unfortunately failed the phase III clinical trials because of lack of significant improvement in cognitive function (Hebert, 2007; Blazer and Neubig, 2008). Despite the failure in human trials, the data acquired provided evidence that targeting specific subregions of Aβ with small molecule inhibitors may be a therapeutic approach for the treatment of AD (Blazer and Neubig, 2008). Other inhibitors of Aβ aggregation have been reported. These include clioquinol, an antibiotic that chelates copper and zinc, cucurmin, a phenolic natural product with antioxidant and antiinflammatory action, rifampicin, an antitubercular drug, and fullerene (Tomiyama et al., 1994; Cherny et al., 2001; Frautschy et al., 2001; Kim and Lee, 2003).

α-Secretase Inducers/Activators

α-Secretase cleaves within the Aβ peptide sequence region of APP, breaking the lysine 16 and leucine 17 peptide bond, to produce sAPPα and the membrane-tethered C83, which is subsequently processed by γ-secretase to produce p3 and AICD (Esch et al., 1990; Anderson et al., 1991; Wang et al., 1991). sAPPα is known to be a neurotrophic and neuroprotective factor. Studies have shown a positive correlation between CSF levels of sAPPα and cognitive performance in rats (Anderson et al., 1999; Sennvik et al., 2000; Colciaghi et al., 2002). Therefore α-secretase cleavage of APP is beneficial, not only by precluding the formation of Aβ peptides but also by protecting against neurotoxic agents. A decrease in α-secretase activity is seen in AD patients (Sennvik et al., 2000; Colciaghi et al., 2002). Therefore increased activation of α-secretase could restore the balance in favor of the nonamyloidogenic pathway and should favorably alter the progression of AD.

α-Secretase activity resides among members of a family of proteins known as a disintegrin and metalloproteinase (ADAM). These are membrane-anchored or -secreted proteins that have a prodomain, a metalloproteinase domain, a disintegrin domain, a cysteine-rich region, and an epidermal growth factor repeat region. Members of the ADAM family of proteins are involved in activation of several signaling pathways. ADAM10 and ADAM17 are primarily responsible for the α-secretase activity. ADAM17 is believed to be responsible for the inducible α-secretase activity while ADAM10 is responsible for the constitutive activity and may also contribute to the inducible activity.

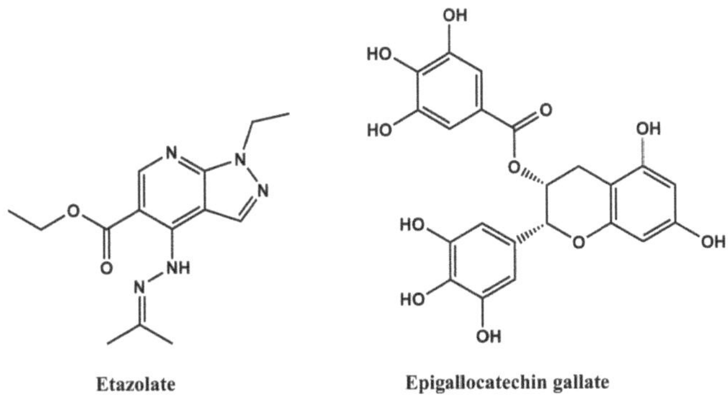

FIGURE 7.4 Structures of α-secretase activators etazolate and epigallocatechin gallate.

Several compounds including phorbol esters, activators of protein kinase A and C (PKC), muscarinic agonists, neuropeptides, statins, and retinoids have been reported to increase α-secretase processing of APP (Xu et al., 1995, 1996; Zhang and Xu, 2007; Fahrenholz, 2007; Postina, 2012). However, because of the lack of selectivity for α-secretase and issues with toxicity, most of these compounds are currently not being developed for the treatment of AD. Etazolate and epigallocatechin gallate (EGCG) (Fig. 7.4) are two promising α-secretase activators that are being developed for AD treatment.

Etazolate (EHT0202) is a pyrazolopyridine-based $GABA_A$ receptor modulator that activates α-secretase in a $GABA_A$ receptor-dependent manner (Marcade et al., 2008). It also inhibits phosphodiesterase-4 and can cause memory improvement because of an increase in cyclic AMP levels (Gong et al., 2004). Treatment with etazolate increased sAPPα in both in vitro and in vivo experiments, protected against the neurotoxic effects of aggregated Aβ42, and improved age-related cognitive decline in animals (Marcade et al., 2008; Drott et al., 2010). In a phase IIa clinical trial that stared in Apr. 2009, etazolate was well tolerated and relatively safe (Vellas et al., 2011). However, phase III clinical trials have yet to be initiated for this drug.

EGCG is a polyphenolic, neuroprotective compound that is abundant in green tea. It enhances the maturation of ADAM10, causes an increase in sAPPα, and decreases both Aβ production and aggregation (Obregon et al., 2006; Sommer et al., 2012). EGCG also scavenges free radicals and activates of PKC, which leads to increased α-secretase activity (Mandel et al., 2008). Other effects include inhibition of APP translation and modulation of mitochondrial function. A phase III clinical trial to study the effect of EGCG in patients with early-stage AD is currently recruiting participants (clinicaltrial.gov ID: NCT00951834).

It should be noted that α-secretase has other substrates and is not specific for APP. These substrates include notch, cadherin, and tumor necrosis factor-α (Vingtdeux and Marambaud, 2012). The impact of increased α-secretase activity on these pathways needs to be evaluated, as altering the functions of these substrates may lead to untoward physiological effects. α-Secretase activation continues to be a plausible target for AD; however, more interest and efforts have been dedicated to the other two secretase enzymes, β- and γ-secretases.

β-Secretase Inhibitors

β-Secretase [also referred as β-site APP cleaving enzyme (BACE), Asp-2, or memapsin-2] is an aspartyl protease that catalyzes the rate-limiting step in the formation of Aβ peptide.

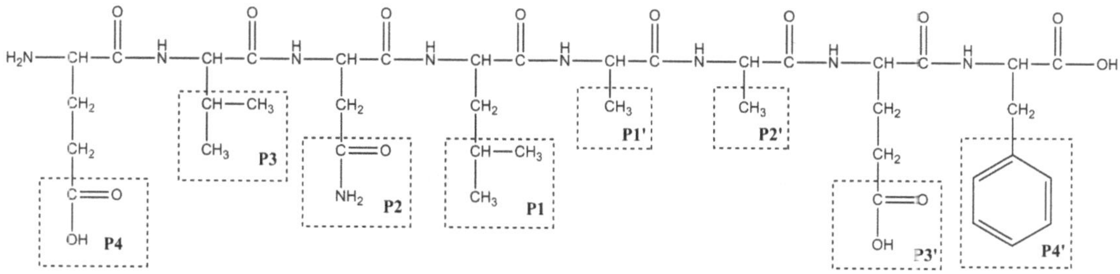

FIGURE 7.5 First reported peptidomimetic inhibitor of β-secretase, an octapeptide (Glu-Val-Asn-Leu*Ala-Ala-Glu-Phe).

It cleaves APP to generate a soluble N-terminal fragment (sAPPβ) and a membrane-bound fragment (C99) (Evin et al., 2010; Butini et al., 2013; Gilbert, 2013). The membrane-bound fragment is subsequently processed by γ-secretase to produce the Aβ peptide (Evin et al., 2010; Gilbert, 2013). BACE-1 expression and activity are increased in the brain of individuals with AD (Yang et al., 2003; Johnston et al., 2005). Factors such as hypoxia, oxidative stress, traumatic brain injury, and the herpes simplex virus increase β-secretase activity, which could lead to increased Aβ peptide and onset of AD (Blasko et al., 2004; Sun et al., 2006; Xue et al., 2006; Wozniak et al., 2007; Tamagno et al., 2008). Also mice carrying loss-of-function mutation of β-secretase are deficient in Aβ production, indicating the lack of a compensatory mechanism for the production of Aβ peptide in the absence of β-secretase (Butini et al., 2013; Luo et al., 2001; Cai et al., 2001). Additionally, the loss of β-secretase in knockout mice did not affect their productivity as the animals were found to be healthy and fertile. This enzyme thus provides us with a unique target for the design of the novel therapeutic agents for the treatment of AD (Butini et al., 2013; Luo et al., 2001; Roberds et al., 2001; Huang et al., 2013).

Structurally, β-secretase has a very large binding site (1000 Å) with fewer hydrophobic domains, making drug discovery efforts challenging. Despite these challenges, several promising inhibitors have now been identified, with most of the early compounds being peptidomimetics. Because of the large catalytic site, the peptidomimetic inhibitors require 6–10 amino acids for enhanced selectively (Turner et al., 2001; Ghosh et al., 2008, 2012; Yuan et al., 2013). Compounds this large usually exhibit poor pharmacokinetic properties and low CNS penetration because of the inability to cross the blood–brain barrier (BBB). β-Secretase also shares close substrate similarity with other aspartyl proteases such as renin and more specifically cathepsin D (CatD). This similarity presents a challenge in developing more BACE-1-specific inhibitors.

The first reported peptidomimetic inhibitor of β-secretase, an octapeptide (Glu-Val-Asn-Leu*Ala-Ala-Glu-Phe, also known as OM99-2, Fig. 7.5) showed a very high specificity (K_i = 1.6 nM) for β-secretase. The crystal structure of this inhibitor complexed with β-secretase demonstrated that the inhibitor incorporated a noncleavable hydroxyethylene isostere (*) into the cleavage site (Hong et al., 2000). Moreover, the crystal structure also showed that β-secretase preferred more acidic or polar amino acids at specific positions (P2 and P1′, Fig. 7.7) as compared to CatD, which exhibits selectivity for more hydrophobic substituents. This difference between CatD and β-secretase has been exploited to design and develop more selective and effective peptidomimetic β-secretase inhibitors.

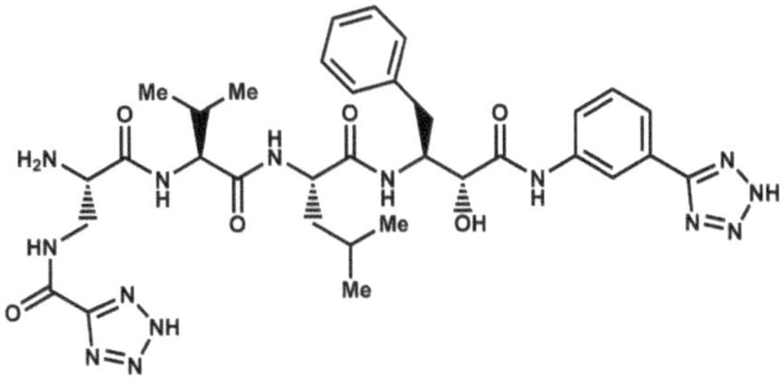

Phenylnorstatin Contaning Inhibitor
(Freskos et al., 2007)
(Ki = 1.2 nM)

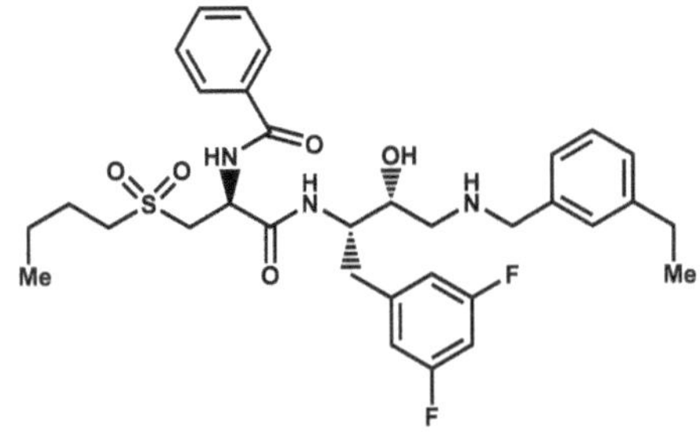

Hydroethyamine Contaning Inhibitor
(Iserloh et al., 2008)
(Ki = 2nM)

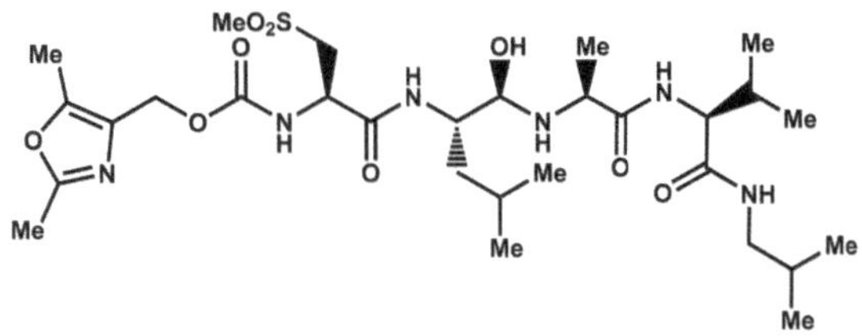

Hydroethylene Contaning Inhibitor
(Rajapakse et al., 2006)
(Ki = 0.12 nM)

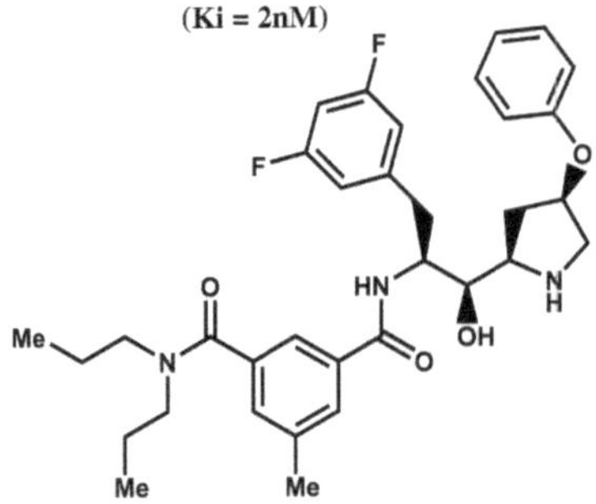

Constrained Hydroethyamine Contaning Inhibitor
(Cole et al., 2006)
(Ki = 3nM)

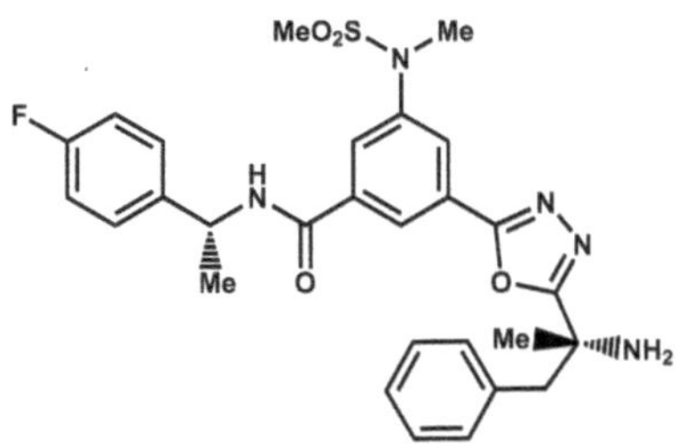

Carbinamine and Reduced Amide Contaning Inhibitor
(Gerritz et al., 2012)
(Ki = 1.2 nM)

FIGURE 7.6 Peptidomimetic beta-site APP cleaving enzyme-1 (BACE-1) inhibitors with different isosteres along with their K_i values (Kimura et al., 2006; Ghosh et al., 2006; Freskos et al., 2007; Iserloh et al., 2008; Rajapakse et al., 2006).

PEPTIDOMIMETIC BACE-1 INHIBITORS

Fig. 7.6 shows some of the most potent peptidomimetic BACE-1 inhibitors that have been synthesized. All of these agents exhibited excellent in vitro properties but their large size and polarity resulted in unfavorable in vivo pharmacological properties and limited their potential therapeutic use. As a consequence, investigators have turned toward designing small molecule BACE-1 inhibitors.

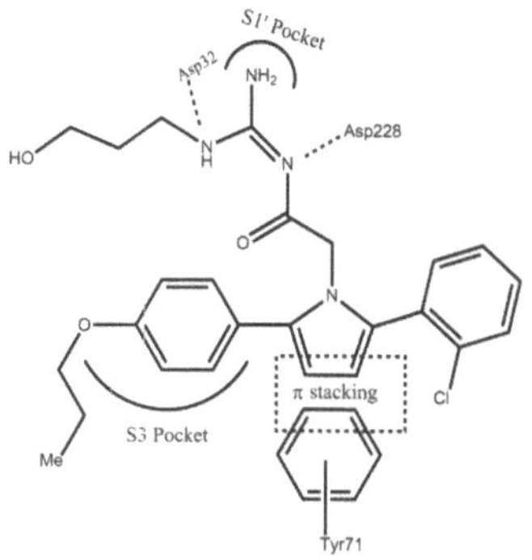

FIGURE 7.7 Predicted interactions of the lead acylaminoguanidines with β-secretase.

SMALL MOLECULE BACE-1 INHIBITORS

Because of the large catalytic core, the discovery of small molecule BACE-1 inhibitors has been challenging. However, extensive validation and use of high-throughput screening has led to numerous inhibitors with various chemotypes such as acylguanidines, amino, and aminoimidazoles containing heterocycles. The acylguanidines were among the first classes of the lead compounds that were discovered by fluorescence resonance energy transfer assay (Cole et al., 2006; Gerritz et al., 2012). As shown in Fig. 7.7, the pyrrole ring of the acylguanidines forms a π stacking interaction with tyrosine 71 of BACE-1 whereas the *p*-propyloxyphenyl group has significant binding interactions with the protein. In addition, the acylguanidine moiety directly binds to Asp32 and Asp228 of the beta secretase, whereas the third nitrogen fits well in the S1′ pocket (Cole et al., 2006; Gerritz et al., 2012). The acylguanidine inhibitors are polar in nature, which results in poor BBB penetration. Molecular modeling studies suggest that the amino pyridine moiety could replace the acylguanidine moiety and bind satisfactorily to BACE-1 at Asp32 and Asp228. Similarly, addition of pyridine or pyrimidine ring also increases the ability of the compound to fit into the S3 pocket of β-secretase.

Eli Lilly developed LY2886721 (Fig. 7.8), an orally bioavailable compound by introducing pyridine substituents. LY2886721 had acceptable BBB penetration and showed no in vivo toxicity as compared to its predecessor LY2811376 (Vassar, 2014). The molecule LY2886721 also showed acceptable pharmacokinetic and pharmacodynamic characteristics in in vivo studies using rodent models. In a phase I clinical trial, LY2886721 demonstrated dose-dependent decreases in CSF Aβ42 and sAPPβ levels. Levels of Aβ40 in the both plasma and CSF were also reduced by LY2886721 (Willis et al., 2012). The positive evaluation from the phase I trials led to the 6-month phase II clinical trial (clinicaltrial.gov ID: NCT01561430) in which 130 patients with prodromal AD or mild AD were dosed with either 35 or 70 mg of LY2886721 once a day. However, the phase II clinical trial was terminated because some patients developed abnormal liver biochemistries after taking LY2886721.

AstraZeneca synthesized the novel amino imidazole derivative AZD3293 (Fig. 7.8) as a BACE-1 inhibitor (Vassar, 2014; Alexander et al., 2014). In single- and multidose randomized, double-blind, placebo-controlled phase I clinical trials (clinicaltrial.gov ID: NCT01739647, and NCT01795339) in patients with mild AD, AZD3293 also showed a dose-dependent reduction in CSF levels of Aβ40, Aβ42, and sAPPβ. Combined phase II/III trials in the AMARANTH trial (clinicaltrials.gov ID: NCT02245737) for 104 weeks are ongoing.

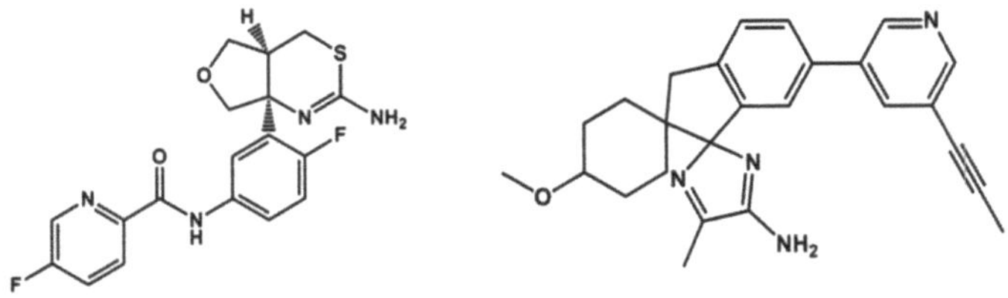

FIGURE 7.8 Structures of two β-secretase inhibitors LY2886721 and AZD3293.

TABLE 7.1 List of β-Secretase Inhibitors in Clinical Trials for the Treatment of Alzheimer's Disease (AD) (Vassar, 2014)

Company	Drug	Phase
AstraZeneca/Lilly	AZD3293	Phase II/III
Merck	MK-8931	Phase II/III
Pfizer	PF-05297909	Phase I
Takeda	TAK-070	Phase I
Vitae/Boehringer Ingelheim	VTP-37948	Phase I
CoMentis	CTS-21166	Phase I
Eisai/Biogen Idec	E2609	Phase II
High Point	HPP854	Phase I

Another small molecule β-secretase inhibitor, MK-8931, was developed by Merck (Forman et al., 2013). In healthy volunteers, MK-8931 was well tolerated, and no serious adverse events were reported. To determine the feasibility of using MK-8931 as a β-secretase inhibitor, biomarkers of BACE-1 activity were measured in CSF, including Aβ40, Aβ42, and sAPPβ. MK-8931 treatment was associated with reduced levels of Aβ40, Aβ42, and sAPPβ in the CSF. Moreover, it has a plasma half-life of ~20h, making it amenable to once-daily dosing. Encouraged by the positive results, a 78-week, randomized, placebo-controlled, parallel-group, double-blind phase II/III combined clinical trial was started in late 2012. The phase III efficacy study for MK-8931 (clinicaltrials.gov ID: NCT01739348) is expected to conclude in 2017.

A number of other small molecule inhibitors of β-secretase with reasonably good BBB penetration are currently in clinical trials (Table 7.1).

γ-Secretase Inhibitors and Modulators

γ-Secretase is a large multiprotein enzyme complex that catalyzes the intramembranous proteolysis of several type 1 proteins including APP, notch, ErbB4, and sortilin (Haapasalo and Kovacs, 2011). The active protein complex consists of presenilin (PS1 or PS2), aph-1, nicastrin, and PEN-2 (Kimberly et al., 2003; Sato et al., 2007; Tolia and De Strooper, 2009). While PS houses the catalytic activity of this enzyme, all four proteins are obligatory for optimal enzymatic activity (Wolfe et al., 1999a,b; Kimberly et al., 2000). γ-Secretase functions as an aspartyl protease and acts on C83 and C99 to produce p3 and Aβ peptide, respectively.

γ-Secretase is a processive enzyme that catalyzes multiple consecutive reactions following substrate binding (Takami et al., 2009; Chavez-Gutierrez, 2013). First, its endopeptidase activity cleaves APP-CTFβ at the ε-site to liberate AICD into the cytosol. The second step involves the excision of tripeptides and/or tetrapeptides from the remaining membrane-bound fragment to give Aβ peptides (Takami et al., 2009; Chavez-Gutierrez, 2013). Because of its key role in producing Aβ peptide, γ-secretase continues to be a focus of intense research both in academia and in the pharmaceutical industry. However, the large number of potential substrates for γ-secretase (>80) presents a significant challenge to targeting γ-secretase (Haapasalo and Kovacs, 2011; Rochette and Murphy, 2002). With the exception of notch, the physiological consequence of inhibiting the processing of other substrates has not been extensively studied. Notch is involved in cell development and differentiation of hematopoietic, immune, mucosal, and skin cells. Indeed, hematological, gastrointestinal, and skin toxicity has been associated with usage of nonselective GSIs (Shearman et al., 2000; Milano et al., 2004; Doody et al., 2013).

Although there is currently no GSI approved for AD treatment, several promising leads have been identified and these compounds have served as invaluable tools to study the structure and function of this enzyme over the last two decades (Olson and Albright, 2008; Wolfe, 2008). The first compounds to be reported as GSIs were peptide aldehydes, which were originally designed as calpain inhibitors (Higaki et al., 1995; Klafki et al., 1996; Schmidt, 2003). These compounds inhibited Aβ peptide production in transfected cells with micromolar potency. However, they lack specificity and also inhibit serine and cysteine proteases. Early efforts at designing GSIs were focused on peptidomimetic compounds with isosteres of the scissile bond in APP. The importance of γ-secretase in notch signaling was not readily obvious at that time and most of these compounds were not tested for notch inhibition. The substrate-based difluoroketone peptidomimetic MW167 (Fig. 7.9) was the first selective GSI reported (Wolfe et al., 1998). It mimicked the transition state of the APP-CTFβ during proteolysis and was specifically designed to model the Aβ42–43 bond. While it reduced the total Aβ peptide with an IC_{50} of 13 μM, it was more potent at reducing Aβ40 relative to Aβ42 and even increased the latter at low concentrations (Wolfe et al., 1998, 1999).

Several peptidomimetic compounds were subsequently developed to inhibit γ-secretase. L-685458 (Fig. 7.9), which contains the hydroxyethylene dipeptide isostere, inhibits γ-secretase with an IC_{50} of 17 nM and displays similar potency for both Aβ40 and Aβ42 inhibition (Shearman et al., 2000). The potential therapeutic usefulness and development of most of the peptidomimetic GSIs was invariably hampered by the pharmacokinetic challenges associated with peptide analogs, much like the challenges encountered with peptide-based inhibitors of β-secretase and Aβ aggregation. However, these peptidomimetic GSIs and their photoaffinity-labeled analogs are invaluable probes that have been used to significantly increase our understanding of γ-secretase structure, properties, and catalytic activity (Schmidt, 2003; Wolfe et al., 1999a,b; Li et al., 2000; Esler et al., 2000; Weihofen et al., 2003; Fuwa et al., 2007).

DAPT and compound E (Fig. 7.9) represent a new class of potent, structurally similar, and nontransition state GSIs that inhibit the production of Aβ40/Aβ42 (Seiffert et al., 2000; Dovey et al., 2001; Tian et al., 2002, 2003). Both compounds are dipeptide analogs with compound E formed by the introduction of a benzodiazepine moiety on one end of DAPT. Unlike the peptidomimetic isosteres, these compounds are noncompetitive inhibitors, and display

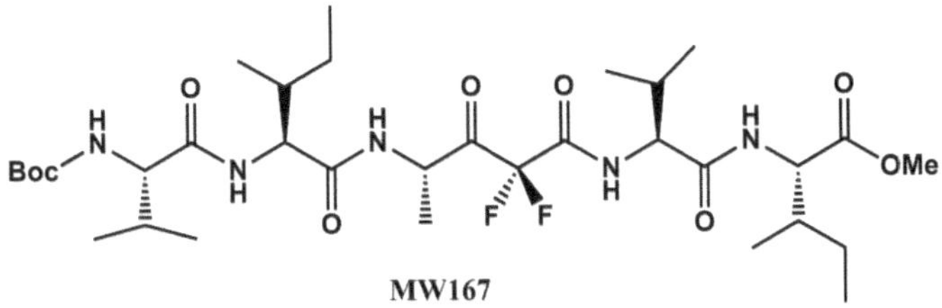

MW167

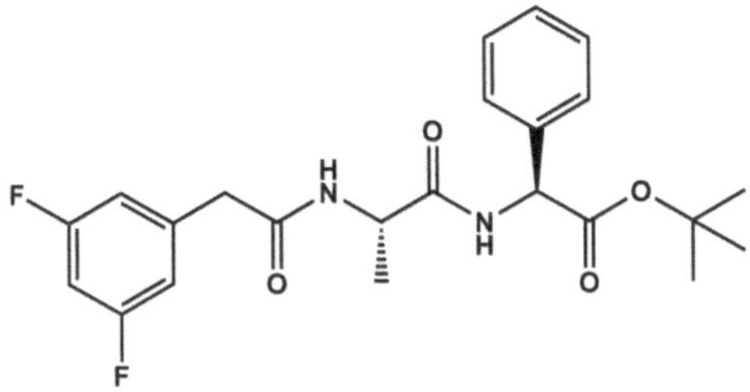

DAPT

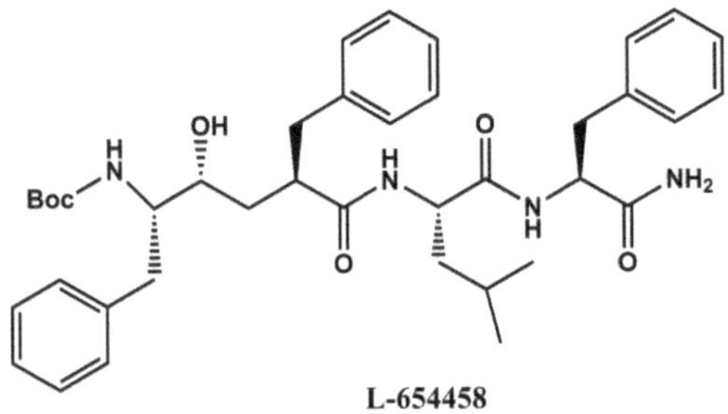

L-654458

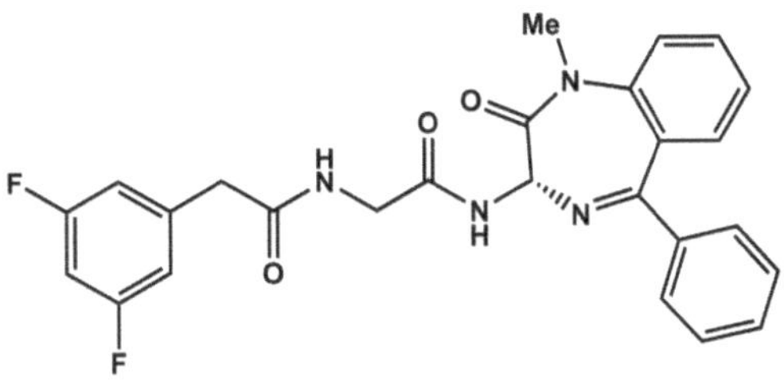

Compound E

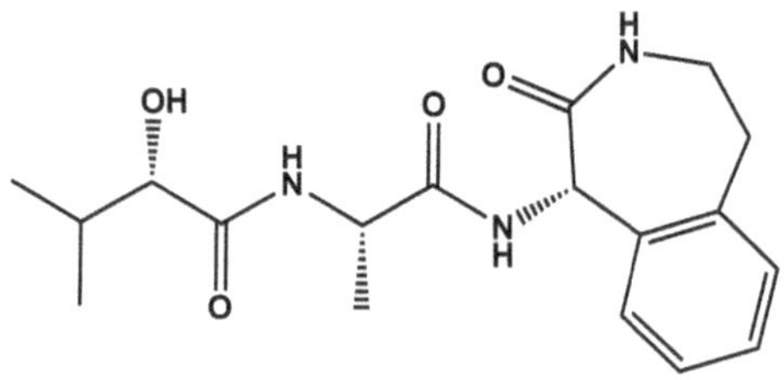

Semagacestat

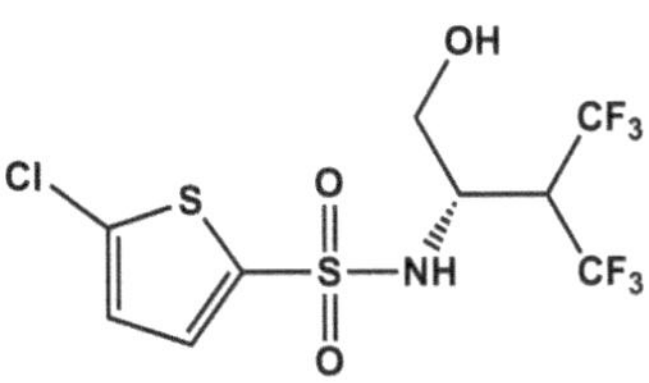

Begacestat

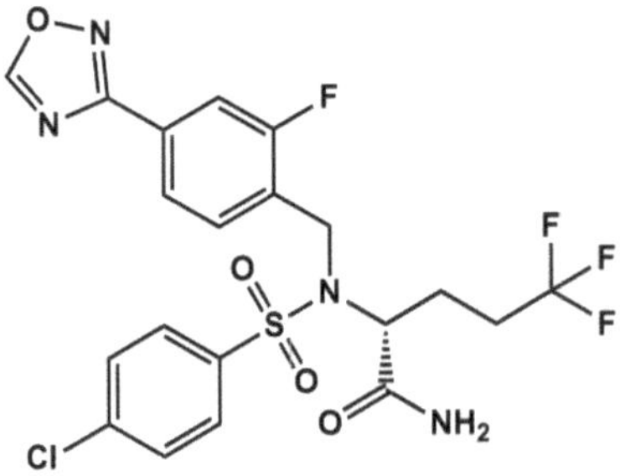

Avagacestat

FIGURE 7.9 Structures of γ-secretase inhibitors (GSIs).

significantly improved in vivo activities (Tian et al., 2002, 2003). DAPT (IC_{50} = 20 nM) was the first GSI with reported in vivo activity. In PDAPP and Tg2576 transgenic mice models of AD, DAPT significantly reduced the Aβ load in the plasma and CSF (Dovey et al., 2001; Lanz et al., 2003). Compound E (IC_{50} = 0.3 nM) remains one of the most potent GSIs reported in literature.

Further structural modifications led to the development of another dipeptide analog, LY450139 (semagacestat) (Fig. 7.9). LY450139 inhibited γ-secretase activity (IC_{50} = 11–15 nM), reduced Aβ40/Aβ42 production in PDAPP transgenic mice, and had an improved pharmacokinetic profile justifying its advancement into clinical trials (Gitter et al., 2004; Henley et al., 2009; Ness et al., 2004; Mitani et al., 2012). Semagacestat was not selective for APP and may even preferentially inhibit notch processing as shown by the Aβ/notch ratio of 0.1 in a cell-free assay (Chavez-Gutierrez et al., 2012). In phase II safety studies, semagacestat was well tolerated when given in once-daily escalating doses that peaked at 100 mg or 140 mg by week 8 of a 14-week treatment period (Fleisher et al., 2008). However, increased adverse events including skin rash and hair discoloration were observed in patients taking semagacestat. Furthermore, there was a decline in cognitive and functional abilities in patients taking semagacestat relative to placebo. These effects were more pronounced in patients given the higher dose of the drug and led to the termination of the clinical trial. Interestingly, in patients given the higher dose of semagacestat, there was a 50% and 18% reduction in plasma Aβ40 and Aβ42, respectively, relative to placebo-treated patients; yet, there were no significant changes in the levels of both Aβ peptides in the CSF. This was despite adequate CNS penetration and levels of semagacestat in the CSF being several-fold higher than the IC_{50} value obtained from in vitro experiments (Doody et al., 2013; Siemers et al., 2006).

Other GSIs that are devoid of dipeptide linkages have since been developed by us and others, with most of these compounds having the arylsulfonamide moiety. As part of research efforts into GSIs in our lab, we synthesized and evaluated novel adamantine-based arylsulfonamides (Adeniji A.O., PhD Dissertation). These adamantine-based compounds inhibited Aβ peptide production in cell lines stably overexpressing APP but displayed no selectivity between APP and notch (Adeniji et al., 2012).

Begacestat (GSI-953) (Mayer et al., 2008; Martone et al., 2009; Hopkins, 2012) and avagacestat (BMS-708163) (Gillman et al., 2010) are notch-sparing GSIs that have the arylsulfonamide moiety (Fig. 7.9). These agents displayed 20- and 190-fold selectivity, respectively, for inhibiting APP processing over notch. The major benefit of these compounds is their ability to inhibit γ-secretase processing of APP at concentrations that do not affect notch processing. This selectivity should translate to reduction or absence of notch-related toxicity in vivo (Martone et al., 2009; Dockens et al., 2012; Tong et al., 2012). Both compounds are low nanomolar potency inhibitors of γ-secretase and significantly reduced Aβ levels in the plasma, brain, and CSF of treated animal models of AD. Despite the improved safety profile, avagacestat was not advanced to phase III clinical trials because of lack of adequate clinical efficacy (Squibb, 2012). There is absence of data on begacestat following the completion of a phase I study where it was used in combination with donepezil.

Given the challenges with GSIs, there has been an interest in γ-secretase modulators (GSM). GSMs are compounds that selectively reduce production of the amyloidogenic Aβ42 in favor of shorter, less pathogenic Aβ species without affecting total Aβ production and have little to no effect on γ-secretase processing of notch and other substrates (Weggen et al., 2001, 2003). By selectively targeting the pathogenic Aβ42, GSMs have the potential to be safer and equally or perhaps more efficacious than GSIs. Indeed, recent studies suggest that complete inhibition of γ-secretase may actually be deleterious in AD. First, the age of onset of FAD was inversely correlated with both the Aβ42/Aβ40 ratio and Aβ42 levels in the CSF but directly correlated with levels of Aβ40 (Kumar-Singh et al., 2006). Second, overexpression of Aβ40 in a transgenic animal model resulted in reduced amyloid deposition (Kim et al., 2007). Third, APP-CTFβ accumulation can lead to increase of Aβ42/Aβ40, endosome dysfunction, and synaptotoxicity (Mitani et al., 2012; Yin et al., 2007; Jiang et al., 2010). These data suggest that Aβ40 may prevent Aβ42 aggregation and that increased Aβ42/Aβ40 ratio resulting from increased Aβ42 and/or decreased Aβ40 is an important driver of the pathogenic cascade in AD, making the total γ-secretase inhibition undesirable.

The very first GSMs were nonsteroidal antiinflammatory drugs including indomethacin, sulindac sulfide, and flurbiprofen (Fig. 7.10) although their γ-secretase modulatory activity did not correlate with the inhibitory potency on cyclooxygenase (COX) enzymes and appeared to be independent of their effects on the latter (Weggen et al., 2001, 2003). One of the most extensively studied GSMs is *R*-flurbiprofen (tarenflurbil), which is devoid of COX inhibitory activity. This compound was shown to inhibit Aβ42 production ($IC_{50} > 100\,\mu M$), increase Aβ38 production, and lack significant effect on Aβ40 production (Eriksen et al., 2003). Tarenflurbil was subsequently advanced to clinical trials. Despite promising data from phase I and II studies, tarenflurbil did not show significant clinical efficacy compared to placebo in phase III clinical trials. The lack of efficacy has partly been attributed to low potency, issues with BBB penetration, and target engagement within the CNS.

Second-generation GSMs, such as GSM-2 and E2012 (Fig. 7.10), which exhibit vastly increased potency and CNS penetration, have been developed (Mitani et al., 2012; Lu et al., 2012; Crump et al., 2013; Golde et al., 2013). GSM-2 is a piperidine acetic acid that blocked Aβ42 production ($IC_{50} = 65\,nM$), increased Aβ38 (EC_{50} of 81 nM) and lacked any significant effect on Aβ40 production and notch processing. It also produced significantly greater improvement of cognitive deficits in treated transgenic Tg2576 mice compared to semagacestat and avagacestat (Mitani et al., 2012). E2012, unlike GSM-2 and the first-generation GSMs, does not have the carboxylic acid moiety and has a different Aβ peptide inhibition profile. It reduced both Aβ42 and Aβ40 production ($IC_{50} = 92\,nM$ and 330 nM, respectively) and increased the levels of Aβ37 and Aβ38 (Crump et al., 2013; Hashimoto et al., 2010; Portelius et al., 2010; Borgegard et al., 2012). Of the second-generation GSMs, E2012 was the first to be advanced to clinical trials although its development was ultimately terminated because of increase in the incidence of cataract and the development of a more potent compound (E2212) with an improved safety profile (Crump et al., 2013; Nakano-Ito et al., 2014). GSMs represent the safest way of interfering with γ-secretase activity and constitute an area of intense research. Several GSMs with varying chemical structures and Aβ peptide inhibition profile have been developed and are in various phases of clinical development.

Aβ Peptide Immunotherapy

Removal of Aβ peptides from the brain represents an interesting approach to combating AD that had not attracted much interest until the pioneering work of Schenk et al. (1999). The authors showed that immunization of the PDAPP transgenic mice with synthetic Aβ42 led to production of antibodies against the peptide. This resulted in significant reduction

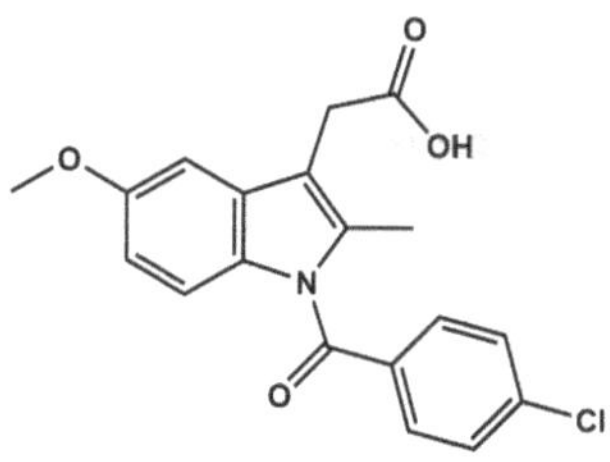

Indomethacin

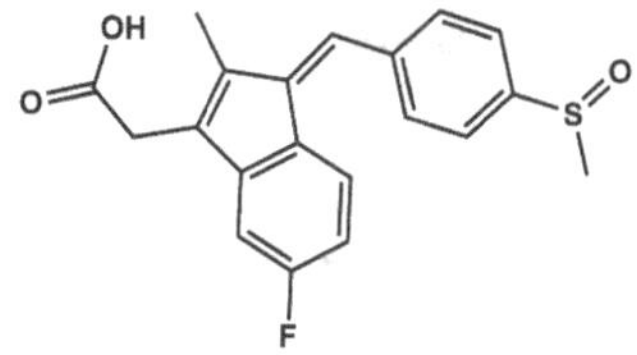

Sulindac Sulfide

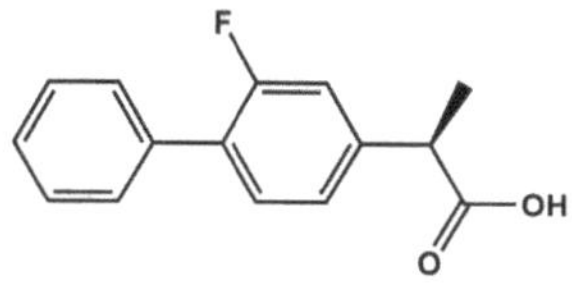

R-Flurbiprofen

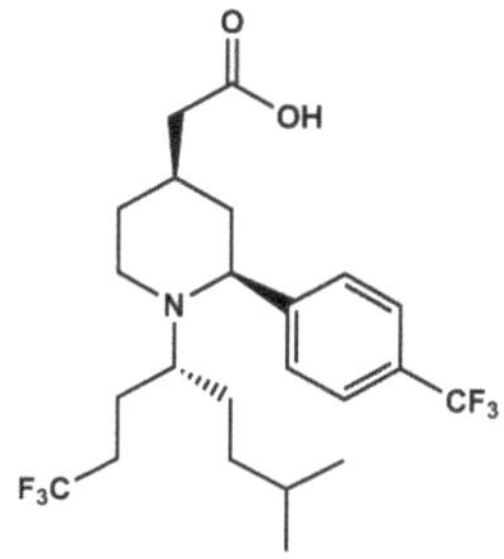

GSM-2

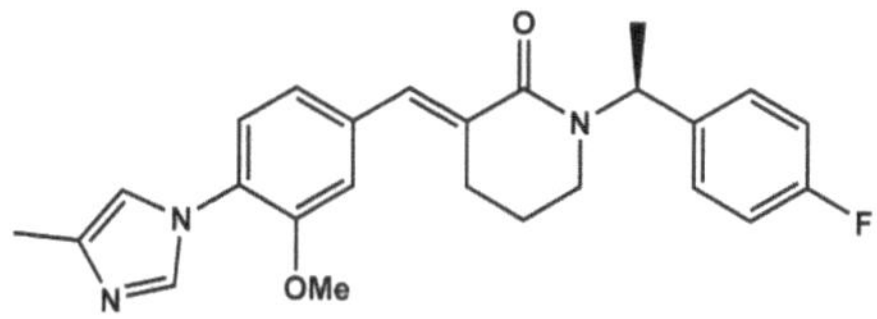

E2012

FIGURE 7.10 Structures of γ-secretase modulators (GSMs).

in brain Aβ peptide, neuritic lesions, and brain plaque burden as well as the other pathological events associated with AD. This effect was seen in all animals immunized with Aβ42 regardless of whether the animals were immunized before or after development of AD pathology. This successful proof-of-concept study highlighted the potential therapeutic benefit of active or passive immunization to induce clearance of Aβ peptides from the CNS before or after the formation of the neurotoxic Aβ oligomers and/or plaques. The interest in immunotherapy resulted in the first active vaccination trial with human Aβ42 (AN1972) and the immunological adjuvant QS-21 in patients with mild-to-moderate AD (Orgogozo et al., 2003; Gilman et al., 2005). Of 300 patients treated with AN1972, only about 20% produced a significant amount of anti-AN1972 IgG (responders). Although improvements in some cognitive scores were observed among the responders, the phase II trial was discontinued following the development of meningoencephalitis in 6% of the patients that were given AN1972. The authors attributed the meningoencephalitis to T-cell activation probably resulting from change in the formulation (Gilman et al., 2005). The use of Aβ fragments rather the full length peptide was proposed as a way of limiting T-cell activation, and a subsequent immunization study conducted with the shorter Aβ peptide CAD-106 ($A\beta_{1-6}$) reported no incidence of meningoencephalitis (Winblad et al., 2012). The choice of adjuvants as well as the route of administration may also influence T-cell activation (Fu et al., 2010). Several other active immunizations studies are being pursued (Fu et al., 2010; Lemere and Masliah, 2010; Jia et al., 2014).

Passive immunization through administration of antibodies against Aβ is another immunotherapy approach that produces similar results without the concern over low response rates and attendant risk of T-cell activation (Bard et al., 2000; Buttini et al., 2005). Bard et al. (2000) showed that anti-Aβ antibodies administered to PDAPP mice were able to cross the BBB and attain therapeutically relevant concentrations in the CNS. The antibodies also reduced Aβ42 levels and amyloid plaque burden by inducing phagocytosis of the plaques. Importantly, they were unable to detect any T-cell activation in immunized animals. Some of these mouse antibodies have been humanized and evaluated in human subjects.

Bapinezumab is a humanized form of the murine monoclonal antibody 3D6 that recognizes the Aβ N-terminus ($A\beta_{1-5}$) and preferentially binds to the aggregated Aβ peptide (Bard et al., 2000; Kerchner and Boxer, 2010). It produces reduction in Aβ peptide and amyloid plaque levels, prevents degeneration of the synapse, and improves memory in transgenic mice (Shankar et al., 2008; Bard et al., 2000; Buttini et al., 2005). Although bapinezumab failed to produce a significant change in levels of Aβ42 and tau within the CSF of immunized patients in a phase II trial, there was an indication that it may offer some therapeutic benefits in noncarriers of the APOE ε4 allele (Salloway et al., 2009). However, two phase III clinical trials of bapinezumab in mild-to-moderate AD patients did not show any significant clinical benefit in either the noncarriers or the carriers of the APOE ε4 allele (Salloway et al., 2014). There was also an increased incidence (10%) of vasogenic edema in patients given bapinezumab, which resolved following discontinuation of the drug.

Another monoclonal antibody that has been evaluated in human subjects is solanezumab. Solanezumab is a humanized analog of the murine monoclonal antibody m266.2 that recognizes the mid region of the Aβ ($A\beta_{13-28}$) (Kerchner and Boxer, 2010). It differs from bapinezumab by preferentially targeting the soluble rather than the aggregated form of Aβ (Seubert et al., 1992). In preclinical studies, it reduced Aβ deposition in the CNS by altering the Aβ equilibrium between the CNS and the periphery in favor of a significant increase in plasma levels of Aβ peptide ("peripheral sink" mechanism) (DeMattos et al., 2001). Despite the decrease in amyloid deposition, it produced an increase in total Aβ in the CSF presumably caused by leakage of Aβ peptides from the amyloid plaques. This effect on plasma and CSF Aβ levels was replicated in human studies. In phase II and III clinical trials, solanezumab was relatively well tolerated and did not increase the risk of vasogenic edema (Farlow et al., 2012; Doody et al., 2014). Nevertheless, solanezumab did not produce a significant improvement of cognitive or functional abilities in patients with mild-to-moderate AD compared to placebo. Another phase III trial (EXPEDITION 3, clinicaltrials.gov ID: NCT01900665) was started in July 2013 to evaluate the effects of solanezumab on patients with mild AD. Despite the failure of the aforementioned antibodies in clinical trials, efforts are ongoing to develop more efficacious products. Some of the antibodies that are currently in clinical development for the treatment of AD include gantenerumab, crenezumab, SAR228810, and GSK933776 (Jia et al., 2014; Panza et al., 2014; Pradier et al., 2013; Leyhe et al., 2014).

DISCUSSION

AD continues to be a major public health concern in the United States and around the world. While our knowledge of the disease has increased exponentially over the last three decades, questions still remain about the pathological process(es) leading to AD and consequently rational therapeutic approaches that might alter the progression of the disease. The prevailing scientific opinion on AD pathogenesis for the last three decades has been the Aβ hypothesis with Aβ aggregates being the key neurotoxic moieties that lead to development of AD. Numerous clinical and genetic studies show that Aβ accumulation is associated with AD and provide strong support for this hypothesis. However, the exact place and role of Aβ in the pathological cascade of AD, in particular LOAD, has not been conclusively established. Moreover, several clinical observations that are not consistent with the hypothesis have now being reported (reviewed in Drachman, 2014). These observations have led researchers to question the veracity of the Aβ hypothesis, suggest that other prominent players are involved in AD pathology, or propose that the link between Aβ peptide and AD pathogenesis is not as direct as many had predicted or hoped.

One of the more widespread concerns about the Aβ hypothesis is the observation that the amyloid plaque deposition and neurofibrillary tangles that are hallmarks of AD are often seen in older individuals who are cognitively normal (Bennett et al., 2006; Price et al., 2009; Mathis et al., 2013). In a study on geriatric individuals without cognitive impairment, postmortem analysis showed that 50 out of 134 individuals met the neuropathological criteria for likelihood of AD (Bennett et al., 2006). In another similar study conducted in seven centers across America, 20–40% of nondemented individuals met the neuropathological criteria for AD (Price et al., 2009). It should be noted that this is not entirely inconsistent with the Aβ hypothesis since individuals with chronic diseases often have substantial pathological changes before clinical symptoms become apparent. Because these studies were conducted postmortem, it is difficult to know whether the individuals would have eventually developed clinical AD.

Mathis et al. (2013) conducted a study in nondemented individuals using in vivo imaging with labeled Pittsburgh compound B (PiB), a compound used to image amyloid plaques. They found that 55% of nondemented individuals aged 80 and older had amyloid plaque deposition as measured by PiB positivity. Cognitively normal individuals that have substantial plaque deposition are now referred to as being in the "preclinical or presymptomatic stage of AD" (Price et al., 2009; Sperling et al., 2011a,b; Snitz et al., 2013). It is instructive to note that higher Aβ deposition in these nondemented individuals was associated with subtle cognitive deficits. The cohort from Mathis et al. are being followed to see how many eventually develop AD. These observations are also supported by the finding that not all individuals with trisomy 21 develop AD despite the constant and substantial Aβ deposition (Krinsky-McHale et al., 2008; Zigman et al., 2008). This would suggest the existence of other factors that act independent of or in concert with Aβ peptide to trigger the neurotoxic events that lead to AD.

The failure of several anti-Aβ agents to produce improvement in cognition in human trials is probably the biggest challenge to the standing of the Aβ hypothesis. Compounds targeting various steps in Aβ peptide production (α-secretase activators, β- and γ-secretase inhibitors), aggregation, and clearance (passive and active Aβ immunization) have so far not shown significant therapeutic benefits when tested in individuals with AD. This is despite the fact that most of these agents had good CNS penetration and some were able to reduce Aβ peptide levels and amyloid plaque burden in the CNS. Notable examples include AN1972 and semagacestat. In a follow-up study of patients from the AN1972 active immunization study, Aβ42 immunization with AN1972 did not prevent disease progression or improve survival even in patients that had complete plaque removal (Holmes et al., 2008). The worsening of cognitive function in patients taking the GSI semagacestat was particular significant (Doody et al., 2013). The cognitive decline has been partly attributed to the ability of the drug to interfere with the processing of notch and perhaps other γ-secretase substrates. However, the notch-sparing GSI avagacestat did not show any improvement in cognitive function of patients (Dockens et al., 2012; Squibb, 2012).

Despite the setbacks and disappointing results from clinical trials, there are plausible explanations in support of the Aβ hypothesis that justify the failure of these anti-Aβ drugs. First, there are questions about the appropriate time to use these anti-Aβ agents that relate specifically to whether these drugs are likely to be more effective prior to the onset of dementia. It is now known that Aβ aggregation and neuronal damage occur many years, even decades, prior to the onset of clinical symptoms of AD (Bateman et al., 2012; Reiman et al., 2012; Fleisher et al., 2012; Jack Jr. et al., 2013). This observation suggests that the appropriate approach may be to use these anti-Aβ agents in at-risk individuals, as a preventive therapy, or at the earliest sign of Aβ deposition since the agents may no longer be effective once the damage is done and dementia starts (Sperling et al., 2011a,b). Secondary prevention trials with anti-Aβ agents (solanezumab and gantenerumab) in individuals at risk of having EOAD are currently ongoing (clinicaltrials.gov ID: NCT01760005). The outcome of these trials will be important in our understanding of AD.

Second, the failure of these agents has also been attributed to the quality of the compounds as well as the design of the clinical trials (Selkoe, 2011; De Strooper, 2014; Karran and Hardy, 2014). It is suggested that the compounds were not ideal candidates for testing the Aβ hypothesis and were not thoroughly validated nor rigorously tested before being advanced into clinical trials, particularly phase III trials. For example, the failure of tarenflurbil in clinical trial was not totally unpredictable given its low potency (>100 μM), poor penetration, and lack of target engagement in the CNS. The monoclonal antibody solanezumab was also found to display significant cross-reactivity with non-Aβ proteins, which makes it less effective at targeting Aβ in human tissue compared to human Aβ overexpressed in mouse models (Watt et al., 2014). This apparent lack of target engagement would explain the lack of efficacy seen in human testing.

The GSI semagacestat, like a number of other GSIs, also stimulates γ-secretase, albeit under conditions of low inhibitor and substrate concentration (Chavez-Gutierrez et al., 2012; Burton et al., 2008). This stimulation leads to increase in Aβ production as the levels of the drug go down in the CSF, which may negate any reduction in Aβ caused by the administration of a high dose of the compound. In a kinetic study, a single dose of semagacestat administered to healthy individuals with a dose range of 100–280 mg produced 47–84% reduction in CSF Aβ production over a 12-h period (Bateman et al., 2009). Interestingly, the Aβ levels were above baseline 36 h after dosing. This observation is consistent with the short half-life (1.96–3.04 h) of the compound in the CSF as well as the concentration-dependent stimulatory/inhibitory effect on γ-secretase (Chavez-Gutierrez et al., 2012; Burton et al., 2008; Bateman et al., 2009). The design of the clinical trial is thought to be one of many reasons for the failure of the compound in clinical trials

(De Strooper, 2014; Karran and Hardy, 2014). To preclude notch-related toxicity, the phase III clinical trial was conducted at 140mg once daily, a dosing regimen that was never shown to reduce Aβ production in the CSF and still caused significant notch-related toxicities in the trials (Doody et al., 2013; Fleisher et al., 2008). Based on the properties of semagacestat outlined earlier, the dosing regimen utilized in the phase III trial cannot be expected to produce a sustained reduction in Aβ levels in the CSF nor offer any therapeutic benefit.

CONCLUSIONS

Giant strides have been and continue to be made in the development of agents that can arrest the neuropathological process driving AD. Most, if not all, of these agents have been based on the Aβ hypothesis, which places aberrant Aβ peptide production and aggregation at the center of the pathological cascade that leads to AD. Several anti-Aβ agents have now been tested in human trials without clinical success and questions continue to be raised about the Aβ hypothesis, the drug candidates, and the design of the trials.

Given all these findings, there is clear need for a better and more precise understanding of the pathophysiology of AD especially as it involves the role of Aβ either as the single or one out of many interdependent villains in the AD script, or perhaps an innocent bystander. This is probably the most important need as it serves as a foundation for future drug discovery efforts. Lead compounds will likewise need to be rigorously tested and evaluated before commencement of large-scale human trials. Animal models that recapitulate a greater degree of the features of AD on a timeline and sequence that correlate to the human disease as well as biomarkers that accurately reflect changes or alteration of the pathological process will be essential to this task. With the accomplishments of the last several decades in the field of AD and the extensive scientific tools that can be put to bear, it is hoped that a disease-modifying treatment will be developed in the near future, whether based on the Aβ hypothesis, a modified form of Aβ hypothesis, or a yet to be articulated explanation for AD pathology.

References

Adeniji, A.O., Wells, R.M., Adejare, A., 2012. Syntheses and in-vitro evaluation of novel adamantane based gamma-secretase inhibitors. Curr. Med. Chem. 19, 2458–2471.

Alexander, R., Budd, S., Russell, M., Kugler, A., Cebers, G., Ye, N., Olsson, T., Burdette, D., Maltby, J., Paraskos, J., Elsby, K., Han, D., Goldwater, R., Ereshefsky, L., 2014. AZD3293 A novel BACE1 inhibitor: safety, tolerability, and effects on plasma and CSF Aβ peptides following single- and multiple-dose administration. Neurobiol. Aging 35, S2.

Alzheimer's, A., 2014. 2014 Alzheimer's disease facts and figures. Alzheimers Dement. 10, e47–92.

Anderson, J.P., Esch, F.S., Keim, P.S., Sambamurti, K., Lieberburg, I., Robakis, N.K., 1991. Exact cleavage site of Alzheimer amyloid precursor in neuronal PC-12 cells. Neurosci. Lett. 128, 126–128.

Anderson, J.J., Holtz, G., Baskin, P.P., Wang, R., Mazzarelli, L., Wagner, S.L., Menzaghi, F., 1999. Reduced cerebrospinal fluid levels of alpha-secretase-cleaved amyloid precursor protein in aged rats: correlation with spatial memory deficits. Neuroscience 93, 1409–1420.

Bard, F., Cannon, C., Barbour, R., Burke, R.L., Games, D., Grajeda, H., Guido, T., Hu, K., Huang, J., Johnson-Wood, K., Khan, K., Kholodenko, D., Lee, M., Lieberburg, I., Motter, R., Nguyen, M., Soriano, F., Vasquez, N., Weiss, K., Welch, B., Seubert, P., Schenk, D., Yednock, T., 2000. Peripherally administered antibodies against amyloid beta-peptide enter the central nervous system and reduce pathology in a mouse model of Alzheimer disease. Nat. Med. 6, 916–919.

Bate, C., Williams, A., 2010. Amyloid-β_{1-40} inhibits amyloid-β_{1-42} induced activation of cytoplasmic phospholipase A2 and synapse degeneration. J. Alzheimers Dis. 21, 985–993.
Bateman, R.J., Siemers, E.R., Mawuenyega, K.G., Wen, G., Browning, K.R., Sigurdson, W.C., Yarasheski, K.E., Friedrich, S.W., Demattos, R.B., May, P.C., Paul, S.M., Holtzman, D.M., 2009. A gamma-secretase inhibitor decreases amyloid-beta production in the central nervous system. Ann. Neurol. 66, 48–54.
Bateman, R.J., Xiong, C., Benzinger, T.L., Fagan, A.M., Goate, A., Fox, N.C., Marcus, D.S., Cairns, N.J., Xie, X., Blazey, T.M., Holtzman, D.M., Santacruz, A., Buckles, V., Oliver, A., Moulder, K., Aisen, P.S., Ghetti, B., Klunk, W.E., McDade, E., Martins, R.N., Masters, C.L., Mayeux, R., Ringman, J.M., Rossor, M.N., Schofield, P.R., Sperling, R.A., Salloway, S., Morris, J.C., Dominantly Inherited Alzheimer Network, 2012. Clinical and biomarker changes in dominantly inherited Alzheimer's disease. N. Engl. J. Med. 367, 795–804.
Bennett, D.A., Schneider, J.A., Arvanitakis, Z., Kelly, J.F., Aggarwal, N.T., Shah, R.C., Wilson, R.S., 2006. Neuropathology of older persons without cognitive impairment from two community-based studies. Neurology 66, 1837–1844.
Blasko, I., Beer, R., Bigl, M., Apelt, J., Franz, G., Rudzki, D., Ransmayr, G., Kampfl, A., Schliebs, R., 2004. Experimental traumatic brain injury in rats stimulates the expression, production and activity of Alzheimer's disease beta-secretase (BACE-1). J. Neural Transm. 111, 523–536.
Blazer, L.L., Neubig, R.R., 2008. Small molecule protein-protein interaction inhibitors as CNS therapeutic agents: current progress and future hurdles. Neuropsychopharmacology 34, 126–141.
Bloom, G.S., 2014. Amyloid-beta and tau: the trigger and bullet in Alzheimer disease pathogenesis. JAMA Neurol. 71, 505–508.
Borgegard, T., Jureus, A., Olsson, F., Rosqvist, S., Sabirsh, A., Rotticci, D., Paulsen, K., Klintenberg, R., Yan, H., Waldman, M., Stromberg, K., Nord, J., Johansson, J., Regner, A., Parpal, S., Malinowsky, D., Radesater, A.C., Li, T., Singh, R., Eriksson, H., Lundkvist, J., 2012. First and second generation γ-secretase modulators (GSMs) modulate amyloid-β (Aβ) peptide production through different mechanisms. J. Biol. Chem. 287, 11810–11819.
Burton, C.R., Meredith, J.E., Barten, D.M., Goldstein, M.E., Krause, C.M., Kieras, C.J., Sisk, L., Iben, L.G., Polson, C., Thompson, M.W., Lin, X.A., Corsa, J., Fiedler, T., Pierdomenico, M., Cao, Y., Roach, A.H., Cantone, J.L., Ford, M.J., Drexler, D.M., Olson, R.E., Yang, M.G., Bergstrom, C.P., McElhone, K.E., Bronson, J.J., Macor, J.E., Blat, Y., Grafstrom, R.H., Stern, A.M., Seiffert, D.A., Zaczek, R., Albright, C.F., Toyn, J.H., 2008. The amyloid-β rise and γ-secretase inhibitor potency depend on the level of substrate expression. J. Biol. Chem. 283, 22992–23003.
Butini, S., Brogi, S., Novellino, E., Campiani, G., Ghosh, A.K., Brindisi, M., Gemma, S., 2013. The structural evolution of β-secretase inhibitors: a focus on the development of small-molecule inhibitors. Curr. Top. Med. Chem. 13, 1787–1807.
Buttini, M., Masliah, E., Barbour, R., Grajeda, H., Motter, R., Johnson-Wood, K., Khan, K., Seubert, P., Freedman, S., Schenk, D., Games, D., 2005. β-amyloid immunotherapy prevents synaptic degeneration in a mouse model of Alzheimer's disease. J. Neurosci. 25, 9096–9101.
Cai, H., Wang, Y., McCarthy, D., Wen, H., Borchelt, D.R., Price, D.L., Wong, P.C., 2001. BACE1 is the major β-secretase for generation of Aβ peptides by neurons. Nat. Neurosci. 4, 233–234.
Castellano, J.M., Kim, J., Stewart, F.R., Jiang, H., DeMattos, R.B., Patterson, B.W., Fagan, A.M., Morris, J.C., Mawuenyega, K.G., Cruchaga, C., Goate, A.M., Bales, K.R., Paul, S.M., Bateman, R.J., Holtzman, D.M., 2011. Human apoE isoforms differentially regulate brain amyloid-β peptide clearance. Sci. Transl. Med. 3, 89ra57.
Chartier-Harlin, M.C., Crawford, F., Houlden, H., Warren, A., Hughes, D., Fidani, L., Goate, A., Rossor, M., Roques, P., Hardy, J., et al., 1991. Early-onset Alzheimer's disease caused by mutations at codon 717 of the β-amyloid precursor protein gene. Nature 353, 844–846.
Chavez-Gutierrez, L., Bammens, L., Benilova, I., Vandersteen, A., Benurwar, M., Borgers, M., Lismont, S., Zhou, L., Van Cleynenbreugel, S., Esselmann, H., Wiltfang, J., Serneels, L., Karran, E., Gijsen, H., Schymkowitz, J., Rousseau, F., Broersen, K., De Strooper, B., 2012. The mechanism of γ-Secretase dysfunction in familial Alzheimer disease. EMBO J. 31, 2261–2274.
Chavez-Gutierrez, L., 2013. Dissecting γ-secretase function. J. Neurochem. 125, 1–3.
Cheng, A.C., Coleman, R.G., Smyth, K.T., Cao, Q., Soulard, P., Caffrey, D.R., Salzberg, A.C., Huang, E.S., 2007. Structure-based maximal affinity model predicts small-molecule druggability. Nat. Biotechnol. 25, 71–75.
Cherny, R.A., Atwood, C.S., Xilinas, M.E., Gray, D.N., Jones, W.D., McLean, C.A., Barnham, K.J., Volitakis, I., Fraser, F.W., Kim, Y., Huang, X., Goldstein, L.E., Moir, R.D., Lim, J.T., Beyreuther, K., Zheng, H., Tanzi, R.E., Masters, C.L., Bush, A.I., 2001. Treatment with a copper-zinc chelator markedly and rapidly inhibits beta-amyloid accumulation in Alzheimer's disease transgenic mice. Neuron 30, 665–676.

Cohen, S.I., Linse, S., Luheshi, L.M., Hellstrand, E., White, D.A., Rajah, L., Otzen, D.E., Vendruscolo, M., Dobson, C.M., Knowles, T.P., 2013. Proliferation of amyloid-beta42 aggregates occurs through a secondary nucleation mechanism. Proc. Natl. Acad. Sci. U.S.A. 110, 9758–9763.

Colciaghi, F., Borroni, B., Pastorino, L., Marcello, E., Zimmermann, M., Cattabeni, F., Padovani, A., Di Luca, M., 2002. α-Secretase ADAM10 as well as αAPPs is reduced in platelets and CSF of Alzheimer disease patients. Mol. Med. 8, 67–74.

Cole, D.C., Manas, E.S., Stock, J.R., Condon, J.S., Jennings, L.D., Aulabaugh, A., Chopra, R., Cowling, R., Ellingboe, J.W., Fan, K.Y., Harrison, B.L., Hu, Y., Jacobsen, S., Jin, G., Lin, L., Lovering, F.E., Malamas, M.S., Stahl, M.L., Strand, J., Sukhdeo, M.N., Svenson, K., Turner, M.J., Wagner, E., Wu, J., Zhou, P., Bard, J., 2006. Acylguanidines as small-molecule β-secretase inhibitors. J. Med. Chem. 49, 6158–6161.

Crump, C.J., Johnson, D.S., Li, Y.M., 2013. Development and mechanism of gamma-secretase modulators for Alzheimer's disease. Biochemistry 52, 3197–3216.

D'Andrea, M.R., Nagele, R.G., Wang, H.Y., Peterson, P.A., Lee, D.H., 2001. Evidence that neurons accumulating amyloid can undergo lysis to form amyloid plaques in Alzheimer's disease. Histopathology 38, 120–134.

De Strooper, B., 2014. Lessons from a failed γ-secretase Alzheimer trial. Cell 159, 721–726.

DeMattos, R.B., Bales, K.R., Cummins, D.J., Dodart, J.C., Paul, S.M., Holtzman, D.M., 2001. Peripheral anti-A beta antibody alters CNS and plasma A beta clearance and decreases brain A beta burden in a mouse model of Alzheimer's disease. Proc. Natl. Acad. Sci. U.S.A. 98, 8850–8855.

Dockens, R., Wang, J.S., Castaneda, L., Sverdlov, O., Huang, S.P., Slemmon, R., Gu, H., Wong, O., Li, H., Berman, R.M., Smith, C., Albright, C.F., Tong, G., 2012. A placebo-controlled, multiple ascending dose study to evaluate the safety, pharmacokinetics and pharmacodynamics of avagacestat (BMS-708163) in healthy young and elderly subjects. Clin. Pharmacokinet. 51, 681–693.

Doody, R.S., Raman, R., Farlow, M., Iwatsubo, T., Vellas, B., Joffe, S., Kieburtz, K., He, F., Sun, X., Thomas, R.G., Aisen, P.S., Alzheimer's Disease Cooperative Study Steering Committee, Siemers, E., Sethuraman, G., Mohs, R., Semagacestat Study Group, 2013. A phase 3 trial of semagacestat for treatment of Alzheimer's disease. N. Engl. J. Med. 369, 341–350.

Doody, R.S., Thomas, R.G., Farlow, M., Iwatsubo, T., Vellas, B., Joffe, S., Kieburtz, K., Raman, R., Sun, X., Aisen, P.S., Siemers, E., Liu-Seifert, H., Mohs, R., Alzheimer's Disease Cooperative Study Steering Committee, Solanezumab Study Group, 2014. Phase 3 trials of solanezumab for mild-to-moderate Alzheimer's disease. N. Engl. J. Med. 370, 311–321.

Dovey, H.F., John, V., Anderson, J.P., Chen, L.Z., de Saint Andrieu, P., Fang, L.Y., Freedman, S.B., Folmer, B., Goldbach, E., Holsztynska, E.J., Hu, K.L., Johnson-Wood, K.L., Kennedy, S.L., Kholodenko, D., Knops, J.E., Latimer, L.H., Lee, M., Liao, Z., Lieberburg, I.M., Motter, R.N., Mutter, L.C., Nietz, J., Quinn, K.P., Sacchi, K.L., Seubert, P.A., Shopp, G.M., Thorsett, E.D., Tung, J.S., Wu, J., Yang, S., Yin, C.T., Schenk, D.B., May, P.C., Altstiel, L.D., Bender, M.H., Boggs, L.N., Britton, T.C., Clemens, J.C., Czilli, D.L., Dieckman-McGinty, D.K., Droste, J.J., Fuson, K.S., Gitter, B.D., Hyslop, P.A., Johnstone, E.M., Li, W.Y., Little, S.P., Mabry, T.E., Miller, F.D., Audia, J.E., 2001. Functional γ-secretase inhibitors reduce β-amyloid peptide levels in brain. J. Neurochem. 76, 173–181.

Drachman, D.A., 2014. The amyloid hypothesis, time to move on: amyloid is the downstream result, not cause, of Alzheimer's disease. Alzheimers Dement. 10, 372–380.

Drott, J., Desire, L., Drouin, D., Pando, M., Haun, F., 2010. Etazolate improves performance in a foraging and homing task in aged rats. Eur. J. Pharmacol. 634, 95–100.

Eriksen, J.L., Sagi, S.A., Smith, T.E., Weggen, S., Das, P., McLendon, D.C., Ozols, V.V., Jessing, K.W., Zavitz, K.H., Koo, E.H., Golde, T.E., 2003. NSAIDs and enantiomers of flurbiprofen target γ-secretase and lower Aβ 42 in vivo. J. Clin. Invest. 112, 440–449.

Esch, F.S., Keim, P.S., Beattie, E.C., Blacher, R.W., Culwell, A.R., Oltersdorf, T., McClure, D., Ward, P.J., 1990. Cleavage of amyloid β peptide during constitutive processing of its precursor. Science 248, 1122–1124.

Esler, W.P., Kimberly, W.T., Ostaszewski, B.L., Diehl, T.S., Moore, C.L., Tsai, J.Y., Rahmati, T., Xia, W., Selkoe, D.J., Wolfe, M.S., 2000. Transition-state analogue inhibitors of γ-secretase bind directly to presenilin-1. Nat. Cell Biol. 2, 428–434.

Evans, C.G., Wisen, S., Gestwicki, J.E., 2006. Heat shock proteins 70 and 90 inhibit early stages of amyloid β-(1–42) aggregation in vitro. J. Biol. Chem. 281, 33182–33191.

Evin, G., Barakat, A., Masters, C.L., 2010. BACE: therapeutic target and potential biomarker for Alzheimer's disease. Int. J. Biochem. Cell Biol. 42, 1923–1926.

Fahrenholz, F., 2007. Alpha-secretase as a therapeutic target. Curr. Alzheimer Res. 4, 412–417.

Farlow, M., Arnold, S.E., van Dyck, C.H., Aisen, P.S., Snider, B.J., Porsteinsson, A.P., Friedrich, S., Dean, R.A., Gonzales, C., Sethuraman, G., DeMattos, R.B., Mohs, R., Paul, S.M., Siemers, E.R., 2012. Safety and biomarker effects of solanezumab in patients with Alzheimer's disease. Alzheimers Dement. 8, 261–271.

Fernandez-Vizarra, P., Fernandez, A.P., Castro-Blanco, S., Serrano, J., Bentura, M.L., Martinez-Murillo, R., Martinez, A., Rodrigo, J., 2004. Intra- and extracellular Aβ and PHF in clinically evaluated cases of Alzheimer's disease. Histol. Histopathol. 19, 823–844.

Fleisher, A.S., Raman, R., Siemers, E.R., Becerra, L., Clark, C.M., Dean, R.A., Farlow, M.R., Galvin, J.E., Peskind, E.R., Quinn, J.F., Sherzai, A., Sowell, B.B., Aisen, P.S., Thal, L.J., 2008. Phase 2 safety trial targeting amyloid β production with a γ-secretase inhibitor in Alzheimer disease. Arch. Neurol. 65, 1031–1038.

Fleisher, A.S., Chen, K., Quiroz, Y.T., Jakimovich, L.J., Gomez, M.G., Langois, C.M., Langbaum, J.B., Ayutyanont, N., Roontiva, A., Thiyyagura, P., Lee, W., Mo, H., Lopez, L., Moreno, S., Acosta-Baena, N., Giraldo, M., Garcia, G., Reiman, R.A., Huentelman, M.J., Kosik, K.S., Tariot, P.N., Lopera, F., Reiman, E.M., 2012. Florbetapir PET analysis of amyloid-β deposition in the presenilin 1 E280A autosomal dominant Alzheimer's disease kindred: a cross-sectional study. Lancet Neurol. 11, 1057–1065.

Fonte, V., Kapulkin, W.J., Taft, A., Fluet, A., Friedman, D., Link, C.D., 2002. Interaction of intracellular β amyloid peptide with chaperone proteins. Proc. Natl. Acad. Sci. U.S.A. 99, 9439–9444.

Forman, M., Kleijn, H.-J., Dockendorf, M., Palcza, J., Tseng, J., Canales, C., Egan, M., Kennedy, M., Laterza, O., Ma, L., Scott, J., Tanen, M., Apter, J., Backonja, M., Ereshefsky, L., Gevorkyan, H., Jhee, S., Rynders, R., Zari, A., Bryan, E., Wagner, J., Troyer, M., Stone, J., 2013. The novel BACE inhibitor MK-8931 dramatically lowers CSF β-amyloid in patients with mild-to-moderate Alzheimer's disease. Alzheimers Dement. J. Alzheimers Assoc. 9, P139.

Fornicola, W., Pelcovits, A., Li, B.X., Heath, J., Perry, G., Castellani, R.J., 2014. Alzheimer disease pathology in middle age reveals a spatial-temporal disconnect between amyloid-β and phosphorylated tau. Open Neurol. J. 8, 22–26.

Fradinger, E.A., Monien, B.H., Urbanc, B., Lomakin, A., Tan, M., Li, H., Spring, S.M., Condron, M.M., Cruz, L., Xie, C.-W., Benedek, G.B., Bitan, G., 2008. C-terminal peptides coassemble into Aβ42 oligomers and protect neurons against Aβ42-induced neurotoxicity. Proc. Natl. Acad. Sci. U.S.A. 105, 14175–14180.

Frautschy, S.A., Hu, W., Kim, P., Miller, S.A., Chu, T., Harris-White, M.E., Cole, G.M., 2001. Phenolic anti-inflammatory antioxidant reversal of Aβ-induced cognitive deficits and neuropathology. Neurobiol. Aging 22, 993–1005.

Freskos, J.N., Fobian, Y.M., Benson, T.E., Moon, J.B., Bienkowski, M.J., Brown, D.L., Emmons, T.L., Heintz, R., Laborde, A., McDonald, J.J., Mischke, B.V., Molyneaux, J.M., Mullins, P.B., Bryan Prince, D., Paddock, D.J., Tomasselli, A.G., Winterrowd, G., 2007. Design of potent inhibitors of human β-secretase. Part 2. Bioorg. Med. Chem. Lett. 17, 78–81.

Fu, H.J., Liu, B., Frost, J.L., Lemere, C.A., 2010. Amyloid-β immunotherapy for Alzheimer's disease. CNS Neurol. Disord. Drug Targets 9, 197–206.

Fuwa, H., Takahashi, Y., Konno, Y., Watanabe, N., Miyashita, H., Sasaki, M., Natsugari, H., Kan, T., Fukuyama, T., Tomita, T., Iwatsubo, T., 2007. Divergent synthesis of multifunctional molecular probes to elucidate the enzyme specificity of dipeptidic γ-secretase inhibitors. ACS Chem. Biol. 2, 408–418.

Games, D., Adams, D., Alessandrini, R., Barbour, R., Berthelette, P., Blackwell, C., Carr, T., Clemens, J., Donaldson, T., Gillespie, F., et al., 1995. Alzheimer-type neuropathology in transgenic mice overexpressing V717F β-amyloid precursor protein. Nature 373, 523–527.

Gandy, S., 2005. The role of cerebral amyloid beta accumulation in common forms of Alzheimer disease. J. Clin. Invest. 115, 1121–1129.

Gardberg, A.S., Dice, L.T., Ou, S., Rich, R.L., Helmbrecht, E., Ko, J., Wetzel, R., Myszka, D.G., Patterson, P.H., Dealwis, C., 2007. Molecular basis for passive immunotherapy of Alzheimer's disease. Proc. Natl. Acad. Sci. U.S.A. 104, 15659–15664.

Gerritz, S.W., Zhai, W., Shi, S., Zhu, S., Toyn, J.H., Meredith, J.E., Iben, L.G., Burton, C.R., Albright, C.F., Good, A.C., Tebben, A.J., Muckelbauer, J.K., Camac, D.M., Metzler, W., Cook, L.S., Padmanabha, R., Lentz, K.A., Sofia, M.J., Poss, M.A., Macor, J.E., Thompson, L.A., 2012. Acyl guanidine inhibitors of β-secretase (BACE-1): optimization of a micromolar hit to a nanomolar lead via iterative solid- and solution-phase library synthesis. J. Med. Chem. 55, 9208–9223.

Ghosh, A.K., Kumaragurubaran, N., Hong, L., Lei, H., Hussain, K.A., Liu, C.-F., Devasamudram, T., Weerasena, V., Turner, R., Koelsch, G., Bilcer, G., Tang, J., 2006. Design, synthesis and X-ray structure of protein–ligand complexes: important insight into selectivity of memapsin 2 (β-secretase) inhibitors. J. Am. Chem. Soc. 128, 5310–5311.

Ghosh, A., Gemma, S., Tang, J., 2008. β-Secretase as a therapeutic target for Alzheimer's disease. Neurotherapeutics 5, 399–408.

Ghosh, A.K., Brindisi, M., Tang, J., 2012. Developing beta-secretase inhibitors for treatment of Alzheimer's disease. J. Neurochem. 120 (Suppl. 1), 71–83.

Gilbert, E.J., 2013. 1,3-Oxazines as BACE1 and/or BACE2 inhibitors: a patent evaluation (WO2012156284). Expert Opin. Ther. Pat. 23, 1069–1073.

Gillman, K.W., Starrett Jr., J.E., Parker, M.F., Xie, K., Bronson, J.J., Marcin, L.R., McElhone, K.E., Bergstrom, C.P., Mate, R.A., Williams, R., Meredith Jr., J.E., Burton, C.R., Barten, D.M., Toyn, J.H., Roberts, S.B., Lentz, K.A., Houston, J.G., Zaczek, R., Albright, C.F., Decicco, C.P., Macor, J.E., Olson, R.E., 2010. Discovery and evaluation of BMS-708163, a potent, selective and orally bioavailable γ-secretase inhibitor. ACS Med. Chem. Lett. 1, 120–124.

Gilman, S., Koller, M., Black, R.S., Jenkins, L., Griffith, S.G., Fox, N.C., Eisner, L., Kirby, L., Rovira, M.B., Forette, F., Orgogozo, J.M., 2005. Clinical effects of Aβ immunization (AN1792) in patients with AD in an interrupted trial. Neurology 64, 1553–1562.

Gitter, B.D., Czilli, D.L., Li, W., Dieckman, D.K., Bender, M.H., Nissen, J.S., Mabry, T.E., Yin, T., Boggs, L.N., McClure, D.B., Little, S.P., Johnstone, E.M., Audia, J.E., May, P.C., Hyslop, P.A., 2004. P4-339 Stereoselective inhibition of amyloid β peptide secretion by LY450139, a novel functional gamma secretase inhibitor. Neurobiol. Aging 25 (Suppl. 2), S571.

Glenner, G.G., Wong, C.W., 1984a. Alzheimer's disease and Down's syndrome: sharing of a unique cerebrovascular amyloid fibril protein. Biochem. Biophys. Res. Commun. 122, 1131–1135.

Glenner, G.G., Wong, C.W., 1984b. Alzheimer's disease: initial report of the purification and characterization of a novel cerebrovascular amyloid protein. Biochem. Biophys. Res. Commun. 120, 885–890.

Goate, A., Chartier-Harlin, M.C., Mullan, M., Brown, J., Crawford, F., Fidani, L., Giuffra, L., Haynes, A., Irving, N., James, L., et al., 1991. Segregation of a missense mutation in the amyloid precursor protein gene with familial Alzheimer's disease. Nature 349, 704–706.

Golde, T.E., Koo, E.H., Felsenstein, K.M., Osborne, B.A., Miele, L., 2013. γ-Secretase inhibitors and modulators. Biochim. Biophys. Acta 1828, 2898–2907.

Gong, B., Vitolo, O.V., Trinchese, F., Liu, S., Shelanski, M., Arancio, O., 2004. Persistent improvement in synaptic and cognitive functions in an Alzheimer mouse model after rolipram treatment. J. Clin. Invest. 114, 1624–1634.

Gotz, J., Chen, F., van Dorpe, J., Nitsch, R.M., 2001. Formation of neurofibrillary tangles in P301l tau transgenic mice induced by Aβ 42 fibrils. Science 293, 1491–1495.

Gouras, G.K., Tsai, J., Naslund, J., Vincent, B., Edgar, M., Checler, F., Greenfield, J.P., Haroutunian, V., Buxbaum, J.D., Xu, H., Greengard, P., Relkin, N.R., 2000. Intraneuronal Aβ42 accumulation in human brain. Am. J. Pathol. 156, 15–20.

Haapasalo, A., Kovacs, D.M., 2011. The many substrates of presenilin/γ-secretase. J. Alzheimers Dis. 25, 3–28.

Haass, C., Selkoe, D.J., 2007. Soluble protein oligomers in neurodegeneration: lessons from the Alzheimer's amyloid β-peptide. Nat. Rev. Mol. Cell Biol. 8, 101–112.

Haass, C., Hung, A.Y., Schlossmacher, M.G., Teplow, D.B., Selkoe, D.J., 1993. β-Amyloid peptide and a 3-kDa fragment are derived by distinct cellular mechanisms. J. Biol. Chem. 268, 3021–3024.

Hamilton, A., Zamponi, G.W., Ferguson, S.S., 2015. Glutamate receptors function as scaffolds for the regulation of β-amyloid and cellular prion protein signaling complexes. Mol. Brain 8, 18.

Hardy, J., Allsop, D., 1991. Amyloid deposition as the central event in the aetiology of Alzheimer's disease. Trends Pharmacol. Sci. 12, 383–388.

Hardy, J.A., Higgins, G.A., 1992. Alzheimer's disease: the amyloid cascade hypothesis. Science 256, 184–185.

Hardy, J., Selkoe, D.J., 2002. The amyloid hypothesis of Alzheimer's disease: progress and problems on the road to therapeutics. Science 297, 353–356.

Hashimoto, T., Ishibashi, A., Hagiwara, H., Murata, Y., Takenaka, O., Miyagawa, T., 2010. E2012: a novel γ-secretase modulator-pharmacology part. Alzheimer's Dement. J. Alzheimer's Assoc. 6, S242.

Hebert, L., 2007. American College of Neuropsychopharmacology.

Henley, D.B., May, P.C., Dean, R.A., Siemers, E.R., 2009. Development of semagacestat (LY450139), a functional γ-secretase inhibitor, for the treatment of Alzheimer's disease. Expert Opin. Pharmacother. 10, 1657–1664.

Higaki, J., Quon, D., Zhong, Z., Cordell, B., 1995. Inhibition of β-amyloid formation identifies proteolytic precursors and subcellular site of catabolism. Neuron 14, 651–659.

Holmes, C., Boche, D., Wilkinson, D., Yadegarfar, G., Hopkins, V., Bayer, A., Jones, R.W., Bullock, R., Love, S., Neal, J.W., Zotova, E., Nicoll, J.A., 2008. Long-term effects of Aβ42 immunisation in Alzheimer's disease: follow-up of a randomised, placebo-controlled phase I trial. Lancet 372, 216–223.

Hong, L., Koelsch, G., Lin, X., Wu, S., Terzyan, S., Ghosh, A.K., Zhang, X.C., Tang, J., 2000. Structure of the protease domain of memapsin 2 (β-secretase) complexed with inhibitor. Science 290, 150–153.

Hopkins, C.R., 2012. ACS chemical neuroscience molecule spotlight on Begacestat (GSI-953). ACS Chem. Neurosci. 3, 3–4.
Huang, D., Liu, Y., Shi, B., Li, Y., Wang, G., Liang, G., 2013. Comprehensive 3D-QSAR and binding mode of BACE-1 inhibitors using R-group search and molecular docking. J. Mol. Graph. Model. 45, 65–83.
Hubin, E., van Nuland, N.A., Broersen, K., Pauwels, K., 2014. Transient dynamics of Aβ contribute to toxicity in Alzheimer's disease. Cell Mol. Life Sci. 71, 3507–3521.
Hudry, E., Dashkoff, J., Roe, A.D., Takeda, S., Koffie, R.M., Hashimoto, T., Scheel, M., Spires-Jones, T., Arbel-Ornath, M., Betensky, R., Davidson, B.L., Hyman, B.T., 2013. Gene transfer of human Apoe isoforms results in differential modulation of amyloid deposition and neurotoxicity in mouse brain. Sci. Transl. Med. 5, 212ra161.
Iserloh, U., Wu, Y., Cumming, J.N., Pan, J., Wang, L.Y., Stamford, A.W., Kennedy, M.E., Kuvelkar, R., Chen, X., Parker, E.M., Strickland, C., Voigt, J., 2008. Potent pyrrolidine- and piperidine-based BACE-1 inhibitors. Bioorg. Med. Chem. Lett. 18, 414–417.
Iulita, M.F., Allard, S., Richter, L., Munter, L.M., Ducatenzeiler, A., Weise, C., Do Carmo, S., Klein, W.L., Multhaup, G., Cuello, A.C., 2014. Intracellular Aβ pathology and early cognitive impairments in a transgenic rat overexpressing human amyloid precursor protein: a multidimensional study. Acta Neuropathol. Commun. 2, 61.
Jack Jr., C.R., Knopman, D.S., Jagust, W.J., Petersen, R.C., Weiner, M.W., Aisen, P.S., Shaw, L.M., Vemuri, P., Wiste, H.J., Weigand, S.D., Lesnick, T.G., Pankratz, V.S., Donohue, M.C., Trojanowski, J.Q., 2013. Tracking pathophysiological processes in Alzheimer's disease: an updated hypothetical model of dynamic biomarkers. Lancet Neurol. 12, 207–216.
Jan, A., Adolfsson, O., Allaman, I., Buccarello, A.L., Magistretti, P.J., Pfeifer, A., Muhs, A., Lashuel, H.A., 2011. Aβ42 neurotoxicity is mediated by ongoing nucleated polymerization process rather than by discrete Aβ42 species. J. Biol. Chem. 286, 8585–8596.
Jia, Q., Deng, Y., Qing, H., 2014. Potential therapeutic strategies for Alzheimer's disease targeting or beyond β-amyloid: insights from clinical trials. BioMed. Res. Int. 2014, 837157.
Jiang, Y., Mullaney, K.A., Peterhoff, C.M., Che, S., Schmidt, S.D., Boyer-Boiteau, A., Ginsberg, S.D., Cataldo, A.M., Mathews, P.M., Nixon, R.A., 2010. Alzheimer's-related endosome dysfunction in Down syndrome is Aβ-independent but requires APP and is reversed by BACE-1 inhibition. Proc. Natl. Acad. Sci. U.S.A. 107, 1630–1635.
Johnston, J.A., Liu, W.W., Todd, S.A., Coulson, D.T., Murphy, S., Irvine, G.B., Passmore, A.P., 2005. Expression and activity of β-site amyloid precursor protein cleaving enzyme in Alzheimer's disease. Biochem. Soc. Trans. 33, 1096–1100.
Jones, S., Thornton, J.M., 1996. Principles of protein-protein interactions. Proc. Natl. Acad. Sci. U.S.A. 93, 13–20.
Kang, J., Lemaire, H.G., Unterbeck, A., Salbaum, J.M., Masters, C.L., Grzeschik, K.H., Multhaup, G., Beyreuther, K., Muller-Hill, B., 1987. The precursor of Alzheimer's disease amyloid A4 protein resembles a cell-surface receptor. Nature 325, 733–736.
Karch, C.M., Goate, A.M., 2015. Alzheimer's disease risk genes and mechanisms of disease pathogenesis. Biol. Psychiatry 77, 43–51.
Karran, E., Hardy, J., 2014. A critique of the drug discovery and phase 3 clinical programs targeting the amyloid hypothesis for Alzheimer disease. Ann. Neurol. 76, 185–205.
Kerchner, G.A., Boxer, A.L., 2010. Bapineuzumab. Expert Opin. Biol. Ther. 10, 1121–1130.
Keskin, O., Gursoy, A., Ma, B., Nussinov, R., 2008. Principles of protein-protein interactions: what are the preferred ways for proteins to interact? Chem. Rev. 108, 1225–1244.
Kim, J.E., Lee, M., 2003. Fullerene inhibits β-amyloid peptide aggregation. Biochem. Biophys. Res. Commun. 303, 576–579.
Kim, J., Onstead, L., Randle, S., Price, R., Smithson, L., Zwizinski, C., Dickson, D.W., Golde, T., McGowan, E., 2007. Aβ40 inhibits amyloid deposition in vivo. J. Neurosci. 27, 627–633.
Kim, J., Castellano, J.M., Jiang, H., Basak, J.M., Parsadanian, M., Pham, V., Mason, S.M., Paul, S.M., Holtzman, D.M., 2009. Overexpression of low-density lipoprotein receptor in the brain markedly inhibits amyloid deposition and increases extracellular A β clearance. Neuron 64, 632–644.
Kim, J., Jiang, H., Park, S., Eltorai, A.E., Stewart, F.R., Yoon, H., Basak, J.M., Finn, M.B., Holtzman, D.M., 2011. Haploinsufficiency of human APOE reduces amyloid deposition in a mouse model of amyloid-β amyloidosis. J. Neurosci. 31, 18007–18012.
Kim, J., Eltorai, A.E., Jiang, H., Liao, F., Verghese, P.B., Kim, J., Stewart, F.R., Basak, J.M., Holtzman, D.M., 2012. Anti-apoE immunotherapy inhibits amyloid accumulation in a transgenic mouse model of Aβ amyloidosis. J. Exp. Med. 209, 2149–2156.

Kimberly, W.T., Xia, W., Rahmati, T., Wolfe, M.S., Selkoe, D.J., 2000. The transmembrane aspartates in presenilin 1 and 2 are obligatory for γ-secretase activity and amyloid β-protein generation. J. Biol. Chem. 275, 3173–3178.
Kimberly, W.T., LaVoie, M.J., Ostaszewski, B.L., Ye, W., Wolfe, M.S., Selkoe, D.J., 2003. γ-secretase is a membrane protein complex comprised of presenilin, nicastrin, Aph-1, and Pen-2. Proc. Natl. Acad. Sci. U.S.A. 100, 6382–6387.
Kimura, T., Hamada, Y., Stochaj, M., Ikari, H., Nagamine, A., Abdel-Rahman, H., Igawa, N., Hidaka, K., Nguyen, J.-T., Saito, K., Hayashi, Y., Kiso, Y., 2006. Design and synthesis of potent β-secretase (BACE1) inhibitors with carboxylic acid bioisosteres. Bioorg. Med. Chem. Lett. 16, 2380–2386.
King, M.E., Kan, H.M., Baas, P.W., Erisir, A., Glabe, C.G., Bloom, G.S., 2006. Tau-dependent microtubule disassembly initiated by prefibrillar β-amyloid. J. Cell Biol. 175, 541–546.
Klafki, H., Abramowski, D., Swoboda, R., Paganetti, P.A., Staufenbiel, M., 1996. The carboxyl termini of β-amyloid peptides 1-40 and 1-42 are generated by distinct γ-secretase activities. J. Biol. Chem. 271, 28655–28659.
Koffie, R.M., Meyer-Luehmann, M., Hashimoto, T., Adams, K.W., Mielke, M.L., Garcia-Alloza, M., Micheva, K.D., Smith, S.J., Kim, M.L., Lee, V.M., Hyman, B.T., Spires-Jones, T.L., 2009. Oligomeric amyloid β associates with postsynaptic densities and correlates with excitatory synapse loss near senile plaques. Proc. Natl. Acad. Sci. U.S.A. 106, 4012–4017.
Krinsky-McHale, S.J., Devenny, D.A., Gu, H., Jenkins, E.C., Kittler, P., Murty, V.V., Schupf, N., Scotto, L., Tycko, B., Urv, T.K., Ye, L., Zigman, W.B., Silverman, W., 2008. Successful aging in a 70-year-old man with down syndrome: a case study. Intellect. Dev. Disabil. 46, 215–228.
Kumar-Singh, S., Theuns, J., Van Broeck, B., Pirici, D., Vennekens, K., Corsmit, E., Cruts, M., Dermaut, B., Wang, R., Van Broeckhoven, C., 2006. Mean age-of-onset of familial Alzheimer disease caused by presenilin mutations correlates with both increased Aβ42 and decreased Aβ40. Hum. Mutat. 27, 686–695.
Kuperstein, I., Broersen, K., Benilova, I., Rozenski, J., Jonckheere, W., Debulpaep, M., Vandersteen, A., Segers-Nolten, I., Van Der Werf, K., Subramaniam, V., Braeken, D., Callewaert, G., Bartic, C., D'Hooge, R., Martins, I.C., Rousseau, F., Schymkowitz, J., De Strooper, B., 2010. Neurotoxicity of Alzheimer's disease Aβ peptides is induced by small changes in the Aβ42 to Aβ40 ratio. EMBO J. 29, 3408–3420.
Ladiwala, A.R., Litt, J., Kane, R.S., Aucoin, D.S., Smith, S.O., Ranjan, S., Davis, J., Van Nostrand, W.E., Tessier, P.M., 2012. Conformational differences between two amyloid beta oligomers of similar size and dissimilar toxicity. J. Biol. Chem. 287, 24765–24773.
Lanz, T.A., Himes, C.S., Pallante, G., Adams, L., Yamazaki, S., Amore, B., Merchant, K.M., 2003. The γ-secretase inhibitor N-[N-(3,5-difluorophenacetyl)-L-alanyl]-S-phenylglycine t-butyl ester reduces A β levels in vivo in plasma and cerebrospinal fluid in young (plaque-free) and aged (plaque-bearing) Tg2576 mice. J. Pharmacol. Exp. Ther. 305, 864–871.
Lauren, J., Gimbel, D.A., Nygaard, H.B., Gilbert, J.W., Strittmatter, S.M., 2009. Cellular prion protein mediates impairment of synaptic plasticity by amyloid-β oligomers. Nature 457, 1128–1132.
Lemere, C.A., Masliah, E., 2010. Can Alzheimer disease be prevented by amyloid-β immunotherapy? Nat. Rev. Neurol. 6, 108–119.
Leon, W.C., Canneva, F., Partridge, V., Allard, S., Ferretti, M.T., DeWilde, A., Vercauteren, F., Atifeh, R., Ducatenzeiler, A., Klein, W., Szyf, M., Alhonen, L., Cuello, A.C., 2010. A novel transgenic rat model with a full Alzheimer's-like amyloid pathology displays pre-plaque intracellular amyloid-beta-associated cognitive impairment. J. Alzheimers Dis. 20, 113–126.
Leroy, K., Ando, K., Laporte, V., Dedecker, R., Suain, V., Authelet, M., Heraud, C., Pierrot, N., Yilmaz, Z., Octave, J.N., Brion, J.P., 2012. Lack of tau proteins rescues neuronal cell death and decreases amyloidogenic processing of APP in APP/PS1 mice. Am. J. Pathol. 181, 1928–1940.
Lesne, S., Koh, M.T., Kotilinek, L., Kayed, R., Glabe, C.G., Yang, A., Gallagher, M., Ashe, K.H., 2006. A specific amyloid-beta protein assembly in the brain impairs memory. Nature 440, 352–357.
Levy-Lahad, E., Wasco, W., Poorkaj, P., Romano, D.M., Oshima, J., Pettingell, W.H., Yu, C.E., Jondro, P.D., Schmidt, S.D., Wang, K., et al., 1995. Candidate gene for the chromosome 1 familial Alzheimer's disease locus. Science 269, 973–977.
Leyhe, T., Andreasen, N., Simeoni, M., Reich, A., von Arnim, C.A., Tong, X., Yeo, A., Khan, S., Loercher, A., Chalker, M., Hottenstein, C., Zetterberg, H., Hilpert, J., Mistry, P., 2014. Modulation of β-amyloid by a single dose of GSK933776 in patients with mild Alzheimer's disease: a phase I study. Alzheimer's Res. Ther. 6, 19.
Li, Y.M., Xu, M., Lai, M.T., Huang, Q., Castro, J.L., DiMuzio-Mower, J., Harrison, T., Lellis, C., Nadin, A., Neduvelil, J.G., Register, R.B., Sardana, M.K., Shearman, M.S., Smith, A.L., Shi, X.P., Yin, K.C., Shafer, J.A., Gardell, S.J., 2000. Photoactivated γ-secretase inhibitors directed to the active site covalently label presenilin 1. Nature 405, 689–694.

Liao, F., Hori, Y., Hudry, E., Bauer, A.Q., Jiang, H., Mahan, T.E., Lefton, K.B., Zhang, T.J., Dearborn, J.T., Kim, J., Culver, J.P., Betensky, R., Wozniak, D.F., Hyman, B.T., Holtzman, D.M., 2014. Anti-ApoE antibody given after plaque onset decreases Aβ accumulation and improves brain function in a mouse model of Aβ amyloidosis. J. Neurosci. 34, 7281–7292.

Lloret, A., Badia, M.C., Giraldo, E., Ermak, G., Alonso, M.D., Pallardo, F.V., Davies, K.J., Vina, J., 2011. Amyloid-β toxicity and tau hyperphosphorylation are linked via RCAN1 in Alzheimer's disease. J. Alzheimers Dis. 27, 701–709.

Lo Conte, L., Chothia, C., Janin, J., 1999. The atomic structure of protein-protein recognition sites. J. Mol. Biol. 285, 2177–2198.

Lu, Y., Riddell, D., Hajos-Korcsok, E., Bales, K., Wood, K.M., Nolan, C.E., Robshaw, A.E., Zhang, L., Leung, L., Becker, S.L., Tseng, E., Barricklow, J., Miller, E.H., Osgood, S., O'Neill, B.T., Brodney, M.A., Johnson, D.S., Pettersson, M., 2012. Cerebrospinal fluid amyloid-β (Aβ) as an effect biomarker for brain Aβ lowering verified by quantitative preclinical analyses. J. Pharmacol. Exp. Ther. 342, 366–375.

Luo, Y., Bolon, B., Kahn, S., Bennett, B.D., Babu-Khan, S., Denis, P., Fan, W., Kha, H., Zhang, J., Gong, Y., Martin, L., Louis, J.C., Yan, Q., Richards, W.G., Citron, M., Vassar, R., 2001. Mice deficient in BACE1, the Alzheimer's β-secretase, have normal phenotype and abolished β-amyloid generation. Nat. Neurosci. 4, 231–232.

Maji, S.K., Ogorzalek Loo, R.R., Inayathullah, M., Spring, S.M., Vollers, S.S., Condron, M.M., Bitan, G., Loo, J.A., Teplow, D.B., 2009. Amino acid position-specific contributions to amyloid β-protein oligomerization. J. Biol. Chem. 284, 23580–23591.

Mandel, S.A., Amit, T., Weinreb, O., Reznichenko, L., Youdim, M.B., 2008. Simultaneous manipulation of multiple brain targets by green tea catechins: a potential neuroprotective strategy for Alzheimer and Parkinson diseases. CNS Neurosci. Ther. 14, 352–365.

Marcade, M., Bourdin, J., Loiseau, N., Peillon, H., Rayer, A., Drouin, D., Schweighoffer, F., Desire, L., 2008. Etazolate, a neuroprotective drug linking GABA(A) receptor pharmacology to amyloid precursor protein processing. J. Neurochem. 106, 392–404.

Martins, I.C., Kuperstein, I., Wilkinson, H., Maes, E., Vanbrabant, M., Jonckheere, W., Van Gelder, P., Hartmann, D., D'Hooge, R., De Strooper, B., Schymkowitz, J., Rousseau, F., 2008. Lipids revert inert Aβ amyloid fibrils to neurotoxic protofibrils that affect learning in mice. EMBO J. 27, 224–233.

Martone, R.L., Zhou, H., Atchison, K., Comery, T., Xu, J.Z., Huang, X., Gong, X., Jin, M., Kreft, A., Harrison, B., Mayer, S.C., Aschmies, S., Gonzales, C., Zaleska, M.M., Riddell, D.R., Wagner, E., Lu, P., Sun, S.C., Sonnenberg-Reines, J., Oganesian, A., Adkins, K., Leach, M.W., Clarke, D.W., Huryn, D., Abou-Gharbia, M., Magolda, R., Bard, J., Frick, G., Raje, S., Forlow, S.B., Balliet, C., Burczynski, M.E., Reinhart, P.H., Wan, H.I., Pangalos, M.N., Jacobsen, J.S., 2009. Begacestat (GSI-953): a novel, selective thiophene sulfonamide inhibitor of amyloid precursor protein γ-secretase for the treatment of Alzheimer's disease. J. Pharmacol. Exp. Ther. 331, 598–608.

Masters, C.L., Simms, G., Weinman, N.A., Multhaup, G., McDonald, B.L., Beyreuther, K., 1985. Amyloid plaque core protein in Alzheimer disease and Down syndrome. Proc. Natl. Acad. Sci. U.S.A. 82, 4245–4249.

Mathis, C.A., Kuller, L.H., Klunk, W.E., Snitz, B.E., Price, J.C., Weissfeld, L.A., Rosario, B.L., Lopresti, B.J., Saxton, J.A., Aizenstein, H.J., McDade, E.M., Kamboh, M.I., DeKosky, S.T., Lopez, O.L., 2013. In vivo assessment of amyloid-β deposition in nondemented very elderly subjects. Ann. Neurol. 73, 751–761.

Mayer, S.C., Kreft, A.F., Harrison, B., Abou-Gharbia, M., Antane, M., Aschmies, S., Atchison, K., Chlenov, M., Cole, D.C., Comery, T., Diamantidis, G., Ellingboe, J., Fan, K., Galante, R., Gonzales, C., Ho, D.M., Hoke, M.E., Hu, Y., Huryn, D., Jain, U., Jin, M., Kremer, K., Kubrak, D., Lin, M., Lu, P., Magolda, R., Martone, R., Moore, W., Oganesian, A., Pangalos, M.N., Porte, A., Reinhart, P., Resnick, L., Riddell, D.R., Sonnenberg-Reines, J., Stock, J.R., Sun, S.C., Wagner, E., Wang, T., Woller, K., Xu, Z., Zaleska, M.M., Zeldis, J., Zhang, M., Zhou, H., Jacobsen, J.S., 2008. Discovery of begacestat, a notch-1-sparing γ-secretase inhibitor for the treatment of Alzheimer's disease. J. Med. Chem.

McLaurin, J., Cecal, R., Kierstead, M.E., Tian, X., Phinney, A.L., Manea, M., French, J.E., Lambermon, M.H., Darabie, A.A., Brown, M.E., Janus, C., Chishti, M.A., Horne, P., Westaway, D., Fraser, P.E., Mount, H.T., Przybylski, M., St George-Hyslop, P., 2002. Therapeutically effective antibodies against amyloid-β peptide target amyloid-β residues 4-10 and inhibit cytotoxicity and fibrillogenesis. Nat. Med. 8, 1263–1269.

McLaurin, J., Kierstead, M.E., Brown, M.E., Hawkes, C.A., Lambermon, M.H., Phinney, A.L., Darabie, A.A., Cousins, J.E., French, J.E., Lan, M.F., Chen, F., Wong, S.S., Mount, H.T., Fraser, P.E., Westaway, D., St George-Hyslop, P., 2006. Cyclohexanehexol inhibitors of Aβ aggregation prevent and reverse Alzheimer phenotype in a mouse model. Nat. Med. 12, 801–808.

Milano, J., McKay, J., Dagenais, C., Foster-Brown, L., Pognan, F., Gadient, R., Jacobs, R.T., Zacco, A., Greenberg, B., Ciaccio, P.J., 2004. Modulation of notch processing by γ-secretase inhibitors causes intestinal goblet cell metaplasia and induction of genes known to specify gut secretory lineage differentiation. Toxicol. Sci. 82, 341–358.

Mitani, Y., Yarimizu, J., Saita, K., Uchino, H., Akashiba, H., Shitaka, Y., Ni, K., Matsuoka, N., 2012. Differential effects between γ-secretase inhibitors and modulators on cognitive function in amyloid precursor protein-transgenic and nontransgenic mice. J. Neurosci. 32, 2037–2050.

Mullan, M., Crawford, F., Axelman, K., Houlden, H., Lilius, L., Winblad, B., Lannfelt, L., 1992. A pathogenic mutation for probable Alzheimer's disease in the *APP gene* at the N-terminus of β-amyloid. Nat. Genet. 1, 345–347.

Nakano-Ito, K., Fujikawa, Y., Hihara, T., Shinjo, H., Kotani, S., Suganuma, A., Aoki, T., Tsukidate, K., 2014. E2012-induced cataract and its predictive biomarkers. Toxicol. Sci. 137, 249–258.

Ness, D.K., Boggs, L.N., Hepburn, D.L., Gitter, B., Long, G.G., May, P.C., Piroozi, K.S., Schafer, K.A., Yang, Z., 2004. P2-053 Reduced β-amyloid burden, increased C-99 concentrations and evaluation of neuropathology in the brains of PDAPP mice given LY450139 dihydrate daily by gavage for 5 months. Neurobiol. Aging 25, S238–S239.

Nie, Q., Du, X.-G., Geng, M.-Y., 2011. Small molecule inhibitors of amyloid β peptide aggregation as a potential therapeutic strategy for Alzheimer's disease. Acta Pharmacol. Sin. 32, 545–551.

Obregon, D.F., Rezai-Zadeh, K., Bai, Y., Sun, N., Hou, H., Ehrhart, J., Zeng, J., Mori, T., Arendash, G.W., Shytle, D., Town, T., Tan, J., 2006. ADAM10 activation is required for green tea (-)-epigallocatechin-3-gallate-induced α-secretase cleavage of amyloid precursor protein. J. Biol. Chem. 281, 16419–16427.

Oliveira, J.M., Henriques, A.G., Martins, F., Rebelo, S., da Cruz e Silva, O.A., 2015. Amyloid-β modulates both AβPP and tau phosphorylation. J. Alzheimers Dis.

Olson, R.E., Albright, C.F., 2008. Recent progress in the medicinal chemistry of γ-secretase inhibitors. Curr. Top. Med. Chem. 8, 17–33.

Orgogozo, J.M., Gilman, S., Dartigues, J.F., Laurent, B., Puel, M., Kirby, L.C., Jouanny, P., Dubois, B., Eisner, L., Flitman, S., Michel, B.F., Boada, M., Frank, A., Hock, C., 2003. Subacute meningoencephalitis in a subset of patients with AD after Aβ42 immunization. Neurology 61, 46–54.

Panza, F., Solfrizzi, V., Imbimbo, B.P., Giannini, M., Santamato, A., Seripa, D., Logroscino, G., 2014. Efficacy and safety studies of gantenerumab in patients with Alzheimer's disease. Expert Rev. Neurother. 14, 973–986.

Permanne, B., Adessi, C., Saborio, G.P., Fraga, S., Frossard, M.J., Van Dorpe, J., Dewachter, I., Banks, W.A., Van Leuven, F., Soto, C., 2002. Reduction of amyloid load and cerebral damage in a transgenic mouse model of Alzheimer's disease by treatment with a β-sheet breaker peptide. FASEB J. 16, 860–862.

Peters, C., Espinoza, M.P., Gallegos, S., Opazo, C., Aguayo, L.G., 2015. Alzheimer's Aβ interacts with cellular prion protein inducing neuronal membrane damage and synaptotoxicity. Neurobiol. Aging 36, 1369–1377.

Portelius, E., Van Broeck, B., Andreasson, U., Gustavsson, M.K., Mercken, M., Zetterberg, H., Borghys, H., Blennow, K., 2010. Acute effect on the Aβ isoform pattern in CSF in response to γ-secretase modulator and inhibitor treatment in dogs. J. Alzheimers Dis. 21, 1005–1012.

Postina, R., 2012. Activation of α-secretase cleavage. J. Neurochem. 120 (Suppl. 1), 46–54.

Pradier, L., Cohen, C., Blanchard, V., Debeir, T., Barneoud, P., Canton, T., Menager, J., Bohme, A., Rooney, T., Guillet, M.-C., Cameron, B., Shi, Y., Naimi, S., Ravetch, J., Claudel, S., Alam, J., 2013. SAR228810: an antiprotofibrillar β-amyloid antibody designed to reduce risk of amyloid-related imaging abnormalities (ARIA). Alzheimers Dement. J. Alzheimers Assoc. 9, P808–P809.

Price, J.L., McKeel Jr., D.W., Buckles, V.D., Roe, C.M., Xiong, C., Grundman, M., Hansen, L.A., Petersen, R.C., Parisi, J.E., Dickson, D.W., Smith, C.D., Davis, D.G., Schmitt, F.A., Markesbery, W.R., Kaye, J., Kurlan, R., Hulette, C., Kurland, B.F., Higdon, R., Kukull, W., Morris, J.C., 2009. Neuropathology of nondemented aging: presumptive evidence for preclinical Alzheimer disease. Neurobiol. Aging 30, 1026–1036.

Rajapakse, H.A., Nantermet, P.G., Selnick, H.G., Munshi, S., McGaughey, G.B., Lindsley, S.R., Young, M.B., Lai, M.-T., Espeseth, A.S., Shi, X.-P., Colussi, D., Pietrak, B., Crouthamel, M.-C., Tugusheva, K., Huang, Q., Xu, M., Simon, A.J., Kuo, L., Hazuda, D.J., Graham, S., Vacca, J.P., 2006. Discovery of oxadiazoyl tertiary carbinamine inhibitors of β-secretase (BACE-1). J. Med. Chem. 49, 7270–7273.

Rapoport, M., Dawson, H.N., Binder, L.I., Vitek, M.P., Ferreira, A., 2002. Tau is essential to β-amyloid-induced neurotoxicity. Proc. Natl. Acad. Sci. U.S.A. 99, 6364–6369.

Reiman, E.M., Quiroz, Y.T., Fleisher, A.S., Chen, K., Velez-Pardo, C., Jimenez-Del-Rio, M., Fagan, A.M., Shah, A.R., Alvarez, S., Arbelaez, A., Giraldo, M., Acosta-Baena, N., Sperling, R.A., Dickerson, B., Stern, C.E., Tirado, V., Munoz, C., Reiman, R.A., Huentelman, M.J., Alexander, G.E., Langbaum, J.B., Kosik, K.S., Tariot, P.N., Lopera, F., 2012. Brain imaging and fluid biomarker analysis in young adults at genetic risk for autosomal dominant Alzheimer's disease in the presenilin 1 E280A kindred: a case-control study. Lancet Neurol. 11, 1048–1056.

Rezaei-Ghaleh, N., Giller, K., Becker, S., Zweckstetter, M., 2011. Effect of zinc binding on β-amyloid structure and dynamics: implications for Aβ aggregation. Biophys. J. 101, 1202–1211.

Roberds, S.L., Anderson, J., Basi, G., Bienkowski, M.J., Branstetter, D.G., Chen, K.S., Freedman, S.B., Frigon, N.L., Games, D., Hu, K., Johnson-Wood, K., Kappenman, K.E., Kawabe, T.T., Kola, I., Kuehn, R., Lee, M., Liu, W., Motter, R., Nichols, N.F., Power, M., Robertson, D.W., Schenk, D., Schoor, M., Shopp, G.M., Shuck, M.E., Sinha, S., Svensson, K.A., Tatsuno, G., Tintrup, H., Wijsman, J., Wright, S., McConlogue, L., 2001. BACE knockout mice are healthy despite lacking the primary beta-secretase activity in brain: implications for Alzheimer's disease therapeutics. Hum. Mol. Genet. 10, 1317–1324.

Roberson, E.D., Scearce-Levie, K., Palop, J.J., Yan, F., Cheng, I.H., Wu, T., Gerstein, H., Yu, G.Q., Mucke, L., 2007. Reducing endogenous tau ameliorates amyloid β-induced deficits in an Alzheimer's disease mouse model. Science 316, 750–754.

Rochette, M.J., Murphy, M.P., 2002. γ-secretase: substrates and inhibitors. Mol. Neurobiol. 26, 81–95.

Rogaev, E.I., Sherrington, R., Rogaeva, E.A., Levesque, G., Ikeda, M., Liang, Y., Chi, H., Lin, C., Holman, K., Tsuda, T., et al., 1995. Familial Alzheimer's disease in kindreds with missense mutations in a gene on chromosome 1 related to the Alzheimer's disease type 3 gene. Nature 376, 775–778.

Salloway, S., Sperling, R., Gilman, S., Fox, N.C., Blennow, K., Raskind, M., Sabbagh, M., Honig, L.S., Doody, R., van Dyck, C.H., Mulnard, R., Barakos, J., Gregg, K.M., Liu, E., Lieberburg, I., Schenk, D., Black, R., Grundman, M., I. Bapineuzumab 201 Clinical Trial, 2009. A phase 2 multiple ascending dose trial of bapineuzumab in mild to moderate Alzheimer disease. Neurology 73, 2061–2070.

Salloway, S., Sperling, R., Fox, N.C., Blennow, K., Klunk, W., Raskind, M., Sabbagh, M., Honig, L.S., Porsteinsson, A.P., Ferris, S., Reichert, M., Ketter, N., Nejadnik, B., Guenzler, V., Miloslavsky, M., Wang, D., Lu, Y., Lull, J., Tudor, I.C., Liu, E., Grundman, M., Yuen, E., Black, R., Brashear, H.R., Bapineuzumab, Clinical Trial Investigators, 2014. Two phase 3 trials of bapineuzumab in mild-to-moderate Alzheimer's disease. N. Engl. J. Med. 370, 322–333.

Sato, T., Diehl, T.S., Narayanan, S., Funamoto, S., Ihara, Y., De Strooper, B., Steiner, H., Haass, C., Wolfe, M.S., 2007. Active γ-secretase complexes contain only one of each component. J. Biol. Chem. 282, 33985–33993.

Schenk, D., Barbour, R., Dunn, W., Gordon, G., Grajeda, H., Guido, T., Hu, K., Huang, J., Johnson-Wood, K., Khan, K., Kholodenko, D., Lee, M., Liao, Z., Lieberburg, I., Motter, R., Mutter, L., Soriano, F., Shopp, G., Vasquez, N., Vandevert, C., Walker, S., Wogulis, M., Yednock, T., Games, D., Seubert, P., 1999. Immunization with amyloid-β attenuates Alzheimer-disease-like pathology in the PDAPP mouse. Nature 400, 173–177.

Schmidt, B., 2003. Aspartic proteases involved in Alzheimer's disease. Chembiochem 4, 366–378.

Seiffert, D., Bradley, J.D., Rominger, C.M., Rominger, D.H., Yang, F., Meredith Jr., J.E., Wang, Q., Roach, A.H., Thompson, L.A., Spitz, S.M., Higaki, J.N., Prakash, S.R., Combs, A.P., Copeland, R.A., Arneric, S.P., Hartig, P.R., Robertson, D.W., Cordell, B., Stern, A.M., Olson, R.E., Zaczek, R., 2000. Presenilin-1 and -2 are molecular targets for γ-secretase inhibitors. J. Biol. Chem. 275, 34086–34091.

Selkoe, D.J., 2001. Alzheimer's disease: genes, proteins, and therapy. Physiol. Rev. 81, 741–766.

Selkoe, D.J., 2011. Resolving controversies on the path to Alzheimer's therapeutics. Nat. Med. 17, 1060–1065.

Sennvik, K., Fastbom, J., Blomberg, M., Wahlund, L.O., Winblad, B., Benedikz, E., 2000. Levels of α- and β-secretase cleaved amyloid precursor protein in the cerebrospinal fluid of Alzheimer's disease patients. Neurosci. Lett. 278, 169–172.

Seubert, P., Vigo-Pelfrey, C., Esch, F., Lee, M., Dovey, H., Davis, D., Sinha, S., Schlossmacher, M., Whaley, J., Swindlehurst, C., et al., 1992. Isolation and quantification of soluble Alzheimer's beta-peptide from biological fluids. Nature 359, 325–327.

Shankar, G.M., Li, S., Mehta, T.H., Garcia-Munoz, A., Shepardson, N.E., Smith, I., Brett, F.M., Farrell, M.A., Rowan, M.J., Lemere, C.A., Regan, C.M., Walsh, D.M., Sabatini, B.L., Selkoe, D.J., 2008. Amyloid-β protein dimers isolated directly from Alzheimer's brains impair synaptic plasticity and memory. Nat. Med. 14, 837–842.

Shearman, M.S., Beher, D., Clarke, E.E., Lewis, H.D., Harrison, T., Hunt, P., Nadin, A., Smith, A.L., Stevenson, G., Castro, J.L., 2000. L-685,458, an aspartyl protease transition state mimic, is a potent inhibitor of amyloid beta-protein precursor gamma-secretase activity. Biochemistry 39, 8698–8704.

Sherrington, R., Rogaev, E.I., Liang, Y., Rogaeva, E.A., Levesque, G., Ikeda, M., Chi, H., Lin, C., Li, G., Holman, K., Tsuda, T., Mar, L., Foncin, J.F., Bruni, A.C., Montesi, M.P., Sorbi, S., Rainero, I., Pinessi, L., Nee, L., Chumakov, I., Pollen, D., Brookes, A., Sanseau, P., Polinsky, R.J., Wasco, W., Da Silva, H.A., Haines, J.L., Perkicak-Vance, M.A., Tanzi, R.E., Roses, A.D., Fraser, P.E., Rommens, J.M., St George-Hyslop, P.H., 1995. Cloning of a gene bearing missense mutations in early-onset familial Alzheimer's disease. Nature 375, 754–760.

Shipton, O.A., Leitz, J.R., Dworzak, J., Acton, C.E., Tunbridge, E.M., Denk, F., Dawson, H.N., Vitek, M.P., Wade-Martins, R., Paulsen, O., Vargas-Caballero, M., 2011. Tau protein is required for amyloid β-induced impairment of hippocampal long-term potentiation. J. Neurosci. 31, 1688–1692.

Siemers, E.R., Quinn, J.F., Kaye, J., Farlow, M.R., Porsteinsson, A., Tariot, P., Zoulnouni, P., Galvin, J.E., Holtzman, D.M., Knopman, D.S., Satterwhite, J., Gonzales, C., Dean, R.A., May, P.C., 2006. Effects of a γ-secretase inhibitor in a randomized study of patients with Alzheimer disease. Neurology 66, 602–604.

Sigurdsson, E.M., Permanne, B., Soto, C., Wisniewski, T., Frangione, B., 2000. In vivo reversal of amyloid-β lesions in rat brain. J. Neuropathol. Exp. Neurol. 59, 11–17.

Smith, R.D., Hu, L., Falkner, J.A., Benson, M.L., Nerothin, J.P., Carlson, H.A., 2006. Exploring protein-ligand recognition with Binding MOAD. J. Mol. Graph. Model. 24, 414–425.

Snitz, B.E., Weissfeld, L.A., Lopez, O.L., Kuller, L.H., Saxton, J., Singhabahu, D.M., Klunk, W.E., Mathis, C.A., Price, J.C., Ives, D.G., Cohen, A.D., McDade, E., Dekosky, S.T., 2013. Cognitive trajectories associated with β-amyloid deposition in the oldest-old without dementia. Neurology 80, 1378–1384.

Sommer, A.P., Bieschke, J., Friedrich, R.P., Zhu, D., Wanker, E.E., Fecht, H.J., Mereles, D., Hunstein, W., 2012. 670 nm laser light and EGCG complementarily reduce amyloid-β aggregates in human neuroblastoma cells: basis for treatment of Alzheimer's disease? Photomed. Laser Surg. 30, 54–60.

Sperling, R.A., Aisen, P.S., Beckett, L.A., Bennett, D.A., Craft, S., Fagan, A.M., Iwatsubo, T., Jack Jr., C.R., Kaye, J., Montine, T.J., Park, D.C., Reiman, E.M., Rowe, C.C., Siemers, E., Stern, Y., Yaffe, K., Carrillo, M.C., Thies, B., Morrison-Bogorad, M., Wagster, M.V., Phelps, C.H., 2011a. Toward defining the preclinical stages of Alzheimer's disease: recommendations from the National Institute on Aging-Alzheimer's Association workgroups on diagnostic guidelines for Alzheimer's disease. Alzheimers Dement. 7, 280–292.

Sperling, R.A., Jack Jr., C.R., Aisen, P.S., 2011b. Testing the right target and right drug at the right stage. Sci. Transl. Med. 3, 111cm133.

Spires-Jones, T.L., Mielke, M.L., Rozkalne, A., Meyer-Luehmann, M., de Calignon, A., Bacskai, B.J., Schenk, D., Hyman, B.T., 2009. Passive immunotherapy rapidly increases structural plasticity in a mouse model of Alzheimer disease. Neurobiol. Dis. 33, 213–220.

Squibb, B.-M., 2012. Statement on Avagacestat Development Status. http://www.bms.com/news/features/2012/Pages/AvagacestatDevelopmentStatus.aspx.

Sun, X., He, G., Qing, H., Zhou, W., Dobie, F., Cai, F., Staufenbiel, M., Huang, L.E., Song, W., 2006. Hypoxia facilitates Alzheimer's disease pathogenesis by up-regulating BACE1 gene expression. Proc. Natl. Acad. Sci. U.S.A. 103, 18727–18732.

Syme, C.D., Nadal, R.C., Rigby, S.E., Viles, J.H., 2004. Copper binding to the amyloid-β (Aβ) peptide associated with Alzheimer's disease: folding, coordination geometry, pH dependence, stoichiometry, and affinity of Aβ-(1-28): insights from a range of complementary spectroscopic techniques. J. Biol. Chem. 279, 18169–18177.

Takahashi, R.H., Milner, T.A., Li, F., Nam, E.E., Edgar, M.A., Yamaguchi, H., Beal, M.F., Xu, H., Greengard, P., Gouras, G.K., 2002. Intraneuronal Alzheimer aβ42 accumulates in multivesicular bodies and is associated with synaptic pathology. Am. J. Pathol. 161, 1869–1879.

Takahashi, R.H., Almeida, C.G., Kearney, P.F., Yu, F., Lin, M.T., Milner, T.A., Gouras, G.K., 2004. Oligomerization of Alzheimer's beta-amyloid within processes and synapses of cultured neurons and brain. J. Neurosci. 24, 3592–3599.

Takami, M., Nagashima, Y., Sano, Y., Ishihara, S., Morishima-Kawashima, M., Funamoto, S., Ihara, Y., 2009. γ-Secretase: successive tripeptide and tetrapeptide release from the transmembrane domain of β-carboxyl terminal fragment. J. Neurosci. 29, 13042–13052.

Tamagno, E., Guglielmotto, M., Aragno, M., Borghi, R., Autelli, R., Giliberto, L., Muraca, G., Danni, O., Zhu, X., Smith, M.A., Perry, G., Jo, D.G., Mattson, M.P., Tabaton, M., 2008. Oxidative stress activates a positive feedback between the γ- and β-secretase cleavages of the β-amyloid precursor protein. J. Neurochem. 104, 683–695.

Tanzi, R.E., Bertram, L., 2005. Twenty years of the Alzheimer's disease amyloid hypothesis: a genetic perspective. Cell 120, 545–555.

Teichmann, S.A., 2002. Principles of protein-protein interactions. Bioinformatics (Oxford, England) 18 (Suppl. 2), S249.

Tian, G., Sobotka-Briner, C.D., Zysk, J., Liu, X., Birr, C., Sylvester, M.A., Edwards, P.D., Scott, C.D., Greenberg, B.D., 2002. Linear non-competitive inhibition of solubilized human γ-secretase by pepstatin A methylester, L685458, sulfonamides, and benzodiazepines. J. Biol. Chem. 277, 31499–31505.

Tian, G., Ghanekar, S.V., Aharony, D., Shenvi, A.B., Jacobs, R.T., Liu, X., Greenberg, B.D., 2003. The mechanism of γ-secretase: multiple inhibitor binding sites for transition state analogs and small molecule inhibitors. J. Biol. Chem. 278, 28968–28975.

Tolia, A., De Strooper, B., 2009. Structure and function of γ-secretase. Semin. Cell Dev. Biol. 20, 211–218.

Tomiyama, T., Asano, S., Suwa, Y., Morita, T., Kataoka, K., Mori, H., Endo, N., 1994. Rifampicin prevents the aggregation and neurotoxicity of amyloid β protein in vitro. Biochem. Biophys. Res. Commun. 204, 76–83.

Tong, G., Wang, J.S., Sverdlov, O., Huang, S.P., Slemmon, R., Croop, R., Castaneda, L., Gu, H., Wong, O., Li, H., Berman, R.M., Smith, C., Albright, C.F., Dockens, R.C., 2012. Multicenter, randomized, double-blind, placebo-controlled, single-ascending dose study of the oral γ-secretase inhibitor BMS-708163 (Avagacestat): tolerability profile, pharmacokinetic parameters, and pharmacodynamic markers. Clin. Ther. 34, 654–667.

Tu, S., Okamoto, S., Lipton, S.A., Xu, H., 2014. Oligomeric Aβ-induced synaptic dysfunction in Alzheimer's disease. Mol. Neurodegener. 9, 48.

Turner, R.T., Koelsch, G., Hong, L., Castenheira, P., Ghosh, A., Tang, J., 2001. Subsite specificity of memapsin 2 (β-secretase): implications for inhibitor design. Biochemistry 40, 10001–10006.

Um, J.W., Nygaard, H.B., Heiss, J.K., Kostylev, M.A., Stagi, M., Vortmeyer, A., Wisniewski, T., Gunther, E.C., Strittmatter, S.M., 2012. Alzheimer amyloid-beta oligomer bound to postsynaptic prion protein activates Fyn to impair neurons. Nat. Neurosci. 15, 1227–1235.

Varga, E., Juhasz, G., Bozso, Z., Penke, B., Fulop, L., Szegedi, V., 2014. Aβ(1-42) enhances neuronal excitability in the CA1 via NR2B subunit-containing NMDA receptors. Neural Plast. 2014, 584314.

Vassar, R., 2014. BACE1 inhibitor drugs in clinical trials for Alzheimer's disease. Alzheimers Res. Ther. 6, 89.

Vellas, B., Sol, O., Snyder, P.J., Ousset, P.J., Haddad, R., Maurin, M., Lemarie, J.C., Desire, L., Pando, M.P., E.H.T. Study Group, 2011. EHT0202 in Alzheimer's disease: a 3-month, randomized, placebo-controlled, double-blind study. Curr. Alzheimer Res. 8, 203–212.

Vingtdeux, V., Marambaud, P., 2012. Identification and biology of α-secretase. J. Neurochem. 120 (Suppl. 1), 34–45.

Vossel, K.A., Zhang, K., Brodbeck, J., Daub, A.C., Sharma, P., Finkbeiner, S., Cui, B., Mucke, L., 2010. Tau reduction prevents Aβ-induced defects in axonal transport. Science 330, 198.

Walsh, D.M., Tseng, B.P., Rydel, R.E., Podlisny, M.B., Selkoe, D.J., 2000. The oligomerization of amyloid β-protein begins intracellularly in cells derived from human brain. Biochemistry 39, 10831–10839.

Walsh, D.M., Klyubin, I., Fadeeva, J.V., Cullen, W.K., Anwyl, R., Wolfe, M.S., Rowan, M.J., Selkoe, D.J., 2002a. Naturally secreted oligomers of amyloid β protein potently inhibit hippocampal long-term potentiation in vivo. Nature 416, 535–539.

Walsh, D.M., Klyubin, I., Fadeeva, J.V., Rowan, M.J., Selkoe, D.J., 2002b. Amyloid-β oligomers: their production, toxicity and therapeutic inhibition. Biochem. Soc. Trans. 30, 552–557.

Wang, R., Meschia, J.F., Cotter, R.J., Sisodia, S.S., 1991. Secretion of the β/A4 amyloid precursor protein. Identification of a cleavage site in cultured mammalian cells. J. Biol. Chem. 266, 16960–16964.

Wasmer, C., Lange, A., Van Melckebeke, H., Siemer, A.B., Riek, R., Meier, B.H., 2008. Amyloid fibrils of the HET-s(218-289) prion form a β solenoid with a triangular hydrophobic core. Science (New York) 319, 1523–1526.

Watt, A.D., Crespi, G.A., Down, R.A., Ascher, D.B., Gunn, A., Perez, K.A., McLean, C.A., Villemagne, V.L., Parker, M.W., Barnham, K.J., Miles, L.A., 2014. Do current therapeutic anti-Aβ antibodies for Alzheimer's disease engage the target? Acta Neuropathol. 127, 803–810.

Weggen, S., Eriksen, J.L., Das, P., Sagi, S.A., Wang, R., Pietrzik, C.U., Findlay, K.A., Smith, T.E., Murphy, M.P., Bulter, T., Kang, D.E., Marquez-Sterling, N., Golde, T.E., Koo, E.H., 2001. A subset of NSAIDs lower amyloidogenic Aβ42 independently of cyclooxygenase activity. Nature 414, 212–216.

Weggen, S., Eriksen, J.L., Sagi, S.A., Pietrzik, C.U., Ozols, V., Fauq, A., Golde, T.E., Koo, E.H., 2003. Evidence that non-steroidal anti-inflammatory drugs decrease amyloid β 42 production by direct modulation of gamma-secretase activity. J. Biol. Chem. 278, 31831–31837.

Weihofen, A., Lemberg, M.K., Friedmann, E., Rueeger, H., Schmitz, A., Paganetti, P., Rovelli, G., Martoglio, B., 2003. Targeting presenilin-type aspartic protease signal peptide peptidase with γ-secretase inhibitors. J. Biol. Chem. 278, 16528–16533.

Williams, T.L., Johnson, B.R., Urbanc, B., Jenkins, A.T., Connell, S.D., Serpell, L.C., 2011. Aβ42 oligomers, but not fibrils, simultaneously bind to and cause damage to ganglioside-containing lipid membranes. Biochem. J. 439, 67–77.

Willis, B., Martenyi, F., Dean, R., Lowe, S., Nakano, M., Monk, S., Gonzales, C., Mergott, D., Daugherty, L., Citron, M., May, P., 2012. Central BACE1 inhibition by LY2886721 produces opposing effects on APP processing as reflected by cerebrospinal fluid sAPP-α and sAPP-β. Alzheimers Dement. J. Alzheimers Assoc. 8, 95.

Winblad, B., Andreasen, N., Minthon, L., Floesser, A., Imbert, G., Dumortier, T., Maguire, R.P., Blennow, K., Lundmark, J., Staufenbiel, M., Orgogozo, J.M., Graf, A., 2012. Safety, tolerability, and antibody response of active Aβ immunotherapy with CAD106 in patients with Alzheimer's disease: randomised, double-blind, placebo-controlled, first-in-human study. Lancet Neurol. 11, 597–604.

Wirths, O., Multhaup, G., Czech, C., Feldmann, N., Blanchard, V., Tremp, G., Beyreuther, K., Pradier, L., Bayer, T.A., 2002. Intraneuronal APP/A β trafficking and plaque formation in β-amyloid precursor protein and presenilin-1 transgenic mice. Brain Pathol. 12, 275–286.

Wogulis, M., Wright, S., Cunningham, D., Chilcote, T., Powell, K., Rydel, R.E., 2005. Nucleation-dependent polymerization is an essential component of amyloid-mediated neuronal cell death. J. Neurosci. 25, 1071–1080.

Wolfe, M.S., Citron, M., Diehl, T.S., Xia, W., Donkor, I.O., Selkoe, D.J., 1998. A substrate-based difluoro ketone selectively inhibits Alzheimer's gamma-secretase activity. J. Med. Chem. 41, 6–9.

Wolfe, M.S., Xia, W., Ostaszewski, B.L., Diehl, T.S., Kimberly, W.T., Selkoe, D.J., 1999a. Two transmembrane aspartates in presenilin-1 required for presenilin endoproteolysis and γ-secretase activity. Nature 398, 513–517.

Wolfe, M.S., Xia, W., Moore, C.L., Leatherwood, D.D., Ostaszewski, B., Rahmati, T., Donkor, I.O., Selkoe, D.J., 1999b. Peptidomimetic probes and molecular modeling suggest that Alzheimer's γ-secretase is an intramembrane-cleaving aspartyl protease. Biochemistry 38, 4720–4727.

Wolfe, M.S., 2008. γ-secretase inhibition and modulation for Alzheimer's disease. Curr. Alzheimer Res. 5, 158–164.

Wozniak, M.A., Itzhaki, R.F., Shipley, S.J., Dobson, C.B., 2007. Herpes simplex virus infection causes cellular β-amyloid accumulation and secretase upregulation. Neurosci. Lett. 429, 95–100.

Xu, H., Greengard, P., Gandy, S., 1995. Regulated formation of Golgi secretory vesicles containing Alzheimer β-amyloid precursor protein. J. Biol. Chem. 270, 23243–23245.

Xu, H., Sweeney, D., Greengard, P., Gandy, S., 1996. Metabolism of Alzheimer β-amyloid precursor protein: regulation by protein kinase A in intact cells and in a cell-free system. Proc. Natl. Acad. Sci. U.S.A 93, 4081–4084.

Xue, S., Jia, L., Jia, J., 2006. Hypoxia and reoxygenation increased BACE1 mRNA and protein levels in human neuroblastoma SH-SY5Y cells. Neurosci. Lett. 405, 231–235.

Xue, W.F., Hellewell, A.L., Hewitt, E.W., Radford, S.E., 2010. Fibril fragmentation in amyloid assembly and cytotoxicity: when size matters. Prion 4, 20–25.

Yang, L.B., Lindholm, K., Yan, R., Citron, M., Xia, W., Yang, X.L., Beach, T., Sue, L., Wong, P., Price, D., Li, R., Shen, Y., 2003. Elevated β-secretase expression and enzymatic activity detected in sporadic Alzheimer disease. Nat. Med. 9, 3–4.

Yang, H., Guan, H., Yang, M., Liu, Z., Takeuchi, S., Yanagisawa, D., Vincent, S.R., Zhao, S., Tooyama, I., 2015. Upregulation of mitochondrial ferritin by proinflammatory cytokines: implications for a role in Alzheimer's disease. J. Alzheimers Dis. 45, 797–811.

Yin, Y.I., Bassit, B., Zhu, L., Yang, X., Wang, C., Li, Y.M., 2007. γ-Secretase substrate concentration modulates the Aβ42/Aβ40 ratio: implications for Alzheimer disease. J. Biol. Chem. 282, 23639–23644.

Yuan, J., Venkatraman, S., Zheng, Y., McKeever, B.M., Dillard, L.W., Singh, S.B., 2013. Structure-based design of β-site APP cleaving enzyme 1 (BACE1) inhibitors for the treatment of Alzheimer's disease. J. Med. Chem. 56, 4156–4180.

Zempel, H., Thies, E., Mandelkow, E., Mandelkow, E.M., 2010. Aβ oligomers cause localized Ca^{2+} elevation, missorting of endogenous Tau into dendrites, Tau phosphorylation, and destruction of microtubules and spines. J. Neurosci. 30, 11938–11950.

Zempel, H., Luedtke, J., Kumar, Y., Biernat, J., Dawson, H., Mandelkow, E., Mandelkow, E.M., 2013. Amyloid-β oligomers induce synaptic damage via Tau-dependent microtubule severing by TTLL6 and spastin. EMBO J. 32, 2920–2937.

Zhang, Y.W., Xu, H., 2007. Molecular and cellular mechanisms for Alzheimer's disease: understanding APP metabolism. Curr. Mol. Med. 7, 687–696.

Zhang, Y., Rempel, D.L., Zhang, J., Sharma, A.K., Mirica, L.M., Gross, M.L., 2013. Pulsed hydrogen-deuterium exchange mass spectrometry probes conformational changes in amyloid β (Aβ) peptide aggregation. Proc. Natl. Acad. Sci. U.S.A. 110, 14604–14609.

Zigman, W.B., Devenny, D.A., Krinsky-McHale, S.J., Jenkins, E.C., Urv, T.K., Wegiel, J., Schupf, N., Silverman, W., 2008. Alzheimer's disease in adults with down syndrome. Int. Rev. Res. Ment. Retard. 36, 103–145.

CHAPTER

8

Tau Proteins

S. Mondragón-Rodríguez, G. Perry, F. Peña-Ortega

OUTLINE

INTRODUCTION

Two proteins are currently the main focus of research of Alzheimer's disease (AD) development: tau and amyloid beta (Aβ) (Figs. 8.1 and 8.2) (Panza et al., 2014; Mondragón-Rodríguez et al., 2012a; Tran and Ha-Duong, 2015; Iqbal et al., 2014). The basis for these research efforts mainly comes from the correlation between AD symptoms and the presence of these two proteins in their aggregated forms: the amyloid plaques and the neurofibrillary tangles (NFTs) (Ogomori et al., 1989; Braak and Braak, 1990). The amyloid plaques, as their name indicates, are mainly comprised of Aβ proteins (Ogomori et al., 1989), whereas the NFTs are mainly constituted of abnormally phosphorylated tau (ptau) proteins (Grundke-Iqbal et al., 1986b; Mena et al., 1996). Both protein aggregates are commonly seen in brain regions that are affected during AD, such as several cortical areas, the isocortex, the entorhinal region, and the hippocampus (Braak and Braak, 1990). Because of its involvement in learning and memory, the hippocampus is a brain area of particular interest for AD pathophysiology (Li et al., 2015).

Drug Discovery Approaches for the Treatment of Neurodegenerative Disorders
http://dx.doi.org/10.1016/B978-0-12-802810-0.00008-8

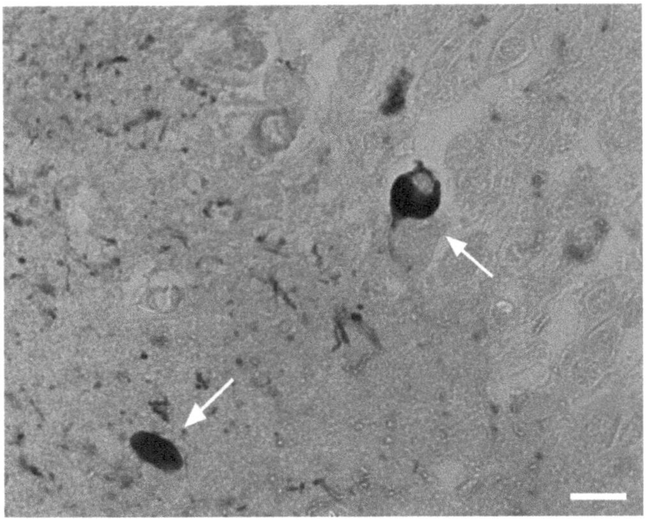

FIGURE 8.1 The brain of AD patients is characterized by neurofibrillary tangles (NFT cytopathology). Immunolabeling (immunoperoxidase) of tau protein revealed the classical NFTs that are comprised of phosphorylated tau (ptau) protein (*white arrows*). As seen in the upper tangle, during late AD stages the abnormal aggregated ptau protein has taken all the intracellular space, therefore prompting the neurons to failure. Scale = 10 μm.

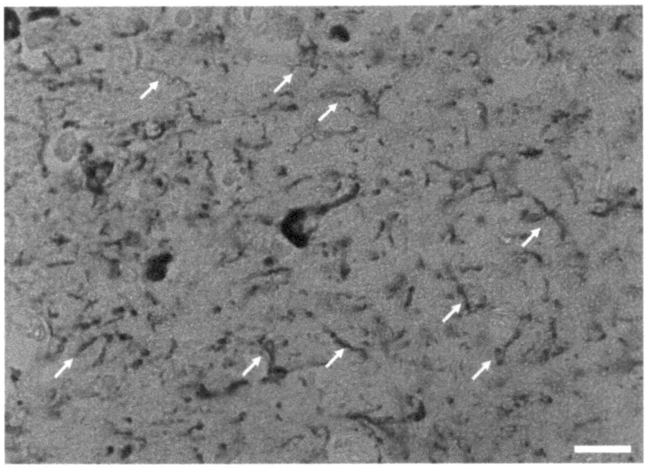

FIGURE 8.2 Phosphorylated tau (ptau) protein in dendrites is a hallmark of AD. Immunolabeling (immunoperoxidase) of ptau reveals a strong signal in several dendrites (*white arrows*) around the affected areas of human AD cases. A neurofibrillary tangle (NFT) is observed in the central area of the picture. Scale = 10 μm.

Of note, the extracellular Aβ and the intraneuronal NFTs are distributed all around the hippocampus (Fig. 8.2) (Kalus et al., 1989). It has been reported that the hippocampus is capable of generating theta activity (Wulff et al., 2009). Critically, alterations in theta activity are significantly correlated with the cognitive deficits observed in AD transgenic (tg) models (Villette et al., 2010; Yue et al., 2014). Not surprisingly, the protein deposition of ptau and Aβ in all hippocampal cell layers is suggested to impair the normal functions of several brain circuits (Kalus et al., 1989; Villette et al., 2010; Peña-Ortega and Bernal-Pedraza, 2012). Indeed, it has been reported that Aβ is responsible for theta activity inhibition and spatial memory alterations as an ultimate consequence (Villette et al., 2010; Yue et al., 2014; Peña-Ortega and Bernal-Pedraza, 2012). Giving support to this hypothesis, we have found accumulation of Aβ plaques in the main hippocampal layers (Fig. 8.3). Importantly, some plaques were found in close proximity to the CA-1 parvalbumin (PV)-positive interneurons (Fig. 8.3, red labeling).

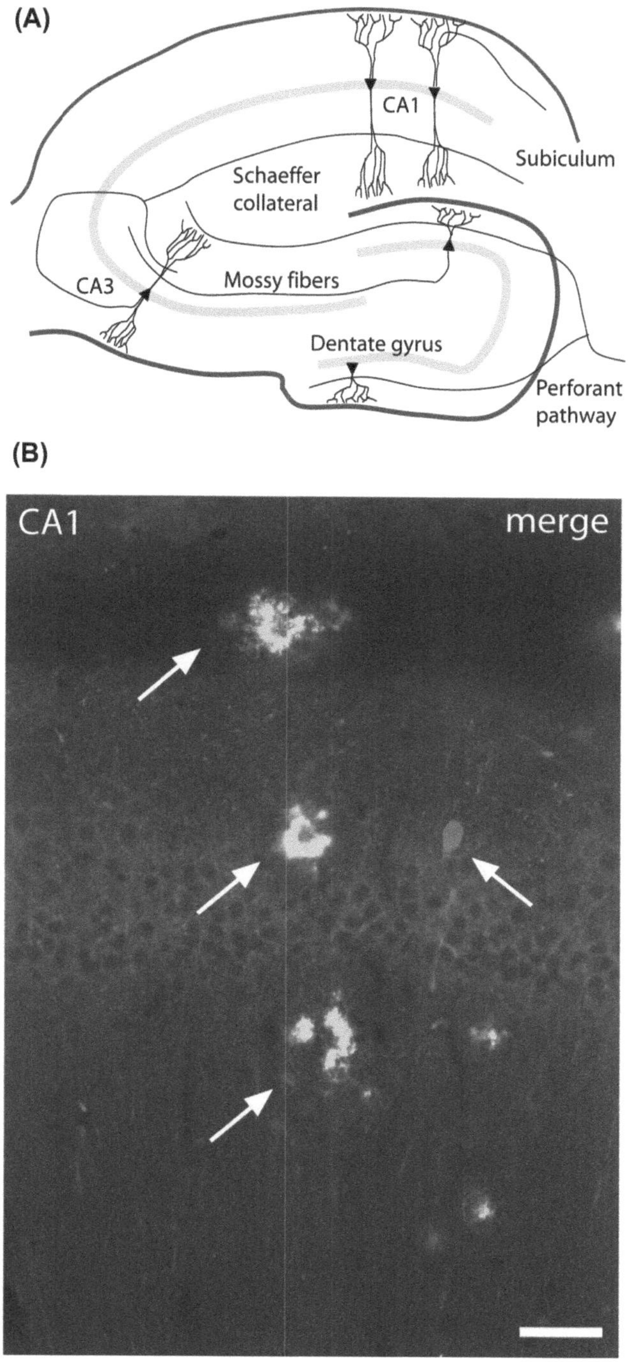

FIGURE 8.3 **Aβ plaques are distributed along the hippocampal cell layers.** Drawing that illustrates the subdivisions of the CA1 somatic layer (A). Aβ plaques (*labeled in green* (light gray in print versions)) are densely located around the stratum oriens (upper plaque, (B)), stratum pyramidale (middle plaque, (B)), and stratum radiatum (lower plaque, (B)). Parvalbumin (PV) hippocampal CA1 interneurons (*red labeling* (gray in print versions)), (B) were found in close proximity to the Aβ plaques. Scale = 20 μm.

Our findings nurture the hypothesis of Aβ reducing theta activity by indirectly affecting PV interneurons (unpublished data). Taken together, data postulate Aβ as critically involved during neurodegeneration, with actions that could be considered either a cause or effect (Mondragón-Rodríguez et al., 2010).

An additional pathological structure that is also commonly seen in the affected areas of AD patients is dystrophic neurites (Onorato et al., 1989) (Fig. 8.2). Importantly, we normally found the dystrophic neurites, mostly containing ptau, in close proximity to the Aβ plaques (unpublished data). This provides foundation for the potential morphological interaction between intracellular tau and extracellular Aβ proteins during AD development. Despite the morphometric proximity between these proteins, the cellular and molecular mechanisms that connect their pathological effects are not fully understood. Aiming to explain these mechanisms underscoring AD development we will explore the phosphorylation of tau protein as the key event that acts as a connector between both proteins. Importantly, we will briefly discuss the physiology of ptau protein related to several important functions such as microtubule stabilization, actin reorganization, and synaptic activity. Additionally, we will examine the contribution of ptau from its pathologic point of view. Overall, this will help to understand the disturbed balance that could be addressed when drug strategies are carried out. In this regard, we will also explore the potential pitfalls of current tau-directed therapeutic strategies. To address this last point it should be established that tau and Aβ are related to AD (Braak and Del Tredici, 2015); however, whether they are responsible for the disease or not remains to be proven. In addition, current therapeutic results for AD treatment are unsuccessful (Mondragón-Rodríguez et al., 2012a; Hyman and Sorger, 2014). Therefore the discussion focuses on what to therapeutically target. According to current lines of thinking, the answer should not be so complicated, and be to eliminate the aggregation of either Aβ or tau proteins (Panza et al., 2014; Mondragón-Rodríguez et al., 2012a; Wischik et al., 2014). However, as previously mentioned, either Aβ or tau-directed therapeutic strategies are failing. The rising question is why are we failing to ameliorate the disease progression? Although the answer is far from easy, two possibilities emerge, either the hypothesis that tau and Aβ are directly causing AD is not accurate, or the therapeutic failure could be attributed to the fact that drug therapy is administrated at late stages rather than early or critical stages of the disease. Tending to support the second possibility, we are finding out that synaptic alterations are occurring long before any histopathological marker is detected in patients (Jansen et al., 2015). In this regard, by studying AD tg models we have found that brain connectivity is altered before any sign of either Aβ or tau deposition (unpublished data). These data call for molecular markers that could help to identify the AD pathology at early stages of the disease. With this in mind, the early marker strategy will provide a better treatment window with a potential better outcome. One event of particular interest is the phosphorylation of tau protein. We have seen that specific phosphorylation events in tau protein can help to identify early stages of the disease progression (Mondragón-Rodríguez et al., 2014). Specifically, early ptau aggregates are well correlated with early stages of AD progression (Mondragón-Rodríguez et al., 2014). Here we firmly believe that identifying and controlling those specific phosphorylation events in tau protein could offer an interesting therapeutic target that may potentially result in restoring cognitive functions.

TAU PROTEIN

In 1975 tau protein was separated from tubulin purified from porcine brain (Weingarten et al., 1975). Because of its capacity in promoting microtubule assembly, tau protein was suggested to act as a major regulator of microtubule formation (Weingarten et al., 1975). Despite this important finding, tau protein did not receive much attention. The watershed moment occurred when tau was related to one of the most prominent structures in AD, the NFTs (Grundke-Iqbal et al., 1986b; Delacourte and Defossez, 1986; Nukina and Ihara, 1986; Wolozin et al., 1986; Wood et al., 1986; Kosik et al., 1986; Ihara et al., 1986). Since then tau protein has been considered one of the main players of AD disease progression and has evolved as one of the principal and current hypotheses that tend to explain AD pathophysiology (Wischik et al., 2014; Wang et al., 2014). Unfortunately, and despite many years of research, we still do not know the exact mechanism by which tau becomes a toxic entity that damages neurons. Mechanistically, what we know is that tau abnormally aggregates in the soma of neurons until it covers the whole cell area and finally, at the last stage, is associated with cell loss (Figs. 8.1 and 8.2) (Ihara et al., 1986). We additionally know that certain posttranslational modifications such as abnormal phosphorylation, structural changes, and cleavage make important contributions to the tau alterations that promote the protein into the aggregation phase (Grundke-Iqbal et al., 1986b; Ihara et al., 1986; Jarero-Basulto et al., 2014; Sui et al., 2015; Garcia-Sierra et al., 2008). We are left to ask: How does tau protein get to an aggregated state? First, we need to know the structural sequence of tau protein. The longest tau isoform has 441 amino acids, two polypeptide sequences that are encoded by exons 2 and 3, two proline-rich regions, and one microtubule-binding domain (Kolarova et al., 2012) (Fig. 8.4). Along its proline and repeat sequences, tau has many sites susceptible to phosphorylation (Kolarova et al., 2012; Petry et al., 2014). Among those sites the most important for AD research are S199/202 labeled by antibody AT8, T212/S214 labeled by antibody AT100, T231/S235 labeled by antibody AT180, and S262 and S393/404 labeled by antibody PHF-1, respectively (Fig. 8.4) (Petry et al., 2014; Mondragón-Rodríguez et al., 2012b). Importantly, the phosphorylation of tau protein is known for affecting its capacity of interactions with the microtubules and promoting the aggregation phase as well (Sui et al., 2015). Thus the phosphorylation of tau protein has

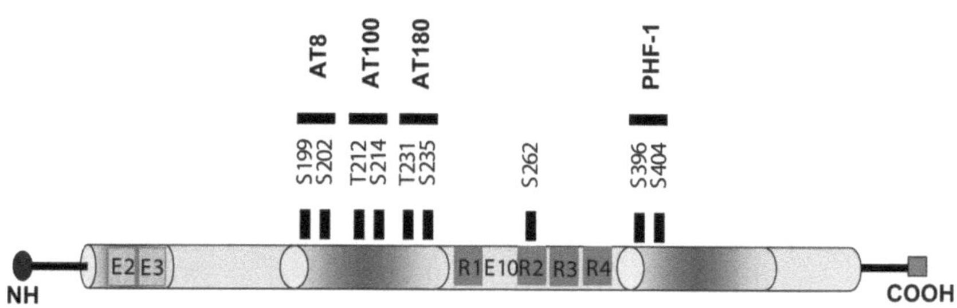

FIGURE 8.4 **Phosphorylation sites of tau protein.** Tau amino acid sequence comprises the polypeptide sequence encoded by exons 2 and 3; microtubule-binding domain R1 to R4. Binding of tau to the microtubules is controlled by phosphorylation and dephosphorylation along the entire sequence. The most studied phosphorylated sites in tau protein are labeled by antibodies AT8 (S199/202), AT100 (T212/S214), AT180 (T231/S235), pS262, and PHF-1 (S396/404).

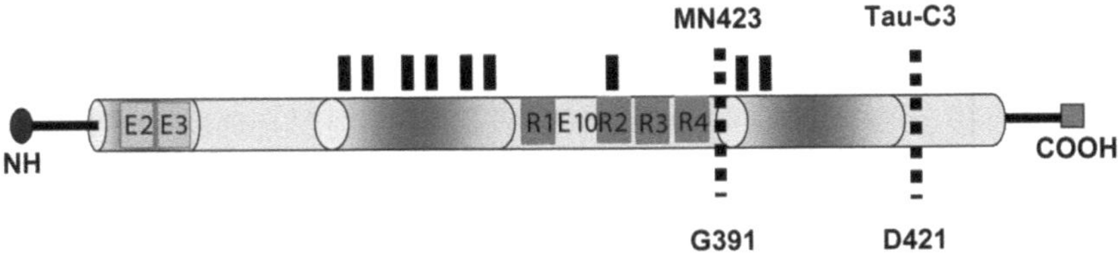

FIGURE 8.5 **Cleavage sites of tau protein.** Tau protein is the target of several proteases that generate cuts along the carboxyl-terminus sequence. The closest cut to the carboxyl-terminus takes place at site D421. This site is labeled by antibody Tau-C3. The canonical cleavage at G391 is labeled by antibody MN423.

been suggested to contribute to both the conformational shifts and the cleavage in the protein, all together promoting the protein to the aggregated stage that gives origin to the NFTs (Garcia-Sierra et al., 2008; Mondragón-Rodríguez et al., 2008a, 2013). However, suggesting a protective roll, it has to be mentioned that some authors have proposed that phosphorylation of tau protein actually prevents abnormal processing of tau protein (Guillozet-Bongaarts et al., 2006). For instance, the phosphorylation of tau protein at site S422 was found to be protective by preventing the cleavage of tau protein at site D421 (Guillozet-Bongaarts et al., 2006). Clearly, these data show that the role of phosphorylation even during abnormal tau processing is far more complex than that of an exclusive disease catalyst.

Regarding the cleavage of tau protein, it was found that it facilitates nucleation-dependent filament formation, therefore promoting NFT formation (Rissman et al., 2004). Although tau protein has many sites susceptible to cleavage, two are the most studied and currently the main focus of AD research: the cleavage at site D421 and the cleavage of G391 (Fig. 8.5) (Rissman et al., 2004; Wischik et al., 1988). Nurturing the pathological role of cleavage, it was reported that cleavage at site D421 also facilitates the conformational changes, suggesting that cleavage was one of the earliest events taking place during tau pathological processing (Rissman et al., 2004). However, we found opposite results: according to our data, early conformational changes were not D421 cleavage dependent (Mondragón-Rodríguez et al., 2008b). Despite this controversy, we firmly believe that chronology of events becomes critical because this information can help to elucidate the earliest events and consequently enable a better therapeutic intervention window. With this in mind, we have analyzed the chronology of the posttranslational events (phosphorylation, conformational changes, and cleavage) (Mondragón-Rodríguez et al., 2008a,b). By using human brains from different AD stages and controls as well we studied the composition of NFTs comprising any of the previous events (phosphorylation, conformational changes, and cleavage). Interestingly, we found different populations of NFTs: (1) some comprising ptau and cleaved tau, (2) some comprising ptau and shifted tau, and (3) some comprising all the events (phosphorylation, conformational changes, and cleavage) (Mondragón-Rodríguez et al., 2008b). Critically, the phosphorylation of tau protein was the only event that we found isolated (Mondragón-Rodríguez et al., 2008b). Indeed, when we analyzed the total amount of NFTs per mm^2 in the affected areas of AD patients, we found that the majority of them were comprised mainly of ptau protein (Mondragón-Rodríguez et al., 2008b). Altogether, our data suggest that ptau was the earliest event happening before either conformational shifts or cleavage (Mondragón-Rodríguez et al., 2008b). Importantly, the presence of altered tau protein was only evaluated in the fibrillar state, which is the conformation that characterized a mature NFT (Fig. 8.1) (Luna-Munoz et al., 2008). Aiming to further

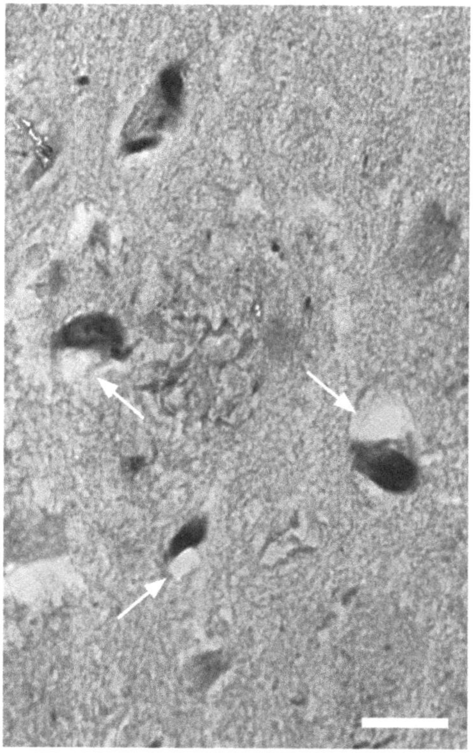

FIGURE 8.6 **Early aggregation of tau protein is found in close proximity to the nucleus.** Phosphorylated tau protein detected by immunoperoxidase was found close to the nuclei (*white arrows*) during early stages of AD development. Scale = 10 μm.

nurture our findings, we decided to study events that happened before the formation of the fibrillar tangle. In other words, identify the tau events occurring in the pretangle stage. Again, we observed that ptau in a nonfibrillar state was the main component (Fig. 8.6) (Mondragón-Rodríguez et al., 2014). Interestingly, we observed that this phosphorylation event was initially located in the proximity of the nuclei, suggesting that an initial aggregation phase required certain nuclear proteins (Fig. 8.6) (Mondragón-Rodríguez et al., 2014). Giving support to these findings, disease-specific oxidative damage to nuclei was found as initial damage in human AD brains (Smith et al., 1996). Although the mechanism is not fully understood, the phosphorylation of tau protein was related to oxidation events (Yan et al., 1995). However, more studies need to be performed to validate this theory. Overall, our data clearly demonstrate that phosphorylation was one of the earliest events taking place before the mature stage of the NFT formation (Mondragón-Rodríguez et al., 2014). Therefore postulating this event as the pivotal posttranslational modification, this central piece of data becomes critical if we think about stopping the disease progression at early stages.

AMYLOID BETA

As previously mentioned, Aβ plaques, mainly comprised of Aβ protein along with the NFTs, constitute the primary hallmark of AD (Ogomori et al., 1989; Grundke-Iqbal et al., 1986a). Opposite to the NFT structure, the Aβ plaques are extracellular aggregates (Fig. 8.3).

Thus for many years it was suggested that the extracellular aggregates were strongly related to AD development (Xiao et al., 2015; Takahashi et al., 2015; Oestereich et al., 2015; Mucke and Selkoe, 2012). However, certain discoveries are showing that the amyloid burden is not necessarily correlated with the disease progression (Jansen et al., 2015). Indeed, the biggest dataset yet, which analyzed brain amyloid deposition, suggested that Aβ decreased with very old age in people clinically diagnosed with AD, while non-AD patients were more likely to harbor Aβ deposits as they get older (Jansen et al., 2015). These data raise a critical point: whatever the contribution of Aβ toward AD development is, it must be at very early stages of the disease. The big problem, however, is to find that early point during the progression of the disease. In the same metaanalysis they confirmed that Aβ deposition starts around 30 years before any cognitive deficit is observed (Jansen et al., 2015). These particular data are being used to explain why the majority of clinical trials, directed against Aβ, have shown little success (Mondragón-Rodríguez et al., 2012a; Gravitz, 2011). As mentioned previously, the key element for AD research is to a prodromal phase of the disease that will help to identify new therapeutic targets. In this regard, current data are focused on finding the initial mechanism of Aβ aggregation (Xiao et al., 2015). It is known that processing of the amyloid precursor protein (APP) generates two major peptides: Aβ40 (1–40) and Aβ42 (1–42), Aβ42 being better related to the toxic cascade that contributes to AD development (Xiao et al., 2015; Kadowaki et al., 2005; Zempel et al., 2010; Salgado-Puga and Peña-Ortega, 2015; Tu et al., 2014). One major finding that tends to support the Aβ42 toxic cascade hypothesis is that Aβ42 can interfere and abolish the hippocampal long-term potentiation (LTP) event (Salgado-Puga and Peña-Ortega, 2015; Shipton et al., 2011). LTP is one of the two major forms of synaptic plasticity currently accepted as the mechanism that underlies learning and memory (Bliss and Collingridge, 2013; Volianskis et al., 2013). Basically, what LTP does to the neuron is to promote the persistent strengthening of synapses, consequently translating into memory and learning (Bliss and Collingridge, 2013; Volianskis et al., 2013). The second big phenomenon that underlies memory and learning is a long-lasting decrease in the synapse strength (long-term depression, LTD) (Collingridge et al., 2010). Although the mechanistic relationship between both events, LTP and LTD, is not fully understood, it is becoming clear that LTP requires LTD to balance the synaptic responses (Collingridge et al., 2010). In addition, certain kinases and receptors are common and interconnect both events (Bradley et al., 2012). Of particular interest, glycogen synthase kinase-3 (GSK-3) and *N*-methyl-D-aspartate receptor (NMDAR) emerge as important LTP/LTD connectors (Bradley et al., 2012). GSK-3 is a critical node in the intracellular cascade that directly modulates the crosstalk between LTP and LTD (Bradley et al., 2012; Peineau et al., 2008). This talk is achieved by modulating the NMDAR response that after the GSK-3 signal activation can direct the synaptic response to either hippocampal LTP or hippocampal LTD (Bradley et al., 2012; Peineau et al., 2008). A further aspect to consider is that the hippocampus is extremely prominent in short-term memory, long-term memory, and spatial navigation (Li et al., 2015; Addante, 2014). Not surprisingly, as mentioned previously, during AD development and other neurodegenerative diseases the hippocampal formation is extremely affected by protein deposition (Braak and Del Tredici, 2015; Mondragón-Rodríguez et al., 2008, 2014; Basurto-Islas et al., 2008). The overall abnormal changes observed in the hippocampal formation of AD patients help to explain the cognitive manifestations seen in AD patients; however, the early relationship between Aβ and tau remains under extensive study.

AMYLOID BETA, TAU, AND SYNAPTIC PLASTICITY: AN INTIMATE RELATIONSHIP

So far we have argued for the involvement of both proteins, tau and Aβ, during AD development, but even more importantly we have discussed data that tend to support the hypothesis that protein deposition could be a catastrophic consequence and not necessarily the cause of the disease. Nevertheless, prodromal events, like either phosphorylation of tau protein or Aβ peptide generation that interact with the critical receptor for synaptic activity (ie, NMDAR), could account for cognitive alterations seen during AD development (Xi et al., 2015). Here the question is: How can we relate the extracellular Aβ peptide and the intracellular ptau protein? Although the exact mechanism that relates both proteins remains under extensive study, by using cellular models it has been reported that the extracellular Aβ is capable of inducing tau intracellular aggregation (Takahashi et al., 2015). In addition, the intracellular aggregation was accompanied by increase in phosphorylation levels in tau protein, specifically at the sites labeled by antibody AT8 (S199/202) and S396 (Takahashi et al., 2015). However, there was a key element that catalyzed the aggregation phenomena, fibrillary samples from human AD brains (Takahashi et al., 2015). These particular data showed that the human brain has a specific environment with elements that help to catalyze the AD pathology and until we unveil all those elements, we will not be able to understand the full mechanism that leads to the pathological stage. Despite this challenge, the data link a very important process: the way extracellular Aβ and the intracellular-aggregated tau couple in AD pathology. In line with these findings, we incubated hippocampal preparations with Aβ42 and evaluated the state of tau phosphorylation. Our data showed that phosphorylation at sites Ser396/404 and T231/S235 were significantly increased post-Aβ42 incubation (Mondragón-Rodríguez et al., 2012b). Our data has further reinforced the hypothesis that alteration in phosphorylation levels is the link between extracellular Aβ42 and intracellular tau. Of note, the sites that we found altered in tau protein are extremely close to the tau repeat domains, the region that binds to microtubules (Fig. 8.4). Aiming to further validate our data, we analyzed human AD brains at different pathological stages and consistently found an increase in phosphorylation levels at sites Ser396/404 (Mondragón-Rodríguez et al., 2014). Overall, these data contribute to explaining the mechanistic actions that extracellular Aβ42 could exert over intracellular tau. Nevertheless, the data do not explain what the consequences to synaptic activity are. With this in mind, we decided to explore the relationship between extracellular Aβ42 and intracellular tau in the synaptic terminal. First, we found that tau protein is physically located in the synaptic terminals (Mondragón-Rodríguez et al., 2012b). Importantly, the total concentration of the protein in the synaptic terminals was as large as the total concentration of the postsynaptic density protein 95 (PSD95), which is a structural protein for postsynaptic terminals (Mondragón-Rodríguez et al., 2012b). Thus our data suggest that tau had a physical role in the synaptic terminal (Mondragón-Rodríguez et al., 2012b). Aiming to unveil the physical function of tau protein, we studied the potential interaction of tau protein with several synaptic proteins such as PSD95, which is also a structural protein for NMDAR activation, NR2B, which is part of the NMDAR complex, and kinases like Fyn that phosphorylates PSD95 and results in NMDAR activation (Mondragón-Rodríguez et al., 2012b). Overall, our data showed for the first time that tau protein binds directly to PSD95 promoting NMDAR activation (Mondragón-Rodríguez et al., 2012b). Thus we also showed that tau protein directly binds to Fyn,

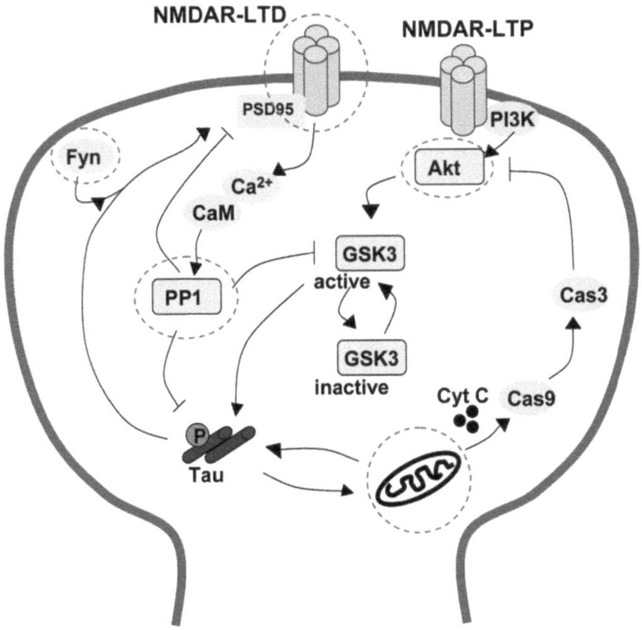

FIGURE 8.7 **Modulation of key effectors for synaptic plasticity (*red circles* (gray in print versions)) could restore events like memory formation.** *N*-Methyl-D-aspartate receptor-long-term depression (NMDAR-LTD) stimulus leads to an increase of intracellular Ca^{2+} that activates PP1, an important enzyme in synaptically induced LTD. PP1 dephosphorylates glycogen synthase kinase-3 (GSK-3) and tau, which determines whether NMDAR inhibits or induces LTD. Tau promotes NMDAR activation by targeting postsynaptic density protein 95 (PSD95) and Fyn. This interaction is regulated through coordinated phosphorylation and dephosphorylation of tau protein. GSK3 under the control of Akt is a critical determinant of the direction of NMDAR-dependent LTD or long-term potentiation (LTP). Modulation of critical check points (*red circles* (gray in print versions)) for synaptic plasticity events (LTP or LTD) could be achieved by multitherapy regimens (cocktail therapy), which in the scope of event restoration could target several check points at the same time.

tau protein forms a complex along with PSD95 to deliver Fyn at the NMDAR complex, and, after activation, tau detaches from the complex liberating Fyn kinase (Fig. 8.7) (Mondragón-Rodríguez et al., 2012b). Not surprisingly, the phenomenon that regulates such interesting tau function was the phosphorylation of tau protein (Mondragón-Rodríguez et al., 2012b). In consequence, knowing that Aβ can alter the phosphorylation of tau protein, therefore affecting the NMDAR response, could explain a potential mechanism for synaptic alterations that later translate into cognitive deficits seen in AD patients. These data also open a new perspective in terms of therapeutic intervention that we will discuss in the next section.

THE THERAPEUTIC TARGET

We have discussed elements that argue in favor of tau protein as an important player for, and during, AD development. Maybe the clearest piece of data that support its involvement, as previously discussed, is the histopathological correlation between NFTs and the clinical state from people who died suffering from AD (Braak and Del Tredici, 2015; Garcia-Sierra et al., 2001). Intuitively, in the scope of stopping disease progression, the general idea is to inhibit the aggregation of abnormally ptau protein (Akoury et al., 2013). Further, the porphyrins group (ie, phthalocyanine tetrasulfonate, PCTS) is probably one of the most important classes of aggregation inhibitors (Akoury et al., 2013). PCTS became popular after knowing its therapeutic effects in scrapie disease (Abdel-Haq et al., 2009; Dee et al., 2012). Basically, the mechanistic explanation is that PCTS inhibits the formation of protease-resistant prion protein aggregates (Akoury et al., 2013; Abdel-Haq et al., 2009; Dee et al., 2012). When the properties of PCTS were evaluated regarding tau aggregation, the data showed that PCTS can interfere with the aggregation process, and beyond, PCTS were able to disaggregate tau filaments (Akoury et al., 2013). In the same line of thought, a select grape seed polyphenol extract (GSPE) has been examined (Santa-Maria et al., 2011; Wang et al., 2010). GSPE administration significantly attenuated the development of tau neuropathology in the brain of mouse models of AD (Santa-Maria et al., 2011; Wang et al., 2010).

Despite the development of an important number of molecules that inhibit aggregation, little is known about the inhibition mechanism. Aiming to explain the potential mechanism, it has been reported that those molecules interfere with tau filament formation by transforming the protein into soluble oligomers (Akoury et al., 2013). These data argue in favor of modulating the structural conformation of tau protein to avoid self-aggregation. In sum, the antiaggregation strategy seems promising; however, one important thing to consider is that these approaches will interfere with normal functioning of tau protein. As we previously discussed, the protein–protein interaction is the mechanism that allows tau protein to participate in several physiological processes such as microtubule stabilization, protein transport, actin-related events, receptor activation, etc.

The second most pursued strategy is elimination of the phosphorylated state in tau protein (Iqbal et al., 2014; Ren et al., 2014). As we already mentioned, the phosphorylated state of tau protein is the main hallmark of NFTs (Mondragón-Rodríguez et al., 2014; Wood et al., 1986). In addition, we discussed that certain kinases (ie, GSK3β) are heavily involved in phosphorylating and therefore, according to the current hypothesis, promoting the self-aggregation phase of tau AD pathology (Forlenza et al., 2010). Moreover, the increased platelet GSK3β activity has been reported in patients with AD (Forlenza et al., 2010). Not surprisingly, aiming to stop AD development, GSK3β inhibitors are in the scope of therapeutic research (Fukunaga et al., 2015). One of particular interest is the 2-(alkylmorpholin-4-yl)-6-(3-fluoropyridin-4-yl)-pyrimidin-4(3H) that has already showed tau phosphorylation inhibitory activity by oral administration (Fukunaga et al., 2015). Of note, this blocking strategy is not taking into consideration that GSK3β is also critically involved in the synaptic events like LTP and LTD (Bradley et al., 2012). Therefore by inhibiting GSK3β activity we will be affecting mechanisms that participate in consolidation and memory formation. In the end, the objective is quite similar to the aggregation inhibitors: eliminate phosphorylation in tau protein and consequently eliminate the autoaggregation events that lead to NFT formation. Again by affecting the phosphorylation levels of tau protein we will also be affecting synaptic activity like NMDAR activation (Fig. 8.7).

Finally, the third and probably the most drastic approach is the idea of completely eliminating tau protein (de Barreda and Avila, 2011). This strategy is based on the fact that tau protein is required for Aβ to impair synaptic plasticity, specifically the hippocampal LTP phenomena

(Shipton et al., 2011). This strategy is not taking into consideration that tau protein is not exclusively part of the AD progression, but instead is modulating several physiological processes. Clearly, the therapeutic strategy is not as simple as one target, one drug. Even more important, tau physiology needs to be taken into consideration when therapeutic strategies are designed. In addition, secondary effects also need to be taken into consideration, that is, some antiaggregation compounds directed against the amyloid plaque structure were found to promote tau self-aggregation (Santa-Maria et al., 2007).

To summarize, we are of the opinion that single drug strategies that are not taking into consideration physiology, secondary effects, and secondary targets are overly simplistic. If this scenario holds true, the potential therapeutic outcome will not be so promising.

DISCUSSION AND FUTURE PERSPECTIVES

In this chapter we have discussed the contribution of Aβ and tau during AD development, but more importantly we focused on its contribution during early stages of the disease progression. Here the phosphorylation of tau protein emerged as an early event that strongly relates to the changes seen during AD development. Consequently, as previously mentioned, it is not difficult to imagine that inhibition of phosphorylation of tau protein is one important therapeutic target for AD treatment. However, as we mentioned earlier, the physiology of tau has not been considered when most of the current therapeutic strategies were designed. Here our opinion is that physiology must be studied and taken into consideration before more and new therapeutic targets are selected. In addition, the AD phenomenon is far more complex than one protein and one event that translate into disease. Altogether, data call for new strategies that consider the bigger picture. With this in mind, we proposed that the combination of drugs that enhance LTP in combination with drugs that reduce the induction of LTD could be beneficial to treat AD at early stages (Mondragón-Rodríguez et al., 2012a). The question is how to achieve this strategy? Our proposal is to simultaneously target critical check points for synaptic plasticity that consequently could improve memory formation (Fig. 8.7). Here we aim to balance the activity of GSK3 by modulating the activity of protein phosphatase-1 and the serine–threonine protein kinase Akt (Fig. 8.7). Both exert signaling control for GSK3 that determines whether NMDAR activations are directed at hippocampal LTD or LTP (Fig. 8.7). Another interesting target is the modulation of Fyn kinase that contributes to NMDAR activation. Therefore to modulate NMDAR activation we can modulate Fyn kinase activity (Fig. 8.7). In addition, we can target caspase activation (ie, Cas-3); therefore indirectly we can modulate Akt activation and consequently GSK3 response (Fig. 8.7). Overall, by selecting either up- or downstream targets, we are not blocking the effects of either GSK3 or tau, but rather we are maintaining the activity of both key targets for NMDAR functioning. More importantly, our multiple target strategy is aimed at restoring important synaptic events (ie, LTP) that hopefully will translate into memory formation improvement (Mondragón-Rodríguez et al., 2012a) (Fig. 8.7). In summary, our data are showing that studying the biology of Aβ and tau could offer new hope for effective therapeutics. Of importance, we believe that approaches that focus on either removing or blocking tau activity have great chances of missing the right outcome. In contrast, restoring events by employing cocktail therapy (directed against critical check points for synaptic events) could be the needed alternative to treating the prodromal stages of AD.

FINANCIAL AND COMPETING INTERESTS DISCLOSURE

George Perry is, or has in the past been, a paid consultant for and/or owns equity or stock options in Neurotez Pharmaceuticals. The authors have no other relevant affiliations or financial involvement with any organization or entity with a financial interest in or financial conflict with the subject matter or materials discussed in this chapter apart from those disclosed.

Acknowledgments

The authors thank Francis A. Manno III and Brittanii Rogers for critical comments and administrative support, respectively. Work in the authors' laboratories is supported by the Canadian Institutes of Health Research (CIHR), Canada, and Fonds de la recherche en sante du QC (FRSQ), Quebec, Canada. Conacyt, DGAPA-UNAM, and NIH-GIZ-MD00791. This project was supported by a grant from the National Institute on Minority Health and Health Disparities (G12MD007591) from the National Institutes of Health and by the Semmes Foundation. Siddhartha Mondragón-Rodríguez was awarded with postdoctoral scholarship support from FRSQ, Canada, and currently holds the position as Conacyt Research Fellow–Institute of Neurobiology, INB, México.

References

Abdel-Haq, H., Lu, M., Cardone, F., Liu, Q.G., Puopolo, M., Pocchiari, M., 2009. Efficacy of phthalocyanine tetrasulfonate against mouse-adapted human prion strains. Arch. Virol. 154, 1005–1007.

Addante, R.J., 2014. A critical role of the human hippocampus in an electrophysiological measure of implicit memory. Neuroimage 109, 515–528.

Akoury, E., Gajda, M., Pickhardt, M., Biernat, J., Soraya, P., Griesinger, C., Mandelkow, E., Zweckstetter, M., 2013. Inhibition of tau filament formation by conformational modulation. J. Am. Chem. Soc. 135, 2853–2862.

Basurto-Islas, G., Luna-Munoz, J., Guillozet-Bongaarts, A.L., Binder, L.I., Mena, R., Garcia-Sierra, F., 2008. Accumulation of aspartic acid421- and glutamic acid391-cleaved tau in neurofibrillary tangles correlates with progression in Alzheimer disease. J. Neuropathol. Exp. Neurol. 67, 470–483.

Bliss, T.V., Collingridge, G.L., 2013. Expression of NMDA receptor-dependent LTP in the hippocampus: bridging the divide. Mol. Brain 6, 5.

Braak, H., Braak, E., 1990. Neurofibrillary changes confined to the entorhinal region and an abundance of cortical amyloid in cases of presenile and senile dementia. Acta Neuropathol. 80, 479–486.

Braak, H., Del Tredici, K., 2015. The pattern of lesions during the transition to the symptomatic phase and in fully developed Alzheimer's disease. Adv. Anat. Embryol. Cell Biol. 215, 95–130.

Bradley, C.A., Peineau, S., Taghibiglou, C., Nicolas, C.S., Whitcomb, D.J., Bortolotto, Z.A., Kaang, B.K., Cho, K., Wang, Y.T., Collingridge, G.L., 2012. A pivotal role of GSK-3 in synaptic plasticity. Front. Mol. Neurosci. 5, 13.

Collingridge, G.L., Peineau, S., Howland, J.G., Wang, Y.T., 2010. Long-term depression in the CNS. Nat. Rev. Neurosci. 11, 459–473.

de Barreda, E.G., Avila, J., 2011. Is tau a suitable therapeutical target in tauopathies? World J. Biol. Chem. 1, 81–84.

Dee, D.R., Gupta, A.N., Anikovskiy, M., Sosova, I., Grandi, E., Rivera, L., Vincent, A., Brigley, A.M., Petersen, N.O., Woodside, M.T., 2012. Phthalocyanine tetrasulfonates bind to multiple sites on natively-folded prion protein. Biochim. Biophys. Acta 1824, 826–832.

Delacourte, A., Defossez, A., 1986. Biochemical characterization of an immune serum which specifically marks neurons in neurofibrillary degeneration in Alzheimer's disease. C R Acad. Sci. 303, 439–444.

Forlenza, O.V., Torres, C.A., Talib, L.L., de Paula, V.J., Joaquim, H.P., Diniz, B.S., Gattaz, W.F., 2010. Increased platelet GSK3B activity in patients with mild cognitive impairment and Alzheimer's disease. J. Psychiatr. Res. 45, 220–224.

Fukunaga, K., Sakai, D., Watanabe, K., Nakayama, K., Kohara, T., Tanaka, H., Sunada, S., Nabeno, M., Okamoto, M., Saito, K., et al., 2015. Discovery of novel 2-(alkylmorpholin-4-yl)-6-(3-fluoropyridin-4-yl)-pyrimidin-4(3H)-ones as orally-active GSK-3beta inhibitors for Alzheimer's disease. Bioorg. Med. Chem. Lett. 25, 1086–1091.

Garcia-Sierra, F., Wischik, C.M., Harrington, C.R., Luna-Munoz, J., Mena, R., 2001. Accumulation of C-terminally truncated tau protein associated with vulnerability of the perforant pathway in early stages of neurofibrillary pathology in Alzheimer's disease. J. Chem. Neuroanat. 22, 65–77.

Garcia-Sierra, F., Mondragón-Rodríguez, S., Basurto-Islas, G., 2008. Truncation of tau protein and its pathological significance in Alzheimer's disease. J. Alzheimers Dis. 14, 401–409.

Gravitz, L., 2011. Drugs: a tangled web of targets. Nature 475, S9–S11.

Grundke-Iqbal, I., Iqbal, K., Tung, Y.C., Quinlan, M., Wisniewski, H.M., Binder, L.I., 1986a. Abnormal phosphorylation of the microtubule-associated protein tau (tau) in Alzheimer cytoskeletal pathology. Proc. Natl. Acad. Sci. U.S.A. 83, 4913–4917.

Grundke-Iqbal, I., Iqbal, K., Quinlan, M., Tung, Y.C., Zaidi, M.S., Wisniewski, H.M., 1986b. Microtubule-associated protein tau. A component of Alzheimer paired helical filaments. J. Biol. Chem. 261, 6084–6089.

Guillozet-Bongaarts, A.L., Cahill, M.E., Cryns, V.L., Reynolds, M.R., Berry, R.W., Binder, L.I., 2006. Pseudophosphorylation of tau at serine 422 inhibits caspase cleavage: in vitro evidence and implications for tangle formation in vivo. J. Neurochem. 97, 1005–1014.

Hyman, B.T., Sorger, P., 2014. Failure analysis of clinical trials to test the amyloid hypothesis. Ann. Neurol. 76, 159–161.

Ihara, Y., Nukina, N., Miura, R., Ogawara, M., 1986. Phosphorylated tau protein is integrated into paired helical filaments in Alzheimer's disease. J. Biochem. 99, 1807–1810.

Iqbal, K., Gong, C.X., Liu, F., 2014. Microtubule-associated protein tau as a therapeutic target in Alzheimer's disease. Expert Opin. Ther. Targets 18, 307–318.

Jansen, W.J., Ossenkoppele, R., Knol, D.L., Tijms, B.M., Scheltens, P., Verhey, F.R., Visser, P.J., Aalten, P., Aarsland, D., Alcolea, D., et al., 2015. Prevalence of cerebral amyloid pathology in persons without dementia: a meta-analysis. JAMA 313, 1924–1938.

Jarero-Basulto, J.J., Luna-Munoz, J., Mena, R., Kristofikova, Z., Ripova, D., Perry, G., Binder, L.I., Garcia-Sierra, F., 2014. Proteolytic cleavage of polymeric tau protein by caspase-3: implications for Alzheimer disease. J. Neuropathol. Exp. Neurol. 72, 1145–1161.

Kadowaki, H., Nishitoh, H., Urano, F., Sadamitsu, C., Matsuzawa, A., Takeda, K., Masutani, H., Yodoi, J., Urano, Y., Nagano, T., et al., 2005. Amyloid beta induces neuronal cell death through ROS-mediated ASK1 activation. Cell Death Differ. 12, 19–24.

Kalus, P., Braak, H., Braak, E., Bohl, J., 1989. The presubicular region in Alzheimer's disease: topography of amyloid deposits and neurofibrillary changes. Brain Res. 494, 198–203.

Kolarova, M., Garcia-Sierra, F., Bartos, A., Ricny, J., Ripova, D., 2012. Structure and pathology of tau protein in Alzheimer disease. Int. J. Alzheimers Dis. 2012:731526.

Kosik, K.S., Joachim, C.L., Selkoe, D.J., 1986. Microtubule-associated protein tau (tau) is a major antigenic component of paired helical filaments in Alzheimer disease. Proc. Natl. Acad. Sci. U.S.A. 83, 4044–4048.

Li, M., Long, C., Yang, L., 2015. Hippocampal-prefrontal circuit and disrupted functional connectivity in psychiatric and neurodegenerative disorders. Biomed. Res. Int 2015:810548.

Luna-Munoz, J., Peralta-Ramirez, J., Chavez-Macias, L., Harrington, C.R., Wischik, C.M., Mena, R., 2008. Thiazin red as a neuropathological tool for the rapid diagnosis of Alzheimer's disease in tissue imprints. Acta Neuropathol. 116, 507–515.

Mena, R., Edwards, P.C., Harrington, C.R., Mukaetova-Ladinska, E.B., Wischik, C.M., 1996. Staging the pathological assembly of truncated tau protein into paired helical filaments in Alzheimer's disease. Acta Neuropathol. 91, 633–641.

Mondragón-Rodríguez, S., Mena, R., Binder, L.I., Smith, M.A., Perry, G., Garcia-Sierra, F., 2008a. Conformational changes and cleavage of tau in Pick bodies parallel the early processing of tau found in Alzheimer pathology. Neuropathol. Appl. Neurobiol. 34, 62–75.

Mondragón-Rodríguez, S., Basurto-Islas, G., Santa-Maria, I., Mena, R., Binder, L.I., Avila, J., Smith, M.A., Perry, G., Garcia-Sierra, F., 2008b. Cleavage and conformational changes of tau protein follow phosphorylation during Alzheimer's disease. Int. J. Exp. Pathol. 89, 81–90.

Mondragón-Rodríguez, S., García-Sierra, F., Smith, M.A., 2010. Cause vs. effect: the increasing complexities of Alzheimer's disease. Neurotherapeutical Experts.

Mondragón-Rodríguez, S., Perry, G., Zhu, X., Boehm, J., 2012a. Amyloid Beta and tau proteins as therapeutic targets for Alzheimer's disease treatment: rethinking the current strategy. Int. J. Alzheimers Dis. 2012:630182.

Mondragón-Rodríguez, S., Trillaud-Doppia, E., Dudilot, A., Bourgeois, C., Lauzon, M., Leclerc, N., Boehm, J., 2012b. Interaction of endogenous tau protein with synaptic proteins is regulated by N-Methyl-D-aspartate receptor-dependent tau phosphorylation. J. Biol. Chem. 287, 32040–32053.

Mondragón-Rodríguez, S., Perry, G., Zhu, X., Moreira, P.I., Acevedo-Aquino, M.C., Williams, S., 2013. Phosphorylation of tau protein as the link between oxidative stress, mitochondrial dysfunction, and connectivity failure: implications for Alzheimer's disease. Oxid. Med. Cell Longev. 2013:940603.

Mondragón-Rodríguez, S., Perry, G., Luna-Munoz, J., Acevedo-Aquino, M.C., Williams, S., 2014. Phosphorylation of tau protein at sites Ser(396–404) is one of the earliest events in Alzheimer's disease and Down syndrome. Neuropathol. Appl. Neurobiol. 40, 121–135.

Mucke, L., Selkoe, D.J., 2012. Neurotoxicity of amyloid beta-protein: synaptic and network dysfunction. Cold Spring Harb. Perspect. Med. 2, a006338.

Nukina, N., Ihara, Y., 1986. One of the antigenic determinants of paired helical filaments is related to tau protein. J. Biochem. 99, 1541–1544.

Oestereich, F., Bittner, H.J., Weise, C., Grohmann, L., Janke, L.K., Hildebrand, P.W., Multhaup, G., Munter, L.M., 2015. Impact of amyloid precursor protein hydrophilic transmembrane residues on amyloid-Beta generation. Biochemistry 54, 2777–2784.

Ogomori, K., Kitamoto, T., Tateishi, J., Sato, Y., Suetsugu, M., Abe, M., 1989. Beta-protein amyloid is widely distributed in the central nervous system of patients with Alzheimer's disease. Am. J. Pathol. 134, 243–251.

Onorato, M., Mulvihill, P., Connolly, J., Galloway, P., Whitehouse, P., Perry, G., 1989. Alteration of neuritic cytoarchitecture in Alzheimer disease. Prog. Clin. Biol. Res. 317, 781–789.

Panza, F., Solfrizzi, V., Imbimbo, B.P., Tortelli, R., Santamato, A., Logroscino, G., 2014. Amyloid-based immunotherapy for Alzheimer's disease in the time of prevention trials: the way forward. Expert Rev. Clin. Immunol. 10, 405–419.

Peineau, S., Bradley, C., Taghibiglou, C., Doherty, A., Bortolotto, Z.A., Wang, Y.T., Collingridge, G.L., 2008. The role of GSK-3 in synaptic plasticity. Br. J. Pharmacol. 153 (Suppl. 1), S428–S437.

Peña-Ortega, F., Bernal-Pedraza, R., 2012. Amyloid Beta Peptide slows down sensory-induced hippocampal oscillations. Int. J. Pept 2012:236289.

Petry, F.R., Pelletier, J., Bretteville, A., Morin, F., Calon, F., Hebert, S.S., Whittington, R.A., Planel, E., 2014. Specificity of anti-tau antibodies when analyzing mice models of Alzheimer's disease: problems and solutions. PLoS One 9, e94251.

Ren, Q.G., Gong, W.G., Wang, Y.J., Zhou, Q.D., Zhang, Z.J., 2014. Citalopram attenuates tau hyperphosphorylation and spatial memory deficit induced by social isolation rearing in middle-aged rats. J. Mol. Neurosci. 56, 145–153.

Rissman, R.A., Poon, W.W., Blurton-Jones, M., Oddo, S., Torp, R., Vitek, M.P., LaFerla, F.M., Rohn, T.T., Cotman, C.W., 2004. Caspase-cleavage of tau is an early event in Alzheimer disease tangle pathology. J. Clin. Invest. 114, 121–130.

Salgado-Puga, K., Peña-Ortega, F., 2015. Cellular and network mechanisms underlying memory impairment induced by amyloid beta protein. Protein Pept. Lett. 22, 303–321.

Santa-Maria, I., Hernandez, F., Del Rio, J., Moreno, F.J., Avila, J., 2007. Tramiprosate, a drug of potential interest for the treatment of Alzheimer's disease, promotes an abnormal aggregation of tau. Mol. Neurodegener 2, 17.

Santa-Maria, I., Diaz-Ruiz, C., Ksiezak-Reding, H., Chen, A., Ho, L., Wang, J., Pasinetti, G.M., 2011. GSPE interferes with tau aggregation in vivo: implication for treating tauopathy. Neurobiol. Aging 33, 2072–2081.

Shipton, O.A., Leitz, J.R., Dworzak, J., Acton, C.E., Tunbridge, E.M., Denk, F., Dawson, H.N., Vitek, M.P., Wade-Martins, R., Paulsen, O., et al., 2011. Tau protein is required for amyloid {beta}-induced impairment of hippocampal long-term potentiation. J. Neurosci. 31, 1688–1692.

Smith, M.A., Perry, G., Richey, P.L., Sayre, L.M., Anderson, V.E., Beal, M.F., Kowall, N., 1996. Oxidative damage in Alzheimer's. Nature 382, 120–121.

Sui, D., Liu, M., Kuo, M.H., 2015. In vitro aggregation assays using hyperphosphorylated tau protein. J. Vis. Exp. e51537.

Takahashi, M., Miyata, H., Kametani, F., Nonaka, T., Akiyama, H., Hisanaga, S., Hasegawa, M., 2015. Extracellular association of APP and tau fibrils induces intracellular aggregate formation of tau. Acta Neuropathol. 129, 895–907.

Tran, L., Ha-Duong, T., 2015. Exploring the Alzheimer amyloid-beta peptide conformational ensemble: a review of molecular dynamics approaches. Peptides 69, 86–91.

Tu, S., Okamoto, S., Lipton, S.A., Xu, H., 2014. Oligomeric Abeta-induced synaptic dysfunction in Alzheimer's disease. Mol. Neurodegener. 9, 48.

Villette, V., Poindessous-Jazat, F., Simon, A., Lena, C., Roullot, E., Bellessort, B., Epelbaum, J., Dutar, P., Stephan, A., 2010. Decreased rhythmic GABAergic septal activity and memory-associated theta oscillations after hippocampal amyloid-beta pathology in the rat. J. Neurosci. 30, 10991–11003.

Volianskis, A., Collingridge, G.L., Jensen, M.S., 2013. The roles of STP and LTP in synaptic encoding. PeerJ 1, e3.

Wang, J., Santa-Maria, I., Ho, L., Ksiezak-Reding, H., Ono, K., Teplow, D.B., Pasinetti, G.M., 2010. Grape derived polyphenols attenuate tau neuropathology in a mouse model of Alzheimer's disease. J. Alzheimers Dis. 22, 653–661.

Wang, J.Z., Gao, X., Wang, Z.H., 2014. The physiology and pathology of microtubule-associated protein tau. Essays Biochem. 56, 111–123.

Weingarten, M.D., Lockwood, A.H., Hwo, S.Y., Kirschner, M.W., 1975. A protein factor essential for microtubule assembly. Proc. Natl. Acad. Sci. U.S.A. 72, 1858–1862.

Wischik, C.M., Novak, M., Edwards, P.C., Klug, A., Tichelaar, W., Crowther, R.A., 1988. Structural characterization of the core of the paired helical filament of Alzheimer disease. Proc. Natl. Acad. Sci. U.S.A. 85, 4884–4888.

Wischik, C.M., Staff, R.T., Wischik, D.J., Bentham, P., Murray, A.D., Storey, J.M., Kook, K.A., Harrington, C.R., 2014. Tau aggregation inhibitor therapy: an exploratory phase 2 study in mild or moderate Alzheimer's disease. J. Alzheimers Dis. 44 (2), 705–720.

Wolozin, B.L., Pruchnicki, A., Dickson, D.W., Davies, P., 1986. A neuronal antigen in the brains of Alzheimer patients. Science 232, 648–650.

Wood, J.G., Mirra, S.S., Pollock, N.J., Binder, L.I., 1986. Neurofibrillary tangles of Alzheimer disease share antigenic determinants with the axonal microtubule-associated protein tau (tau). Proc. Natl. Acad. Sci. U.S.A. 83, 4040–4043.

Wulff, P., Ponomarenko, A.A., Bartos, M., Korotkova, T.M., Fuchs, E.C., Bahner, F., Both, M., Tort, A.B., Kopell, N.J., Wisden, W., et al., 2009. Hippocampal theta rhythm and its coupling with gamma oscillations require fast inhibition onto parvalbumin-positive interneurons. Proc. Natl. Acad. Sci. U.S.A. 106, 3561–3566.

Xi, Y.D., Ding, J., Han, J., Zhang, D.D., Liu, J.M., Feng, L.L., Xiao, R., 2015. The effect of soybean isoflavone on the dysregulation of NMDA receptor signaling pathway induced by beta-amyloid peptides 1–42 in rats. Cell Mol. Neurobiol. 35, 555–562.

Xiao, Y., Ma, B., McElheny, D., Parthasarathy, S., Long, F., Hoshi, M., Nussinov, R., Ishii, Y., 2015. Abeta(1–42) fibril structure illuminates self-recognition and replication of amyloid in Alzheimer's disease. Nat. Struct. Mol. Biol. 22 (6), 499–505.

Yan, S.D., Yan, S.F., Chen, X., Fu, J., Chen, M., Kuppusamy, P., Smith, M.A., Perry, G., Godman, G.C., Nawroth, P., et al., 1995. Non-enzymatically glycated tau in Alzheimer's disease induces neuronal oxidant stress resulting in cytokine gene expression and release of amyloid beta-peptide. Nat. Med. 1, 693–699.

Yue, X.H., Liu, X.J., Wu, M.N., Chen, J.Y., Qi, J.S., 2014. Amyloid beta protein suppresses hippocampal theta rhythm and induces behavioral disinhibition and spatial memory deficit in rats. Sheng Li Xue Bao 66, 97–106.

Zempel, H., Thies, E., Mandelkow, E., Mandelkow, E.M., 2010. Abeta oligomers cause localized Ca(2+) elevation, missorting of endogenous Tau into dendrites, Tau phosphorylation, and destruction of microtubules and spines. J. Neurosci. 30, 11938–11950.

CHAPTER

9

Cholesterol and Fat Metabolism in Alzheimer's Disease

C. Taghibiglou, S. Khalaj

OUTLINE

CHOLESTEROL AND FAT METABOLISM IN ALZHEIMER'S DISEASE

Alzheimer's disease (AD) is the most common cause of dementia in the elderly affecting up to 15 million individuals worldwide. AD is a complex and genetically heterogeneous disease, characterized by progressive memory loss, cognitive impairment, and personality changes. This disease is accompanied by specific structural abnormalities in the brain including senile plaques caused by significant increase in brain β-amyloid levels and hyperphosphorylated tau protein-dependent neurofibrillary tangles. Historically, more than a century ago, Dr. Alois Alzheimer identified three major neuropathological features of a disease later named after him, namely, senile plaques, neurofibrillary tangles, and lipid droplets/granules accumulation (Foley, 2010). The first two microscopic pathological features of AD were widely studied

Drug Discovery Approaches for the Treatment of Neurodegenerative Disorders
http://dx.doi.org/10.1016/B978-0-12-802810-0.00009-X

over the past century. However, the roles of neuronal lipid droplets and granules accumulation in AD have been entirely ignored. A large body of emerging data including the recent genome-wide association studies (GWAS), clinical trials, and epidemiological studies on AD has provided further support for the implication of brain metabolic dysfunction such as insulin resistance (Bedse et al., 2015; de la Monte and Tong, 2014; Lourenco et al., 2015; Ma et al., 2015; Verdile et al., 2015). In addition, perturbed lipid metabolism, particularly dysregulated cholesterol metabolism, has been linked to the pathogenesis of AD (Gamba et al., 2015; Jones et al., 2010; Shepardson et al., 2011a,b). At the molecular level, AD progression has been attributed to inflammation, oxidative stress, and excitotoxicity as well. Here we discuss the role of perturbed lipid/cholesterol metabolism in the progression of AD and how this is linked to the glutamate excitotoxicity-induced activation of lipid transcription factors [sterol regulatory element binding proteins (SREBPs)] leading to neuronal apoptosis.

LIPIDOMICS AS A STRONG TOOL IN DECIPHERING THE ROLE OF LIPID MOIETIES IN AD

There is a large body of evidence connecting aberrant lipid homeostasis with AD. Therefore comparative studies of alterations in brain lipid composition in animal models of AD and postmortem AD brains have been at the center of attention for many research groups. Advancement in biomedical instrumental analysis or so-called "omics" has been an important contributor in better understanding the molecular mechanisms of diseases including AD. Lipidomics or lipid-targeted metabolomics comprehensively characterizes and quantifies all lipid species or "lipidome" in biological systems (Shevchenko and Simons, 2010). Although the lipidome is extremely complex and estimated to comprise more than a million lipid moieties, the lipid species can be categorized based on their chemical structural backbone in the following main categories: fatty acids, steroids, phospholipids [phosphatidic acid, phosphatidylcholine (PC), phosphatidylethanolamine (PE), phosphatidylglycerol, phosphatidylinositol (PI), phosphatidylserine, sphingomyelin (SM), lysophospholipids], sphingolipids (ceramides, sulfatides, gangliosides), glycerolipids [monoacylglycerol, diacylglycerol (DG), triacylglycerol, cardiolipin, cholesterol ester (CE)], glycolipids (monogalactosylDG, digalactosylDG, sulfoquinovosylDG), prenol lipids, and polyketides. Lipid metabolites comprise the majority (~70%) of metabolites recorded in the latest Human Metabolome Database (Wishart et al., 2013). Complexity and diversity of lipid moieties originate from the fact that lipids are defined from alterations in their head and tail groups, which suggests ever-growing possibilities of introducing numerous new lipid moieties in the human metabolome. Mass spectrometry (MS)-based approaches have been widely used to investigate lipidome in cell cultures, animal models, and postmortem specimens (Li et al., 2014; Wang et al., 2015). Among these instrumental analytical techniques, high-throughput and high-sensitivity liquid chromatography and gas chromatography coupled to mass spectrometry are widely being used. These methodologies provide more accurate and comprehensive information on lipid moieties in biological samples for the purposes of biomarker research [blood, cerebrospinal fluid (CSF), and urine] and pathogenesis of diseases (Shevchenko and Simons, 2010; Wenk, 2005). The fundamental challenge in any metabolomics approach is identifying alterations in analyte levels and connecting them with physiopathological events.

Several research groups have investigated lipidome alterations in postmortem AD brain tissues and compared them with age- and sex-matched normal control brains. Chan et al. (2012) studied more than 300 lipid species from 26 lipid subclasses and found significant changes in the diseased prefrontal and entorhinal cortices (PFC and ERC) of patients who suffered from late onset of AD.

They observed more severe lipid alterations in PFC regions with significant reductions in levels of lysophosphatidylcholine (LPC), lyso ether PC (LPCe), and PE as well as elevation in ceramide, glucosyl ceramide, galactosyl ceramide, and diacylglycerol (DAG). Moreover, they reported significant increases in lysobisphosphatidic acid, SM, ganglioside ceramide-lactose-*N*-acetylneuraminic acid (GM3), and CE levels in ERC of AD patients. Based on the overall lipid profile they obtained, it was concluded that the so-called lipid traffic jams exist in the ERC of AD patients. In addition to human postmortem specimens, Chan et al. (2012) analyzed the brain lipid profile of transgenic models of AD such as amyloid precursor protein (APP), presenilin 1 (PS1), and PS1-APP mice and concluded that some of the lipid profile features in these animal models are common with the human AD patients, despite the fact that most aspects were vastly different between mice and human AD specimens. Some of their findings corroborated the molecular and cellular mechanisms and features proposed for AD. For instance, they observed accumulation of SM, ganglioside ceramide-lactose-*N*-acetylneuraminic acid (GM3), and CE in both transgenic mice (APP and PS1-APP models) and in the ERC of postmortem AD specimens. These observations support the hypothesis of endosomal dysfunction and impairment of lysosomal degradation. Several groups also reported an increase in CE content in the vulnerable regions of brains of AD patients and transgenic mouse models (Shibuya et al., 2015; Tajima et al., 2013). An elevated level of cellular CE not only fits well with the accumulation of lipid droplets as a pathologic hallmark of AD (as first described by Alzheimer), but it is in agreement with the reports on therapeutic effects of genetic ablation and pharmacological inhibition of the CE synthesizing enzyme [acetyl-CoA cholesterol acyltransferase (*ACAT1*)] in animal models of AD (Shibuya et al., 2015; Murphy et al., 2013; Shibuya et al., 2014). In fact, the *ACAT1* gene is one of the genes with negative genetic association with AD (Blomqvist et al., 2006; Zhao et al., 2005). Knocking down *ACAT1* gene as well as pharmacological inhibition have decreased amyloid β (Aβ) burden and ameliorated its pathology in animal models of AD (Murphy et al., 2013; Bhattacharyya and Kovacs, 2010; Bryleva et al., 2010). The effects of *ACAT1* inhibitors on signs and symptoms of AD encouraged some to hypothesize that AD and atherosclerosis may have a common cause (Lathe et al., 2014). Although using selective ACAT inhibitors in animal models of AD appeared to be promising (Giovannoni et al., 2003; Ohshiro and Tomoda, 2015), more controlled clinical studies are needed for future application of these pharmacological agents in human AD (Huttunen and Kovacs, 2008).

In a metabolomics study on an APP/PS1 transgenic mice model of AD using direct infusion MS, Gonzalez-Dominguez et al. found an abnormal regional brain metabolism of fatty acids (FA), leading to the accumulation of free FAs as well as alterations in different classes of phospholipids, acylcarnitines, and related compounds. These lipid abnormalities were principally detected in the hippocampus and cortex and mostly attributed to the overactivity of the phospholipase A2 (PLA2) enzyme (Gonzalez-Dominguez et al., 2014a,b, 2015). PLA2 overactivity is also considered as one of the pathological hallmarks of AD (Farooqui et al., 2004; Gentile et al., 2012). Indeed, Aβ partly causes neuronal apoptosis by activating myriad enzymes including cytosolic PLA2 (cPLA2), nicotinamide adenine dinucleotide phosphate (NADPH) oxidase, and sphingomyelinases. Similar to neuroprotective effects of selective cPLA2 inhibitors against Aβ-induced apoptosis in cultured neurons, the reduction of PLA2 activity in an hAPP transgenic mice model of AD also ameliorated Aβ-induced behavioral and cognitive deficits (Sanchez-Mejia et al., 2008). The main function of the PLA2 group of enzymes is to hydrolyze membrane phospholipids present at the sn-2 position into arachidonic acid and lysophospholipids. PLA2 enzymes play a pivotal role in the regulation of lipid droplet biogenesis (Guijas et al., 2014; Pol et al., 2014). Indeed, several enzymes involved in biosynthesis of eicosanoids including cytosolic PLA2α as well as signaling molecules required for cPLA2 activation such as lipin-1, extracellular signal-regulated kinase-1 and -2 (ERK1 and 2) have been associated with lipid droplets (Guijas et al., 2014; Yu et al., 1998). In addition to the role of PLA2 enzymes in the biogenesis of cytosolic lipid droplets (major pathologic hallmarks of AD), they are also involved in oxidative stress and neuroinflammation. Another deleterious consequence of overactivity of PLA2 enzymes is perturbation of membrane biophysical and biochemical properties such as membrane fluidity, thickness, regional curvature, and molecular packing, which may affect receptor trafficking and the activities of membrane-associated enzymes (Hulbert et al., 2013; Ibarguren et al., 2014; Nicolson, 2014). Considering the fact that APP and α-, β-, and γ-secretases are membrane-associated proteins, the membrane composition and its biophysical properties should profoundly affect APP processing (Cecchi and Stefani, 2013; Yang et al., 2014). All these negative features have attracted pharmaceutical companies to search for more selective synthetic and natural inhibitors of PLA2 for the treatment of neurological disorders including AD (Ong et al., 2015).

Lipid analysis in postmortem and animal models of AD also revealed an increase in short-chain lipids whereas polyunsaturated phospholipid levels were found to be reduced (Chan et al., 2012). Similar observations were noted in synaptosome and lipid rafts isolated from brains of AD patients and animal models (Martin et al., 2010; Mateos et al., 2010). It is completely predictable that such alterations in plasma membrane (PM) components will affect membrane thickness as well as rafts/bulk membrane ratio. Sphingolipids and cholesterol contents of lipid rafts favorably interact with short-chain saturated or monosaturated phospholipids when compared with long-chain polyunsaturated phospholipids. Considering the role of lipid rafts in amyloidogenic processing of APP (discussed in more detail in the following section), in AD brain, the rafts/nonrafts (bulk membrane) ratio appears to be increased (Di Paolo and Kim, 2011; Grosgen et al., 2010; Wassall and Stillwell, 2009).

Aberrant metabolism and accumulation of DAG and sphingolipids are other features of brain lipid profile alteration in AD. DAG appears to be involved in a variety of synapse-related functions and features such as synaptic plasticity, regulation of neurotransmitter release, and the regulation of dendritic spine morphology (Haass and Selkoe, 2007; Mucke and Selkoe, 2012) and are some of the processes that are impaired in Alzheimer brain. The pathological accumulation of DAG has been attributed to Aβ oligomer-induced hydrolysis of $PI(4,5)P_2$ by phospholipase C (Berman et al., 2008). It is also suggested that DAG may be responsible for Aβ-induced reduction of sAPPα (prosurvival fragment of APP) through the phospholipase D pathway (Tanabe et al., 2012). Although DAG is involved in the activation of protein kinase C (PKC) or memory kinase, overactivation of this enzyme has been partly involved in memory impairment in AD (Birnbaum et al., 2004; Sun and Alkon, 2014; Lucke-Wold et al., 2015). It is also noteworthy that the physiological function of PKC is required for the modulation of the a disintegrin and metalloproteinase 10 (ADAM10) enzyme intracellular path from Golgi outposts to the excitatory synapses resulting in APP nontoxic ectodomain shedding and preventing amyloid formation in the brain (Saraceno et al., 2014). This process is impaired in the AD brain. In addition to DAG, abnormal accumulation of sphingolipids has also been reported in postmortem AD and transgenic mice brains. Abnormal accumulation of sphingolipids may interfere with the fusion of synaptic vesicles (SVs) and the trafficking of *N*-methyl-D-aspartate (NMDA) subtype of glutamate receptor (GluR) and may contribute to the excitotoxicity-induced neuronal apoptosis in AD (discussed later in more detail) (Haughey et al., 2010; Zadori et al., 2014). Moreover, alterations of sphingolipids as one of the main components of the PM lipid rafts can have profound effects on cellular functions including cell signaling and trafficking (Chakraborty and Jiang, 2013; Fantini and Barrantes, 2009).

Overall, data collected from lipidomic studies strongly suggest brain regional pathologic alterations in lipid profiles, which interfere with physiological function of the CNS and contribute to the pathogenesis of AD. However, it is not known whether lipid alterations are causes or consequences of AD. More studies are warranted to fill the knowledge gaps that exist in the area of pathological lipid droplet accumulation in AD. Advances in technologies and methods for isolating these important subcellular organelles will pave the way in advancing our understanding the role of lipids in AD.

PLASMA MEMBRANE MICRODOMAIN (LIPID RAFTS) AND AD

Numerous studies have implicated a role for lipid rafts in the development of neurodegenerative diseases including AD (Allinquant et al., 2014; Zhou et al., 2014; Williamson and Sutherland, 2011; Sonnino et al., 2014; Kubo et al., 2015; Ben Halima and Rajendran, 2011). In fact, it is generally believed that disarrangement/dysregulation of lipid rafts is linked to the progress of neuropathological diseases (Marin et al., 2013).

The Singer–Nicolson classical fluid mosaic model of PM (Singer and Nicolson, 1972) was modified more than three decades ago. In the fluid mosaic model, PM has been defined as a homogeneous two-dimensional bilayer of glycerophospholipid (liquid disordered phase), which accommodates the lateral movement and floating of its components, mostly proteins (eg, enzymes and receptors) (Nicolson, 2014; Goni, 2014). In the PM microdomain or lipid rafts model (proposed in the 1980s), PM contains small ordered microdomains that are enriched in cholesterol and sphingolipids as well as lipid-interacting proteins such as caveolins and flotillins (Simons and Gerl, 2010). In a simplified definition, one can consider PM as a bilayer ocean of lipids in which islands of sphingolipids and cholesterol (containing some enzymes, receptors, and signaling molecules) are floating. In more technical terms, lipid rafts are dynamic fluctuating nanoscale liquid-ordered assemblies of sphingolipids and cholesterol, associated with proteins that can be stabilized to coalesce, forming platforms that are implicated in several cellular processes, including membrane trafficking, cell adhesion, cortical actin regulation, molecular sorting, and signal transduction (Sebastiao et al., 2013). The self-assembly of sphingolipids and cholesterol with protein in the lipid rafts regulates a variety of membrane functions and bioactivities. In terms of size, membrane rafts are estimated to be between 10 and 20nm, which may become larger platforms through protein–protein and protein–lipid interactions (Pike, 2006). The tight packing of lipid rafts because of the long saturated acyl chains of sphingolipids and compacting filler property of cholesterol molecules in the lipid rafts, in addition to causing phase separation with the rest of the PM (bulk membrane), also make them resistant to solubilization with cold detergents such as Triton-X100 and Brij 96. This further suggests the existence of sterol-dependent sphingolipid and protein association in cell membranes. Despite criticisms, processing crude PM with cold 0.5–1% Triton-X100 and subsequent sucrose gradient ultracentrifugation (and fractionation) is the most common method to isolate detergent-resistant membranes (DRMs) or lipid rafts (Taghibiglou et al., 2009b). Structural proteins of the lipid rafts such as flotillin-1 and caveolin-1 are used as DRMs markers, whereas transferrin receptor serves as nonrafts or bulk membrane marker. Since lipid raft compartments are enriched with gangliosides including ganglioside G_{M1}, which interacts with cholera toxin-B (CTX-B), the PM microdomains can also be visualized and detected with CTX-B conjugated to any reporter molecule such as horseradish peroxidase, fluorophores using a dot-blot (and chemiluminescence), or fluorescent microscopic methods.

An ever-increasing number of receptors and enzymes are reported to be localized to the lipid raft including proteins and enzymes involved in AD. In general, some structural features and posttranslational modifications of proteins, the so-called raft-targeting domains, determine PM microdomain compartmentalization of proteins (Levental et al., 2010). For instance, posttranslation modification by saturated lipids recruits proteins to rafts, whereas raft localization is prevented by short, unsaturated, and/or branched hydrocarbon chain modifications. The glycophosphatidyl inositol (GPI)-anchored proteins, which are saturated lipid-anchored extracellular peripheral proteins, are the best studied and the most well-characterized lipid rafts-associated proteins (Levental et al., 2010; Muniz and Zurzolo, 2014). GPI-anchored proteins include a variety of proteins involved in important cellular functions such as immune system signaling, adhesion, membrane trafficking, and nutrient uptake (Tsai et al., 2012). Cellular prion protein (PrP^C), Thy-1, and placental alkaline phosphatase are some examples of GPI-anchored proteins. Cysteine palmitoylation or S-acylation (double acylation) is another posttranslational modification enabling intracellular proteins to be associated with the lipid rafts. Examples of double acylated proteins include members of the Src-family of kinases and the Ras family of small GTPases. Myristoylation and prenylation are other common lipid modifications of proteins. Both Src-family kinases (eg, Fyn) and PrP^C have been implicated in the pathogenesis of AD (Black et al., 2014; Calella et al., 2010; Hirsch et al., 2014; Kostylev et al., 2015; Lauren et al., 2009; Peters et al., 2015; Um et al., 2012). In some cases, interaction or association with lipid rafts proteins or lipid moieties mediate PM microdomain localization of certain proteins without any of the aforementioned posttranslational modifications.

The number of lipid rafts localized proteins is growing in parallel with new advancement in analytical methods and subcellular imaging techniques. The existence of the cholesterol/sphingolipid-enriched microdomains in CNS in neurons (Suzuki, 2002) and glia cells (Gielen et al., 2006; Hibino and Kurachi, 2007) highlighted possible involvement of neuronal and glial lipid rafts in physiological CNS functions as well as pathophysiological mechanisms of neurological diseases. The connections between cholesterol (a major component of the lipid rafts) and synaptic plasticity, axonal, and neurite outgrowth are well documented, and failure in the brain cholesterol hemostasis has been implicated in synaptic dysfunction and memory loss (Segatto et al., 2014). Depletion of major lipid components of the neuronal microdomains (cholesterol and sphingolipids) resulted in gradual loss of both excitatory and inhibitory synapses indicating the pivotal role of the lipid rafts in synaptic transmission (Hering et al., 2003). Experimental evidence is also suggesting a physical association between postsynaptic membrane rafts and the postsynaptic density structures (PSDs) that could be important in postsynaptic signal integration, synaptic function, and maintenance (Suzuki et al., 2011). Moreover, several members of different neurotransmitter signaling pathways have been identified in the neuronal lipid rafts. In the presynaptic membrane, exocytotic machinery components such as soluble *N*-ethylmaleimide-sensitive factor activating protein receptor proteins (SNAP 25, syntaxin 1, and synaptobrevin2/VAMP2) (Gil et al., 2005), synaptophysin, synaptotagmins, Munc18, neuronal calcium sensor-1, and voltage-dependent Ca^{2+} channels 2.1 (Cav2.1) proteins have been isolated from lipid rafts, and reduction in cholesterol levels (or lipid rafts disruption) impairs presynaptic glutamate release and synaptic plasticity (Linetti et al., 2010; Taverna et al., 2007). In fact, SV membranes are enriched in cholesterol and depletion of presynaptic membrane cholesterol drastically affects release of SVs into the synaptic clefts.

There is increasing evidence indicating that lipid rafts association can also influence neurotransmitter receptor function by affecting transmitter binding, receptor trafficking and clustering, and interacting protein and lipid partner's pattern (Allen et al., 2007). Although several neurotransmitter key signaling components including glutamatergic, GABAergic, dopaminergic, cholinergic, serotoninergic (Bjork et al., 2010), and purinergic systems (Assaife-Lopes et al., 2010, 2014) have been identified in the neuronal lipid rafts (Sebastiao et al., 2013; Korade and Kenworthy, 2008), only those that are more relevant to AD and dementia will be discussed here.

In terms of glutamatergic receptors, ionotropic NMDA, α-amino-3-hydroxy-5-methyl-4-isoxazolepropionic acid (AMPA), kainate subtype receptors, and metabotropic glutamate receptors (mGluRs) have been identified in lipid raft domains. However, one of the important physiological functions of NMDA and AMPA subtypes of GluRs is their participation in induction of long-term potentiation (LTP) and long-term depression (LTD) features of synaptic plasticity and learning and memory. Pathological overactivation of these receptors causes massive influx of Ca^{2+} and triggers a deleterious cycle of events called excitotoxicity. Excitotoxicity plays a major role in the pathogenesis of neurodegenerative diseases including AD, Parkinson's disease (PD), Huntington's disease (HD), amyotrophic lateral sclerosis (ALS), and stroke (Blasco et al., 2014; Gonzalez et al., 2015; Kritis et al., 2015; Lai et al., 2014; Rudy et al., 2015). It is therefore plausible to hypothesize that NMDA and AMPA receptor trafficking and their PM compartment localization may influence both their physiological and pathological functions. Among all glutamate subtype receptors, NMDA receptors (NMDARs) are the ones heavily implicated in neuronal apoptosis in neurodegenerative diseases.

NMDARs are heterotetrameric ligand-gated ion channels composed of two obligatory GluN1 subunits with at least one type of GluN2 (GluN2A–D) and/or GluN3 subunits. The majority of NMDARs in the hippocampus and cerebellar cortex contain GluN2B (NR2B) or GluN2A (NR2A) subunits. Different GluN2 subunits exert specific downstream signaling events and have distinct electrophysiological and pharmacological properties, resulting in different functional consequences for the NMDAR depending on the GluN2 subunit(s) present (Bliss and Collingridge, 1993; Seeburg et al., 1995). NMDARs are essential for brain development and play key physiological roles in neuronal survival and function (Collingridge et al., 2004, 2010; Fan et al., 2014). However, overstimulation of NMDARs, particularly those containing the GluN2B subunit, causes neuronal excitotoxicity because of the accumulation of excessive intraneuronal Ca^{2+}, which contributes to the neuronal death associated with brain ischemia and hypoxia (Arundine and Tymianski, 2004) and chronic neurodegenerative diseases (Kalia et al., 2008; Milnerwood et al., 2010; Milnerwood and Raymond, 2010; Parsons and Raymond, 2014). Paradoxically, the activation of GluN2A-containing NMDAR promotes neuronal survival (Hardingham, 2009; Hardingham and Bading, 2010; Hardingham et al., 2002). Localization and subunit composition appear to determine the physiological/pathological outcomes following their activation (Hardingham, 2009; Gladding and Raymond, 2011; Lai et al., 2011; Paoletti, 2011; Wyllie et al., 2013). Besshoh et al. reported that between 50% and 60% of NMDA receptors as well as 85–90% of Src and Fyn were localized in lipid rafts. They demonstrated that an elevation in the phosphorylation and reduction in protein masses of lipid rafts localized GluN1, GluN2A, and GluN2B following ischemia (Besshoh et al., 2005). The same group later reported developmental and age-dependent changes in NMDAR lipid rafts localization and phosphorylation patterns (Besshoh et al., 2007). Others also reported localization of NMDARs in both rafts and nonrafts compartments (Hering et al., 2003; Guirland et al., 2004; Nothdurfter et al., 2013). We also detected NMDAR major subunits in both rafts and bulk membrane compartments (Taghibiglou, unpublished data). Ponce et al. (2008) demonstrated a connection between lipid rafts-residing NMDARs and excitotoxicity-induced neuronal apoptosis. They reported that the inhibition of neuronal cholesterol synthesis (using simvastatin or AY9944) and disruption of lipid rafts cholesterol contents reduced the number of NMDARs in the lipid rafts and resulted in significant neuroprotection against NMDA excitotoxic insult. Yang et al. (2015) reported a direct interaction between the lipid rafts' structural protein caveolin-1 and GluN2B subunit of NMDAR in the anterior cingulate cortex and implicated this interaction in modulation of chronic neuropathic pain via regulation of GluN2B-dependent Ca^{2+} influx and subsequent activation of ERK/CREB signaling. In line with this finding, Marques-da-Silva and Gutierrez-Merino (2012), who had previously discovered the colocalization of L-type voltage-operated calcium channels, NMDARs, neuronal nitric oxide synthase, and cytochrome b_5 reductase within the lipid rafts of the mature cerebellar granule neurons (Marques-da-Silva et al., 2010), also identified clusters of calcium transport systems in caveolin-1-enriched lipid rafts (Marques-da-Silva and Gutierrez-Merino, 2014). Although knocking out caveolin-1 showed no change in basal glutamatergic transmission and NMDAR-dependent LTD, it altered mGluR1/5-dependent activation (phosphorylation) of MEK and ERK1/2 and affected the induction of mGluR-LTD (Takayasu et al., 2010). There is consensus among neuroscientists on dual prosurvival and prodeath functions of NMDARs, depending on subunit composition of the receptor and/or its localization (synaptic vs extrasynaptic) (Hardingham and Bading, 2010). Head et al. (2008) added caveolin-1 to this paradigm, when it was found that preconditioning cultured neurons with sublethal NMDA or sublethal ischemia triggered the NMDAR-dependent prosurvival signaling pathway by increased expression of phosphorylated caveolin-1, P-Src, and P-ERK1/2 as well as partial localization of GluN2B subunit of NMDAR with caveolin-1 in the lipid rafts. They also concluded that caveolin-1 contributed in part to the prosurvival function of NMDARs. In contrast with this study, del Toro et al. (2010) reported that altered cholesterol hemostasis caused by mutant huntingtin (increased cholesterol, Cav-1, and GM1 levels) resulted in increased presence of NMDAR in the lipid rafts and consequently exacerbated the NMDAR-dependent excitotoxicity and neuronal degeneration in HD. Moreover, reducing cholesterol levels by simvastatin or β-cyclodextrin protected neurons against NMDA-mediated excitotoxicity, suggesting a strong link between cholesterol contents of the lipid rafts and GluR-induced excitotoxicity and neurodegeneration. Similar studies on cell cultures or animal models of AD encouraged and inspired research on clinical application of statins in AD. However, metaanalysis of these studies has not yet reached a solid conclusion (Liang et al., 2015; Mendoza-Oliva et al., 2014; Richardson et al., 2013; Shinohara et al., 2014).

The presence of a fraction of NMDAR in the lipid rafts compartment is required for the physiological functions of the neurons such as memory formation and receptor trafficking. For instance, in rat insular cortex, formation of spatial memory requires rapid recruitment of NMDAR subunits (GluN1, GluN2A, and GluN2B) and PSD-95 to synaptic lipid rafts, whereas in the hippocampus, spatial training induces selective translocation of GluN1 and GluN2A subunits to lipid rafts suggesting rapid translocation of NMDARs from nonrafts to the rafts compartments during spatial memory formation (Delint-Ramirez et al., 2008). An interaction between NMDAR (GluN2A and GluN2B subunits) and different structural proteins of the lipid rafts (flotillin-1 and -2) has also been reported (Swanwick et al., 2009) but its physiological and functional implications remains to be determined.

In cultured neurons, NMDAR activity was found to recruit AMPA receptors (AMPARs) to surface lipid rafts and this effect was NO pathway dependent and CaMKII activity independent (Hou et al., 2008). During membrane targeting, AMPARs insert into or at close proximity of the surface raft domains. Perturbation of lipid rafts dramatically suppresses AMPAR exocytosis, resulting in significant reduction in AMPAR cell surface expression. It is also noteworthy that glutamate has a positive regulatory effect on both mRNA and protein expression of caveolin-1 in cultured hippocampal primary neurons (Bu et al., 2003).

AMPAR subunits GluA1 and GluA2 were found localized in both lipid rafts and nonrafts compartments (Hering et al., 2003; Cole et al., 2010; Huo et al., 2009). Caveolin-1 was also found interfering with AMPAR-related LTP through its inhibitory activity on the enzyme PLA2 (Gaudreault et al., 2004). Although it was reported that PM cholesterol and sphingolipid depletion promoted constitutive AMPAR endocytosis (Hering et al., 2003) or suppressed AMPAR insertion (Hou et al., 2008), in our studies using primary cultured neurons incubated with exogenous cholesterol, we observed enhanced endocytosis of AMPARs (from nonraft compartments) (Taghibiglou, unpublished data). Overall, lipid rafts cholesterol/sphingolipids contents drastically influence ionotropic GluRs trafficking and function.

mGluRs trafficking, signaling, and functions are also affected directly (Takayasu et al., 2010; Francesconi et al., 2009; Hong et al., 2009) or indirectly (Boulware et al., 2013; Meitzen and Mermelstein, 2011; Mermelstein, 2009) by the lipid rafts' lipids and protein components.

Association of excitatory amino acid transporters (EAATs), especially EAAT2, with cholesterol-rich lipid rafts microdomains, has been previously reported. This association appeared to be important for EAAT localization and function, as disruption of lipid rafts by cholesterol depletion significantly reduced Na^+-dependent glutamate uptake in primary cortical cultures (Butchbach et al., 2004). An increased EAAT2 (also known as GLT-1) association with lipid rafts by cytidine diphosphate-choline has been found neuroprotective in experimental stroke (Hurtado et al., 2008). Similarly, the neuroprotective compound riluzole partly exerts its protective function by upregulation of GLT-1 levels in lipid rafts (Carbone et al., 2012). Interestingly, and more relevant with the role of excitotoxicity in pathogenesis of neurodegenerative diseases such as AD, increased expression of cholesterol 24S-hydroxylase resulted in disruption of glial glutamate transporter EAAT2 association with lipid rafts. These observations suggest that disturbance of cholesterol metabolism may contribute to loss of EAAT2 in AD and other neurodegenerative diseases (Cartagena et al., 2008, 2010; Tian et al., 2010).

New emerging evidence indicates that the inhibitory GABAergic neurotransmission is also implicated in pathogenesis of AD. GABA is the main inhibitory neurotransmitter in the brain, which exerts its effects by binding to $GABA_A$ (Cl^- permeable channel) and $GABA_B$ (metabotropic G protein-coupled receptor) receptors (Owens and Kriegstein, 2002; Wang and Kriegstein, 2009). In the rat brain cerebellum, $GABA_B$ receptors ($GABA_BRs$) are exclusively localized in the lipid rafts (Becher et al., 2001). Based on ectopical overexpression of the receptor in the Chinese hamster ovary (CHO) cells, Becher et al. (2004) concluded that the lipid rafts negatively regulate inhibitory function of $GABA_BRs$ following stimulation. $GABA_ARs$ are ionotropic, heteropentameric, ligand-gated ion channels, which are predominantly composed of α, β, and γ_2 subunits. Palmitoylation of $GABA_ARs$ on multiple cysteine residues of γ_2 subunit regulates the clustering of these receptors at synaptic sites (Fang et al., 2006; Rathenberg et al., 2004). Therefore γ_2 subunit-lacking receptors are excluded from synapses (extrasynaptic $GABA_ARs$). γ_2 Subunit is also responsible for ubiquitination and degradation of synaptic $GABA_ARs$ (Jin et al., 2014). It is reported that both extrasynaptic and synaptic $GABA_ARs$ are associated with lipid rafts (Li et al., 2007); however, some inconsistencies still exist mostly because of differences in lipid rafts isolation methodologies. Dalskov et al. (2005) reported lipid rafts association of $GABA_ARs$ in cerebral granular cells using nonionic detergent Brij 98. In our study using cultured primary rat cortical neurons and rat brain slices (cortical and hippocampal) processed with 0.5% cold TritonX-100 and sucrose gradient centrifugation, we detected $GABA_ARs$ in both rafts and nonrafts compartments with the majority localized in the bulk membrane (Taghibiglou, unpublished data). Nothdurfter et al. (2013) reported that depletion of cholesterol and disruption of lipid rafts affected $GABA_AR$ modulation in response to diazepam (Diaz) and enhanced the potentiating effect of Diaz on the $GABA_AR$ at nonsaturating concentrations of GABA, suggesting that the interaction of benzodiazepines with the $GABA_AR$ likely occurs outside of the lipid rafts. It is thus plausible to hypothesize that cholesterol enrichment of PM and expansion of the lipid rafts may have opposite outcomes by reducing $GABA_AR$ population in the nonraft compartment. Since dysregulation of GABA release and compromised function of $GABA_ARs$ have been linked to AD, therefore cholesterol content of PM and lipid raft/bulk membrane ratio may also be implicated in the compromised inhibitory neurotransmission in AD. Here we provide a few reports on this connection. Jo et al. (2014) have reported abnormal release of GABA from reactivated astrocytes in a mouse model of AD, linking it to memory impairment. Moreover, GABA receptors from AD brains appeared to be slightly, but significantly, less sensitive to GABA than receptors from non-AD brains. The reduction of GABA currents in AD was associated with reductions of mRNA and protein of the principal GABA receptor subunits normally present in the temporal cortex (Limon et al., 2012). The downregulation of $GABA_ARs$ has been linked to the weakening effects of Aβ on synaptic inhibition (Paula-Lima et al., 2013; Ulrich, 2015).

Losses of cholinergic tone and acetylcholine (ACh) levels in the brain have been hypothesized to be responsible for the cognitive decline and both nicotinic and muscarinic acetylcholine receptors (nAChRs and mAChRs) are affected in AD (Lombardo and Maskos, 2015). There is a strong body of evidence indicating that acetylcholine receptors (AChRs) interact with lipid rafts (Bruses et al., 2001; Campagna and Fallon, 2006; Marchand et al., 2002; Willmann et al., 2006; Zhu et al., 2006). Cholesterol alteration in the neuronal PM affects trafficking, clustering, stabilization, and function of both nAChRs and mAChRs (Sebastiao et al., 2013; Barrantes, 2007, 2014). For instance, the neuronal-type α7 nicotinic acetylcholine receptor (α7nAChR) is a widely expressed nAChR with a peculiar high Ca^{2+} permeability mediating intracellular cascades involved in both physiological and pathological events. α7nAChR is mainly localized in lipid rafts (Bruses et al., 2001) and acute cholesterol depletion reduces not only cholesterol levels but also the number of cell surface α7nAChRs (Pena et al., 2011). It is noteworthy that a cholesterol-interacting motif for nAChRs has been identified (Baier et al., 2011). Indeed, nonionic lipids such as cholesterol shape activity of nAChRs by modulating the relative proportions of activatable versus nonactivatable conformations and by controlling the transitions between uncoupled and coupled conformations of the receptors (daCosta et al., 2013). In PC12 cells, the nAChR alpha 7-subunit regulates cyclic AMP signaling within the lipid rafts where colocalization with type 6 adenylyl cyclase and cholesterol depletion disrupt this function. In contrast, nAChR alpha 5- and beta 2-subunits were found in the bulk membrane (nonraft) compartment (Oshikawa et al., 2003). The roles of cholesterol content of neuronal lipid rafts play in conjunction with α7nAChRs are more highlighted considering that Aβ oligomers interact with and upregulate α7nAChRs leading to neurotoxicity in hippocampal neurons (Liu et al., 2015) and activation of a7nAChRs elevate presynaptic glutamate release that in turn exacerbates excitotoxicity (McKay et al., 2007).

In terms of mAChRs, Michal et al. (2009, 2014) have reported that experimental alterations of membrane cholesterol concentration exerted various impacts on preferential second messenger signaling mediated by M1, M2, and M3 muscarinic receptors. The same group observed that changes in membrane cholesterol concentration differentially impacted preferential and nonpreferential M1 and M3 receptor signaling (Michal et al., 2014).

Collectively, evidence suggests that lipid rafts and cholesterol, by influencing neurotransmitter receptors trafficking and function as well as neurotransmitter release and uptake (clearance), play an important role in the mediation of neurodegeneration in AD.

CHOLESTEROL AND LIPID RAFTS MODULATE APP PROCESSING AND Aβ MOIETIES GENERATION

In addition to neurotransmitters and their receptor functions, cholesterol and lipid rafts also play a pivotal role in the generation of toxic Aβ peptides and their deleterious signaling in AD.

The Aβ peptide is constantly generated from APP processing by sequential enzymatic cleavage involving β-secretase or β-site APP cleaving enzyme 1 (BACE1) and γ-secretase (Nicolas and Hassan, 2014). There is an alternative nonamyloidogenic, nontoxic APP processing pathway initiated by the enzyme α-secretase (also called ADAM10), which releases αC-terminal truncated fragment and the soluble extracellular domain (sAPPα).

Two major enzymes, BACE1 and γ-secretase, as well as Aβ have been detected in lipid rafts implicating this PM compartment and its lipid components in generating toxic Aβ (Ehehalt et al., 2003; Kalvodova et al., 2005; Lee et al., 1998; Wada et al., 2003). However, α-secretase and most of APP are localized in the bulk membrane outside of lipid rafts, although a small pool of APP has been found in PM microdomain as well (Parkin et al., 1999). It is also known that APP interacts through its C-terminal with flotillin-1, a lipid rafts structural protein, and this interaction is involved in APP clustering, endocytosis, and the amyloidogenic process in neurons (Chen et al., 2006; Schneider et al., 2008). Moreover, APP also directly interacts with cholesterol, a major component of lipid rafts (Beel et al., 2010). In addition, PM cholesterol also plays a pivotal regulatory role in the proteolytic fate of APP or its α or β cleavages. Experimental data suggest that the α-secretase/β-secretase ratio or accessibility of either of these enzymes to APP in the lipid rafts is a major determinant in the generation of toxic Aβ as the targeted expression of α-secretase in the lipid rafts significantly reduced Aβ generation in neuroblastoma SH-SY5Y cells (Harris et al., 2009). In fact, lipid rafts play a profound role not only in the toxic cleavage of APP, but also in its endocytosis and internalization to the acidic endosomes, which is a crucial step in generation of toxic Aβ species (Ehehalt et al., 2003; Saavedra et al., 2007). Accumulation of dimeric Aβ, apolipoprotein E (ApoE), and phosphorylated tau in lipid rafts has also been reported in an animal model of AD and coincided with the beginning of memory loss (Kawarabayashi et al., 2004). We have shown that in cultured hippocampal or cortical neurons, exogenous cholesterol incubation caused expansion of lipid rafts, brain insulin resistance (type III diabetes), and disrupted neuronal receptor trafficking (Taghibiglou et al., 2009b). It is thus plausible to hypothesize that the lipid rafts expansion may potentially work in favor of toxic β cleavage. In fact, epidemiological studies have revealed hypercholesterolemia and insulin resistance as two risk factors for AD (Daviglus et al., 2011; Ledesma and Dotti, 2012; Kalmijn et al., 1997; Gamba et al., 2012; Dawson, 2015; Ong et al., 2013; Simons and Ehehalt, 2002; Vignini et al., 2013; Wood et al., 2014).

Increasing evidence implicates PM microdomain in Aβ aggregation and toxic structural transition, because gangliosides in lipid rafts bind to Aβ and cholesterol facilitates this deleterious event (Kakio et al., 2003; Williams and Serpell, 2011). Among glycosphingolipids of rafts, GM1 has a profound role in regulating proteolysis of APP, interacting and promoting Aβ peptide seeding and toxic aggregation in the brain (Bucciantini et al., 2012; Hayashi et al., 2004; Hoshino et al., 2013; Lemkul and Bevan, 2013; Matsuzaki, 2014; Zha et al., 2004). The interaction between Aβ and GM1 during Aβ aggregation significantly affects the lateral fluidity of membranes and causes enhanced phase separation in lipids as well as provides a less polar environment (Fukunaga et al., 2012; Sasahara et al., 2013). This aggregation occurs prior to the extracellular area release of Aβ and destabilizes neuronal PM. The ganglioside cluster-mediated amyloidogenesis is more prominent and toxic in humans than in rodents (Ueno et al., 2014). GM1–Aβ clustering on PM may cause cell membrane damage partly by uptaking the raft components into Aβ aggregates (Sasahara et al., 2015). There is also a correlation between ganglioside levels (GM1 and GM2) and plaque formation kinetics in both mouse models and AD patients (Chan et al., 2012; Molander-Melin et al., 2005). Furthermore, the role of GM1 and lipid rafts as a platform for seeding toxic Aβ appears to be increasingly important as indicated by the prion-like propagation of neurodegenerative disease including AD (Goedert, 2015).

These reports encouraged several studies based on lipid modulation therapy including using cholesterol-lowering agents such as statins, GM1-lowering agents, and increasing levels of long chain polyunsaturated fatty acids (LCPUFAs). Outcomes from human studies of statins have so far been highly variable and conflicting mostly because of differences in study designs (Shepardson et al., 2011a,b; McGuinness et al., 2010). In terms of GM1, midazolam and leptin have been proposed to exert neuroprotective effects against Aβ-induced neurotoxicity by reducing GM1 levels through $GABA_AR$ and PI3K/Akt/mTOR pathways, respectively (Yamamoto et al., 2014, 2015). Among LCPUFAs, docosahexaenoic acid (DHA; 22:6 n-3) has been at the center of attentions by neuroscientists and nutritionists (Grimm et al., 2013; Lopes da Silva et al., 2014). DHA is the most abundant omega-3 PUFA in the brain and is involved in important CNS learning and memory-related physiological processes such as neurogenesis, synaptogenesis, and synaptic transmission (Salem et al., 2001; Su, 2010). The uptake of DHA into brain phosphatidylethanolamines resulted in exclusion of cholesterol from the DHA-rich membranes (Stillwell et al., 2005). It is noteworthy that inadequacies of DHA have been reported in aging as well as AD patients (Martin et al., 2010; Cunnane et al., 2013; Mohajeri et al., 2015). In addition to its effect on membrane fluidity and other biophysical parameters of lipid rafts as well as alteration in membrane organization (Khmelinskaia et al., 2014), DHA (hydroxyl form) has been shown to reduce the total amyloid load and tau phosphorylation in transgenic mice and in cellular models of AD by affecting the brain lipid membrane composition such as enriching membranes in long PUFAs and PE, as well as reducing the raft-associated sphingomyelin (Torres et al., 2014). In agreement with these observations, Torres et al. (2015) have reported that hydroxyl DHA improved cognition and restored memory loss in a rodent model of AD partly by modulating autophagy and unfolding protein response indicating potential beneficial effects of DHA in AD.

It is strongly believed that molecules involved in restoring and normalizing the membrane lipid composition of PM microdomains (membrane lipid therapy) could potentially be considered as therapeutic tools to treat AD. However, despite promising nutritional and therapeutic approaches (Escriba et al., 2015), nothing has yet been conclusive in clinical trials.

EXCITOTOXICITY-INDUCED LIPID ALTERATION: A POTENTIAL LINK BETWEEN CHOLESTEROL AND AD

Glutamate is the major excitatory transmitter in the mammalian CNS, and it exerts its actions by binding to several types of GluRs (Karakas et al., 2015; Regan et al., 2015). Although multiple pathways and mechanisms may contribute to the synaptic damage and neuronal cell loss in neurodegenerative diseases, the glutamate-mediated excitotoxicity or overactivation of GluRs plays a major role in brain injury and neurodegenerative diseases including typical neuronal dysfunction and cognitive impairment associated with AD (Zadori et al., 2014; Black et al., 2014; Gonzalez et al., 2015; Hu et al., 2012). Among GluRs, NMDARs play a pivotal role in excitotoxicity-induced neuronal death (Parsons and Raymond, 2014; Paula-Lima et al., 2013).

NMDARs are heterotetrameric ligand-gated ion channels composed of two obligatory GluN1 subunits with at least one type of GluN2 (GluN2A–D) and/or GluN3 subunits. The NMDARs are the most abundant in the hippocampus and throughout the forebrain. The majority of NMDARs in the hippocampus and cerebellar cortex contain GluN2B (NR2B) or GluN2A (NR2A) subunits. Different GluN2 subunits exert specific downstream signaling events and have distinct electrophysiological and pharmacological properties, resulting in different functional consequences for the NMDAR depending on the GluN2 subunit(s) present (Seeburg et al., 1995; Fan et al., 2014; Bliss and Schoepfer, 2004). NMDARs are essential for brain development and play key physiological roles in neuronal survival and functions such as regulation of synaptogenesis, neuronal networks, learning, and memory (Bliss and Collingridge, 1993; Collingridge et al., 2004; Thomas and Huganir, 2004). However, overstimulation of NMDARs, particularly those containing the GluN2B (NR2B) subunit, causes neuronal excitotoxicity because of the accumulation of excessive intraneuronal Ca^{2+}, which contributes to neuronal death associated with brain ischemia and hypoxia (Arundine and Tymianski, 2004) and chronic neurodegenerative diseases (Kalia et al., 2008; Milnerwood et al., 2010; Milnerwood and Raymond, 2010; Lipton, 2006; Mehta et al., 2013). Paradoxically, the activation of GluN2A-containing NMDAR promotes neuronal survival (Hardingham et al., 2002; Yano et al., 1998). Localization and subunit composition appear to determine the physiological/pathological outcomes following their activation (Lai et al., 2011, 2014; Hardingham, 2009; Paoletti, 2011; Hanson et al., 2013; Liu et al., 2007; Paoletti and Neyton, 2007; Papouin et al., 2012). In the postsynaptic terminal, most of the GluN2B-containing NMDARs are located in the extrasynaptic area whereas the majority of GluN2A-containing receptors are found in the synaptic cleft. A large body of evidence suggests that the overexcitation of the extrasynaptic GluN2B-containing NMDARs initiates deleterious downstream signaling pathways leading to massive Ca^{2+} influx and activation of calcium-dependent apoptotic/necrotic cascades and neuronal death in stroke and trauma (Liu et al., 2007; Taghibiglou et al., 2009c; Tu et al., 2010; Zhang et al., 2013) as well as the neurotoxic effects of β-amyloid oligomers, and early neuronal dysfunction in AD (Li et al., 2011; Snyder et al., 2005; Rush and Buisson, 2014; Mota et al., 2014; Ronicke et al., 2011). Physiologically, there is a correlation between Aβ production and neuronal activity. Experimental elevation of synaptic activity in brain slices led to increase Aβ generation and secretion in both wild-type and APP transgenic mice, and Aβ in a negative feedback loop inhibits synaptic activity (Kamenetz et al., 2003). Dysregulation of this feedback loop contributes to the pathogenesis of AD. Growing evidence indicates that Aβ oligomers impose their pathologic toxic function mostly through extrasynaptic NMDARs (in a subunit-dependent manner) including generation of reactive oxygen species (ROS) (Decker et al., 2010), loss of dendritic spine, and synaptic connectivity in hippocampal neurons (Shankar et al., 2007; Tackenberg et al., 2013). Moreover, NMDAR was shown to inhibit α-secretase activity and generation of neuroprotective α-cleaved soluble APP in favor of promoting β-secretase function and subsequent $A\beta_{1-42}$ generation (Lesne et al., 2005). On the contrary, targeted activation of synaptic NMDAR resulted in enhanced APP processing by α-secretase and significantly reduced Aβ formation (Bordji et al., 2010; Hoey et al., 2009; Marcello et al., 2007).

Selective antagonists of GluN2B-containing NMDARs have been successfully used to prevent acute exogenous Aβ oligomer-induced LTP impairment and synaptic loss (Li et al., 2011; Ronicke et al., 2011; Hanson et al., 2015; Olsen and Sheng, 2012; Rammes et al., 2011). Increasing evidence also links dysregulation of GluN2B-containing NMDAR remodeling, organization, and trafficking to AD (Ong et al., 2013; Esposito et al., 2013; Leuba et al., 2014). Moreover, blocking the GluN2B subunit of NMDAR also prevented dysregulation of intracellular Ca^{2+} homeostasis and endoplasmic reticulum (ER) oxidative stress associated with exogenous Aβ incubation (Costa et al., 2012; Ferreira et al., 2012). Although these promising results have made the inhibition of extrasynaptic GluN2B-containing NMDAR and its deleterious downstream signaling pathway very attractive targets for novel therapeutics in AD (Zadori et al., 2014; Beinat et al., 2010; Gogas, 2006; Jiang et al., 2012; Mony et al., 2009; Reisberg et al., 2003; Santangelo et al., 2012; Singh et al., 2012; Wang et al., 2014; Xia et al., 2010), unfortunately most of clinical trials failed to produce satisfactory outcomes. Memantine is the only Food and Drug Administration-approved NMDAR blocker. It targets mostly extrasynaptic GluN2B-containing receptors and has found its way into clinical practice being prescribed for the moderate-to-severe stages of AD.

PATHOLOGICAL ACTIVATION OF NEURONAL SREBP1: A COMMON DENOMINATOR IN NEURODEGENERATIVE DISEASES

As shown in Fig. 9.1, NMDAR-induced excitotoxicity alters cellular lipid biogenesis and profile (Taghibiglou and Wang, unpublished data). We have discovered a novel NMDAR-dependent prodeath signaling pathway following excitotoxicity, connecting the

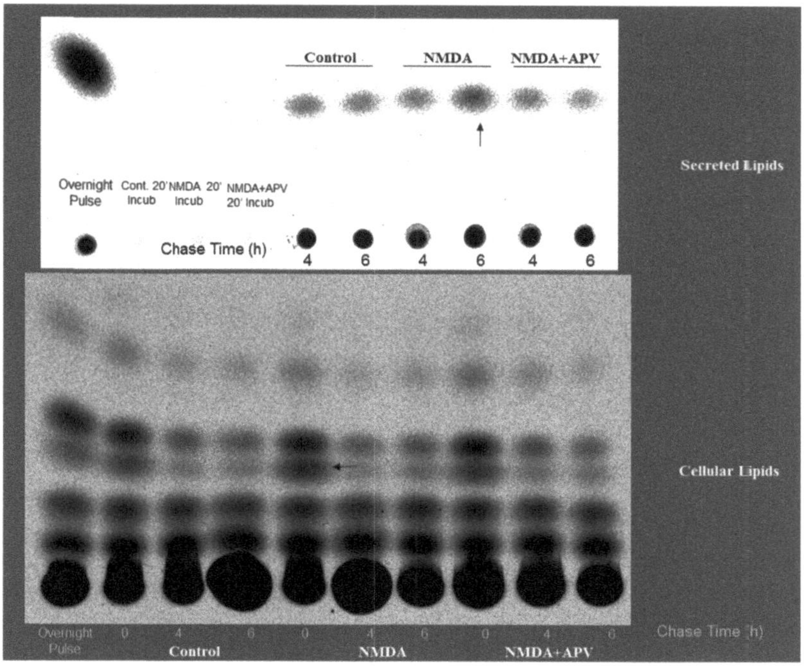

FIGURE 9.1 **NMDAR-dependent excitotoxicity alters cellular and secreted newly synthesized lipid profiles in cultured rat primary cortical neurons.** Cultured rat cortical neurons were metabolically labeled with radiolabeled carbon acetate and incubated with/without 50 μM *N*-methyl-D-aspartate (NMDA) (20 min) and chased up to 6 h in the presence and absence of NMDA receptor (NMDAR) blocker AP5. Both media and cell homogenates were collected and their lipid contents extracted and subjected to the plate chromatography and all the lipid spots were later visualized. The red arrows (gray in print versions) show altered cellular and secreted lipid moieties following NMDA-induced excitotoxicity (Taghibiglou and Wang, unpublished data).

GluN2B subunit to the activation of *SREBP1* and its downstream target genes in both in vitro and in vivo models of stroke and ALS (Taghibiglou et al., 2009c, 2011). The excitotoxicity-induced activation of SREBP1 was Ca^{2+} and calpain dependent, but GluN2A independent. Suppression of SREBP1 expression by siRNA or preventing its activation by a short bioactive peptide (Indip) was found to be profoundly neuroprotective. Similar observations were reported using both in vitro and in vivo G93A mouse models of ALS as well as postmortem sporadic and familial ALS patient samples (Taghibiglou et al., 2011). The inhibition of SREBP1 activation provided significant protection in cultured spinal cord neurons (prepared from wild-type and G93A mice) challenged by glutamate-induced excitotoxicity. Altered cholesterol hemostasis by NMDAR-induced excitotoxicity has also been linked to the pathogenesis of HD using an in vitro cell culture model (del Toro et al., 2010). We have also observed activation of SREBP1 in striatum of a YAC128 transgenic mouse model (Pouladi et al., 2013) of HD (Taghibiglou and Wang, unpublished data). Moreover, web-based GWAS studies have also identified two novel loci, one of them near SREBF1 for PD (Do et al., 2011). A similar observation was made for PD in the Chinese Han population (Li et al., 2012). It is noteworthy that an age-dependent elevation of SREBP1 expression has been reported in rodent brains (Okamoto et al., 2006; Segatto et al., 2012). All the existing evidence suggests a deleterious link between NMDAR excitotoxicity and activation of SREBP1 lipid transcription factor in a variety of aging-related neurodegenerative diseases.

The *SREBPs* are ER-localized transmembrane proteins belonging to the basic helix–loop–helix leucine zipper family of transcription factors, which are best known to regulate a variety of genes mostly involved in lipid metabolism in peripheral tissues. The SREBP family consists of *SREBP1a*, *SREBP1c*, and *SREBP2* and is well conserved from fission yeast to humans (reviewed in Espenshade and Hughes, 2007; Goldstein et al., 2006). Two different promoters of a single gene on chromosome 17 p11.2 are responsible for producing *SREBP1a* and *1c*, whereas a gene on chromosome 22q13 encodes for *SREBP2*. *SREBP1a* and *1c* regulate genes involved in biogenesis and hemostasis of cholesterol and fatty acids, whereas *SREBP2* preferentially activates target genes in cholesterol biosynthesis and metabolism pathways. The full length 125 kDa immature SREBPs are associated with another ER membrane protein called SREBP-cleavage-activating protein (SCAP) through their C-terminal interaction. The N-terminal (sterol-sensing domain) of SCAP interacts with an ER membrane-resident protein, insulin-induced gene-1 (Insig-1). This interaction confines the SCAP–SREBP complex in the ER as a nonactive, immature form. The activation process requires the SCAP–SREBP complex to be transported to the Golgi apparatus, where SREBPs are processed sequentially by two proteases, site 1 protease and site 2 protease. The cleaved 68 kDa N-terminal of SREBPs forms active homodimers, and enters the nucleus in an importin-β-dependent manner and regulates those genes containing sterol response element (*SRE*) and *E-box* in their promoters (Espenshade and Hughes, 2007; Goldstein et al., 2006; Jeon and Osborne, 2012). These genes are mostly involved in lipid biogenesis and homeostasis as well as cellular electron transfer processes (McPherson and Gauthier, 2004).

The feedback inhibition of cholesterol biosynthesis is mediated by Insig-1. When the cholesterol content of membranes increases, Insig-1 retains the SCAP–SREBP complex in the ER or binds to 3-hydroxy-3-methyl-glutaryl coenzyme A (HMG-CoA) reductase resulting in suppression of lipid biosynthesis and uptake (Espenshade and Hughes, 2007; Goldstein et al., 2006). On the contrary, in cases of cellular stress, hypoxia/anoxia, or decrease in membrane cholesterol content, Insig-1 is unable to bind SCAP or HMG-CoA, resulting in immature SREBP delivery to the Golgi apparatus for proteolytic activation and HMG-CoA stability, respectively. In cholesterol-deprived cells or cells under stress, Insig-1 binds to an E3 ubiquitin ligase, gp78 (reviewed in St Pierre and Nabi, 2012) and is destined for degradation via the ER-associated degradation pathway (reviewed in Bernasconi and Molinari, 2011; Smith et al., 2011). After polyubiquitination on Lys156 and Lys158, Insig-1 is degraded by the proteasomal machinery (Gong et al., 2006; Lee et al., 2006a,b). Two other proteins, p97 and Ubxd8, are involved in the proteasomal degradation of polyubiquitinated Insig-1 by facilitating its extraction from ER membrane (Ikeda et al., 2009; Lee et al., 2008). Cellular stress such as hypotonic shock, hypoxia, and ER stress also activate SREBPs using the same pathway (Lee and Ye, 2004; Taghibiglou et al., 2009a). Replenishing cells with cholesterol promotes SCAP binding to Insig-1, displaces gp78 from Insig-1, and prevents its degradation and subsequently SREBP activation is halted (Lee et al., 2006a,b). In the absence of cholesterol, exogenous PUFAs prevent Insig-1 degradation and SREBP1 activation by blocking the Ubxd8/p97 complex association with the polyubiquitinated Insig-1.

Since some compelling evidence indicates that lipid metabolism perturbation favors AD progression, it is therefore quite intriguing to study the potential deleterious role of activation of SREBP lipid transcription factors in AD. Barbero-Camps et al. (2013) generated a triple transgenic mice featuring SREBP2 overexpression in combination with APPswe/PS1ΔE9 mutations (APP/PS1) to examine key biochemical and functional characteristics of AD. Triple transgenic mice displayed increased synaptotoxicity reflected by loss of synaptophysin and neuronal death, resulting in early object-recognition memory impairment associated with deficits in spatial memory. Their data implicated the lipid transcription factor SREBP2 and cholesterol in pathogenesis of AD manifested by Aβ deposition and tauopathy (Barbero-Camps et al., 2013). Their findings are in agreement with reports indicating that excess brain cholesterol regulates APP cleavage and Aβ deposition. In fact, APP fragments also regulate lipid homeostasis, as shown by Pierrot et al. (2013). APP and SREBP1 were colocalized in the Golgi in neurons (and not in astrocytes). There is a feedback regulatory connection between APP and cholesterol biogenesis as the expression of APP decreases HMG-CoA reductase (HMGCR)-mediated cholesterol biosynthesis and SREBP mRNA levels, whereas its downregulation has opposite effects. Pierrot et al. (2013) also showed that neuronal expression of APP decreased both HMGCR and cholesterol 24-hydroxylase mRNA levels and consequently cholesterol turnover, leading to inhibition of neuronal activity and concluded that APP controls cholesterol turnover needed for neuronal activity. Although these observations were made only in neurons and not in astrocytes, Avila-Muñoz and Arias reported that cholesterol exposure induced astrocyte activation, increased APP content, and enhanced the interaction of APP with BACE1. These effects were associated with enrichment of ganglioside GM1-cholesterol patches in the astrocyte membrane and with increased ROS production (Avila-Muñoz and Arias, 2015). Although it has been demonstrated that incubation of cultured neurons

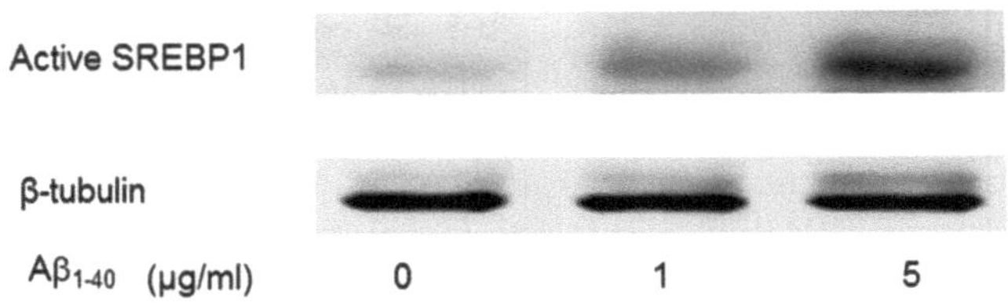

FIGURE 9.2 **Amyloid β (Aβ) oligomers dose dependently activate lipid transcription factor sterol regulatory element binding protein 1 (SREBP1) in cultured hippocampal neurons.** Rat hippocampal neurons were incubated with increasing concentrations of Aβ oligomers overnight. Cell homogenates were subjected to Western blotting and visualized for the active SREBP1 fragment (68 kDa) (Taghibiglou, unpublished data).

with $A\beta_{1-42}$ caused cholesterol sequestration and resulted in the impairment of intracellular cholesterol trafficking and significant reduction of protein prenylation (relevant to AD pathogenesis) because of the inhibition of SREBP2 cleavage (Mohamed et al., 2012), on the contrary we found that the incubation of cultured hippocampal neurons with $A\beta_{1-40}$ dose dependently increased activation of SREBP1 (Fig. 9.2, Taghibiglou, unpublished data). Interestingly, SREBP1a polymorphism has also been linked to the risk of AD in carriers of the ApoE4 allele (Spell et al., 2004). The expression of *SREBP* genes is controlled in part by the transcription regulation retinoid X receptor (RXR)–liver X receptor (LXR) system. Most endogenous oxysterols such as 27-hydroxycholesterol and 24(*S*),25-epoxycholesterol that activate LXRs can also inhibit activation of the SREBP pathway (Hong and Tontonoz, 2014; Noguchi et al., 2014). It is noteworthy that both LXR and RXR are also positively implicated in AD (Boehm-Cagan and Michaelson, 2014; Cramer et al., 2012). Brain is the major source of the circulating endogenous ligand of LXRs, 24*S*-hydroxycholesterol (24*S*-OHC) in the human body (Noguchi et al., 2014). The brain-enriched neuronal ER localized enzyme cholesterol-24*S*-hydroxylase (Cyp46) is responsible for converting cholesterol from the neuronal PM into 24*S*-OHC (Lund et al., 1999; Ramirez et al., 2008). Cyp46 controls cholesterol efflux from the brain and thereby plays a major role in regulating brain cholesterol homeostasis. Both 24*S*-OHC and Cyp46A1 are implicated in the pathogenesis of AD (Noguchi et al., 2015). In fact, serum and CSF concentrations of 24*S*-OHC were found to be significantly higher in Alzheimer and vascular-demented patients than depressed patients and healthy controls (Leoni and Caccia, 2013a,b; Papassotiropoulos et al., 2002). Several lines of evidence suggest that 24*S*-OHC may have both prosurvival and prodeath roles depending on the context and conditions. Adenoviral-mediated suppression of *Cyp46a1* mRNA in wild-type mice increased the cholesterol concentration in hippocampal neurons, followed by cognitive deficits, neuronal apoptosis, and hippocampal atrophy (Djelti et al., 2015). Neuronal cholesterol accumulation recruited more APP to lipid rafts and resulted in enhanced production of β-C-terminal fragment and Aβ peptides (Djelti et al., 2015). Similarly, the genetic ablation of Cyp46a1 reduced cholesterol turnover rate and affected cognition in *Cyp46a1*$^{-/-}$ mouse brain (Kotti et al., 2006). Conversely, adeno-associated virus gene therapy with cholesterol 24-hydroxylase reduced the amyloid pathology before and after the onset of amyloid plaques in mouse models of AD (Hudry et al., 2010). Increased levels of 24*S*-OHC by *ACAT1* gene ablation also ameliorated amyloid pathology in mice with AD (Bryleva et al., 2010). In a different study, treatment of human neuroblastoma SH-SY5Y cells and CHO cells (stably expressing human APP) with 1–10 μM of 24*S*-OHC (equivalent to the concentrations detected in human brain homogenates) diminished Aβ production (Urano et al., 2013).

On the contrary, neurotoxic effects of 24*S*-OHC have been reported in SH-SY5Y (Kolsch et al., 1999) although the exact mechanism of cell death was not well established. *CYP46* gene polymorphism was also linked to an increased 24*S*-OHC/cholesterol ratio in the CSF of AD patients and the *CYP46* gene locus was proposed to predispose to AD by increasing the 24*S*-OHC/cholesterol ratio in the brain (Kolsch et al., 2002).

It was later discovered that depending on the presence of caspase activity in insulted cells, 24*S*-OHC with concentrations of 10 μM or higher can induce either apoptosis or necroptosis, which may contribute to the neuronal loss associated with AD (Yamanaka et al., 2011). The 24*S*-OHC-induced cell death appeared at least in part to be acyl-CoA:cholesterol acyltransferase-1 activity dependent (Yamanaka et al., 2014). Aβ oligomers use this pathway and provide endogenous ligands through the induction of heme oxygenes-1 and cholesterol oxidation leading to the sustained activation of neuronal LXR-α-dependent neuronal death observed in AD (Raina and Kaul, 2010). To corroborate these findings, in a study by Halford and Russel, the cholesterol 24-hydroxylase knockout mice were crossed with a transgenic mice model of AD and resulted in a modest but statistically significant decline in insoluble Aβ42 peptide burden in the hippocampus of 12-month-old knockout/AD male mice. Moreover, the loss of one or both cholesterol 24-hydroxylase alleles increased longevity in AD mice (Halford and Russell, 2009). Ghosh et al. (2015) reported that neuronal infection with chandipura virus causes overexpression of *Cyp46a1* and *Srebf-1* genes leading to 24*S*-OHC-induced neuronal cell death through the FAS-mediated extrinsic apoptosis pathway confirming a concentration-dependent deleterious role of 24*S*-OHC and SREBP1 in neurons.

In the normal healthy adult brain, Cyp46 enzymatic activity is relatively stable whereas significant activity enhancement has been reported in several neuropathological conditions such as traumatic brain injury (Cartagena et al., 2008), kainate-induced excitotoxic hippocampal injury (He et al., 2006), and acute autoimmune encephalomyelitis (Teunissen et al., 2007), which makes inhibition of this enzyme an attractive target for pharmaceutical companies (Uto, 2015). One pathological aspect common in all these injuries is excitotoxicity. Sodero et al. (2011, 2012) have shown that both aging neurons and glutamate-induced excitotoxicity mobilized CYP46A1 toward the PM and resulted in a small but significant loss of membrane cholesterol in a form of released 24*S*-OHC in NMDAR and the NADPH oxidase-dependent pathways. The glutamate-induced neuronal membrane cholesterol loss also required high levels of intracellular Ca^{2+}, which was prevented by CYP46A1 knockdown. These studies highlight the pivotal role of excitotoxicity in the control of membrane lipid composition, and consequently in neuronal membrane organization and function. Maintaining membrane cholesterol content is absolutely vital for the normal function of neurons and is mostly achieved by lipoproteins supplied by neighboring astrocytes (depicted in Fig. 9.3). It appears that following a consistent and prolonged excitotoxic insult similar to what happens in stroke, brain injury, and neurodegenerative diseases, neurons inevitably activate SREBP transcription pathways to compensate for lost membrane lipids (as hypothesized and depicted in Fig. 9.4). We have previously reported that the excitotoxicity-induced neuronal SREBP1 activation was Ca^{2+}, calpain, and GluN2B subunit of NMDAR dependent and disruption of this activation by Indip

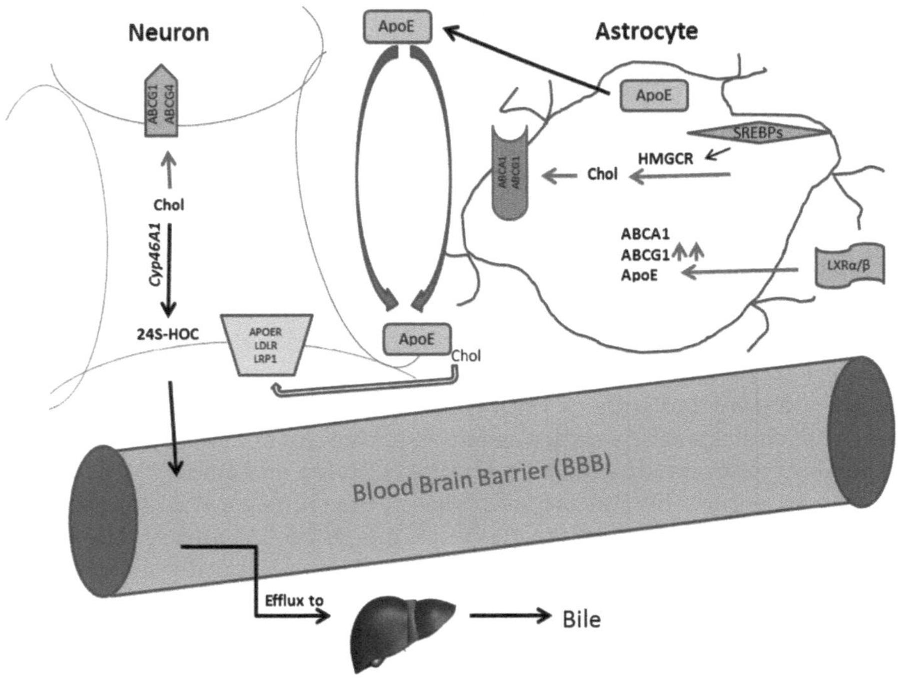

FIGURE 9.3 **Brain cholesterol metabolism and homeostasis.** Astrocytes are the main source of free cholesterol (FC) biosynthesis by using acetate as a precursor. They also participate in exporting synthesized cholesterol to neighboring neurons through apolipoprotein E (ApoE) and the ATP-binding cassette (ABCA1). The low density receptors (LDLRs) on neurons mediate FC uptake, which are later transported to the late endosomes and released. The released FC are supplied to the plasma membrane (PM) and the lipid rafts. The lipid rafts are implicated in cleavage of the amyloid precursor protein (APP) and the amyloid peptide (Aβ) production. The neurons balance their FC contents by either converting excess FC to soluble 24*S*-hydroxycholesterol (24*S*-OHC) and secreted, or esterify it to cholesterol esters (CEs) by acetyl-CoA cholesterol acyltransferase (*ACAT1*) enzymatic reaction and stocked in the cytoplasmic lipid droplets. ABCA1 mediates secretion of a portion of CEs, which are later recaptured and endocytosed by astrocytes. The diffused 24*S*-OHC passes from the blood–brain barrier (BBB) to the peripheral circulation and eventually is excreted by liver in the bile. Another oxysterol 27-hydroxycholesterol (27-OHC) generated from peripheral cholesterol travels in the opposite direction to the brain. Both of these oxysterols are intrinsic ligands for the liver X receptor (LXR). Activation of LXR regulates expression of several cholesterol-related genes such as *ABCA1*, *SREBP1*, and *ApoE*.

peptide proved to be neuroprotective (Taghibiglou et al., 2009c, 2011). Our recently published studies strongly indicate the existence of a deleterious interplay among the overexcitation of GluN2B-containing extrasynaptic NMDARs, massive Ca^{2+} influx, CYP46A1 activation, and PM lipid/cholesterol alteration (and/or lipid rafts expansion), leading to the activation of SREBP1 and neuronal degeneration (Fig. 9.4).

Although more studies are needed to elucidate how NMDAR-dependent activation of *SREBP1* and its downstream genes and/or lipid moieties causes neuronal death, emerging evidence suggests *SREBP1* lipid transcription factor and its upstream and downstream pathways as very promising targets for drug discovery research in neurodegenerative diseases (Luthi-Carter et al., 2010; Taghibiglou, 2013).

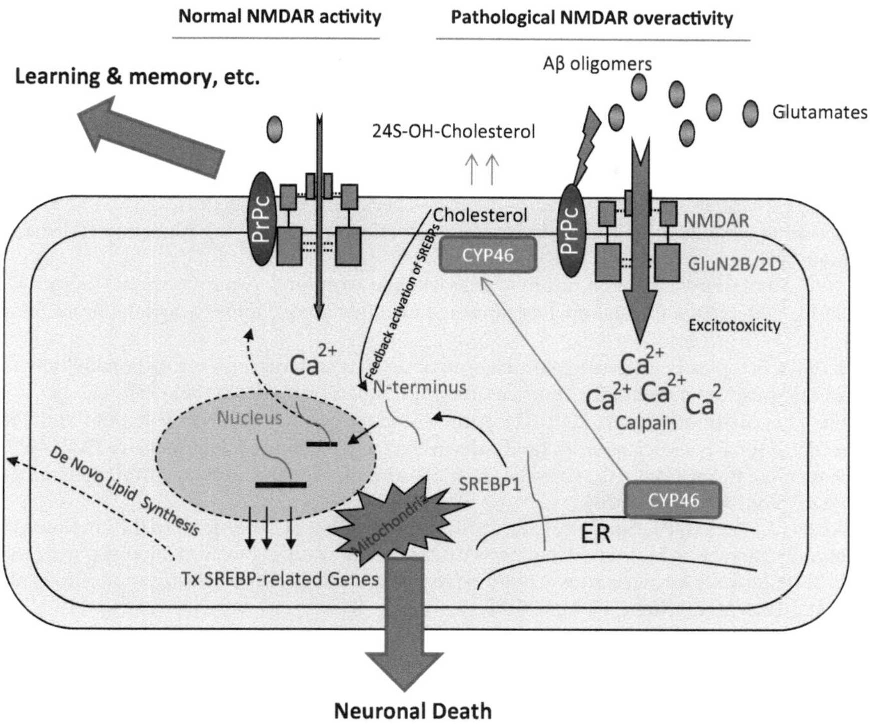

FIGURE 9.4 **Hypothetical mechanism for the sterol regulatory element binding protein 1 (SREBP1) activation-induced neuronal apoptosis in AD.** In the normal physiological conditions the cellular prion protein (PrP^C) interacts with GluN2 subunits of NDMA receptor (NMDAR) and attenuates its excitatory function. At the early stage of Alzheimer's disease (AD), oligomeric Aβ interacts with PrP^C as its receptor affecting PrP^C–NMDAR interactions leading to more potent excitatory function of the glutamate receptor. Excessive glutamate in the synaptic cleft mediates massive Ca^{2+} influx through the GluN2B-containing NMDARs. Following the excitotoxic insult, a portion of the plasma membrane (PM) free cholesterol content is converted to soluble 24*S*-hydroxycholesterol (24*S*-OHC) (mediated by Cyp46A1 activity) and diffused out of the membrane. The decreased PM cholesterol content triggers SREBP1 lipid transcription factor activation in the Golgi apparatus, where the N-terminal of SREBP1 (active form) is cleaved and then transported to the nucleus to regulate sterol response element (*SRE*) and *E-box* containing genes causing apoptosis.

Acknowledgments

The authors thank Dr. Venkat Gopalakrishnan for his critical review of this manuscript.

References

Allen, J.A., Halverson-Tamboli, R.A., Rasenick, M.M., 2007. Lipid raft microdomains and neurotransmitter signalling. Nat. Rev. Neurosci. 8, 128–140.

Allinquant, B., Clamagirand, C., Potier, M.C., 2014. Role of cholesterol metabolism in the pathogenesis of Alzheimer's disease. Curr. Opin. Clin. Nutr. Metab. Care 17, 319–323.

Arundine, M., Tymianski, M., 2004. Molecular mechanisms of glutamate-dependent neurodegeneration in ischemia and traumatic brain injury. Cell Mol. Life Sci. 61, 657–668.

Assaife-Lopes, N., et al., 2010. Activation of adenosine A2A receptors induces TrkB translocation and increases BDNF-mediated phospho-TrkB localization in lipid rafts: implications for neuromodulation. J. Neurosci. 30, 8468–8480.

Assaife-Lopes, N., Sousa, V.C., Pereira, D.B., Ribeiro, J.A., Sebastiao, A.M., 2014. Regulation of TrkB receptor translocation to lipid rafts by adenosine A(2A) receptors and its functional implications for BDNF-induced regulation of synaptic plasticity. Purinergic Signal. 10, 251–267.

Avila-Muñoz, E., Arias, C., 2015. Cholesterol-induced astrocyte activation is associated with increased amyloid precursor protein expression and processing. Glia 63 (11).

Baier, C.J., Fantini, J., Barrantes, F.J., 2011. Disclosure of cholesterol recognition motifs in transmembrane domains of the human nicotinic acetylcholine receptor. Sci. Rep. 1, 69.

Barbero-Camps, E., Fernandez, A., Martinez, L., Fernandez-Checa, J.C., Colell, A., 2013. APP/PS1 mice overexpressing SREBP-2 exhibit combined Aβ accumulation and tau pathology underlying Alzheimer's disease. Hum. Mol. Genet. 22, 3460–3476.

Barrantes, F.J., 2007. Cholesterol effects on nicotinic acetylcholine receptor. J. Neurochem. 103 (Suppl. 1), 72–80.

Barrantes, F.J., 2014. Cell-surface translational dynamics of nicotinic acetylcholine receptors. Front Synaptic Neurosci. 6, 25.

Becher, A., et al., 2004. Ectopically expressed gamma-aminobutyric acid receptor B is functionally down-regulated in isolated lipid raft-enriched membranes. Biochem. Biophys. Res. Commun. 321, 981–987.

Becher, A., White, J.H., McIlhinney, R.A., 2001. The gamma-aminobutyric acid receptor B, but not the metabotropic glutamate receptor type-1, associates with lipid rafts in the rat cerebellum. J. Neurochem. 79, 787–795.

Bedse, G., Di Domenico, F., Serviddio, G., Cassano, T., 2015. Aberrant insulin signaling in Alzheimer's disease: current knowledge. Front Neurosci. 9, 204.

Beel, A.J., Sakakura, M., Barrett, P.J., Sanders, C.R., 2010. Direct binding of cholesterol to the amyloid precursor protein: an important interaction in lipid-Alzheimer's disease relationships? Biochim. Biophys. Acta 1801, 975–982.

Beinat, C., et al., 2010. Insights into structure-activity relationships and CNS therapeutic applications of NR2B selective antagonists. Curr. Med. Chem. 17, 4166–4190.

Ben Halima, S., Rajendran, L., 2011. Membrane anchored and lipid raft targeted beta-secretase inhibitors for Alzheimer's disease therapy. J. Alzheimers Dis. 24 (Suppl. 2), 143–152.

Berman, D.E., et al., 2008. Oligomeric amyloid-beta peptide disrupts phosphatidylinositol-4,5-bisphosphate metabolism. Nat. Neurosci. 11, 547–554.

Bernasconi, R., Molinari, M., 2011. ERAD and ERAD tuning: disposal of cargo and of ERAD regulators from the mammalian ER. Curr. Opin. Cell Biol. 23, 176–183.

Besshoh, S., Bawa, D., Teves, L., Wallace, M.C., Gurd, J.W., 2005. Increased phosphorylation and redistribution of NMDA receptors between synaptic lipid rafts and post-synaptic densities following transient global ischemia in the rat brain. J. Neurochem. 93, 186–194.

Besshoh, S., Chen, S., Brown, I.R., Gurd, J.W., 2007. Developmental changes in the association of NMDA receptors with lipid rafts. J. Neurosci. Res. 85, 1876–1883.

Bhattacharyya, R., Kovacs, D.M., 2010. ACAT inhibition and amyloid beta reduction. Biochim. Biophys. Acta 1801, 960–965.

Birnbaum, S.G., et al., 2004. Protein kinase C overactivity impairs prefrontal cortical regulation of working memory. Science 306, 882–884.

Bjork, K., Sjogren, B., Svenningsson, P., 2010. Regulation of serotonin receptor function in the nervous system by lipid rafts and adaptor proteins. Exp. Cell Res. 316, 1351–1356.

Black, S.A., Stys, P.K., Zamponi, G.W., Tsutsui, S., 2014. Cellular prion protein and NMDA receptor modulation: protecting against excitotoxicity. Front Cell Dev. Biol. 2, 45.

Blasco, H., Mavel, S., Corcia, P., Gordon, P.H., 2014. The glutamate hypothesis in ALS: pathophysiology and drug development. Curr. Med. Chem. 21, 3551–3575.

Bliss, T.V., Collingridge, G.L., 1993. A synaptic model of memory: long-term potentiation in the hippocampus. Nature 361, 31–39.

Bliss, T., Schoepfer, R., 2004. Neuroscience. Controlling the ups and downs of synaptic strength. Science 304, 973–974.

Blomqvist, M.E., et al., 2006. Towards compendia of negative genetic association studies: an example for Alzheimer disease. Hum. Genet. 119, 29–37.

Boehm-Cagan, A., Michaelson, D.M., 2014. Reversal of apoE4-driven brain pathology and behavioral deficits by bexarotene. J. Neurosci. 34, 7293–7301.

Bordji, K., Becerril-Ortega, J., Nicole, O., Buisson, A., 2010. Activation of extrasynaptic, but not synaptic, NMDA receptors modifies amyloid precursor protein expression pattern and increases amyloid-β production. J. Neurosci. 30, 15927–15942.

Boulware, M.I., Heisler, J.D., Frick, K.M., 2013. The memory-enhancing effects of hippocampal estrogen receptor activation involve metabotropic glutamate receptor signaling. J. Neurosci. 33, 15184–15194.

Bruses, J.L., Chauvet, N., Rutishauser, U., 2001. Membrane lipid rafts are necessary for the maintenance of the (alpha)7 nicotinic acetylcholine receptor in somatic spines of ciliary neurons. J. Neurosci. 21, 504–512.

Bryleva, E.Y., et al., 2010. ACAT1 gene ablation increases 24(S)-hydroxycholesterol content in the brain and ameliorates amyloid pathology in mice with AD. Proc. Natl. Acad. Sci. U.S.A. 107, 3081–3086.

Bu, J., Bruckner, S.R., Sengoku, T., Geddes, J.W., Estus, S., 2003. Glutamate regulates caveolin expression in rat hippocampal neurons. J. Neurosci. Res. 72, 185–190.

Bucciantini, M., et al., 2012. Toxic effects of amyloid fibrils on cell membranes: the importance of ganglioside GM1. FASEB J. 26, 818–831.

Butchbach, M.E., Tian, G., Guo, H., Lin, C.L., 2004. Association of excitatory amino acid transporters, especially EAAT2, with cholesterol-rich lipid raft microdomains: importance for excitatory amino acid transporter localization and function. J. Biol. Chem. 279, 34388–34396.

Calella, A.M., et al., 2010. Prion protein and Aβ-related synaptic toxicity impairment. EMBO Mol. Med. 2, 306–314.

Campagna, J.A., Fallon, J., 2006. Lipid rafts are involved in C95 (4,8) agrin fragment-induced acetylcholine receptor clustering. Neuroscience 138, 123–132.

Carbone, M., Duty, S., Rattray, M., 2012. Riluzole elevates GLT-1 activity and levels in striatal astrocytes. Neurochem. Int. 60, 31–38.

Cartagena, C.M., et al., 2008. Cortical injury increases cholesterol 24S hydroxylase (Cyp46) levels in the rat brain. J. Neurotrauma 25, 1087–1098.

Cartagena, C.M., Burns, M.P., Rebeck, G.W., 2010. 24S-hydroxycholesterol effects on lipid metabolism genes are modeled in traumatic brain injury. Brain Res. 1319, 1–12.

Cecchi, C., Stefani, M., 2013. The amyloid-cell membrane system. The interplay between the biophysical features of oligomers/fibrils and cell membrane defines amyloid toxicity. Biophys. Chem. 182, 30–43.

Chakraborty, M., Jiang, X.C., 2013. Sphingomyelin and its role in cellular signaling. Adv. Exp. Med. Biol. 991, 1–14.

Chan, R.B., et al., 2012. Comparative lipidomic analysis of mouse and human brain with Alzheimer disease. J. Biol. Chem. 287, 2678–2688.

Chen, T.Y., Liu, P.H., Ruan, C.T., Chiu, L., Kung, F.L., 2006. The intracellular domain of amyloid precursor protein interacts with flotillin-1, a lipid raft protein. Biochem. Biophys. Res. Commun. 342, 266–272

Cole, A.A., Dosemeci, A., Reese, T.S., 2010. Co-segregation of AMPA receptors with G(M1) ganglioside in synaptosomal membrane subfractions. Biochem. J. 427, 535–540.

Collingridge, G.L., Isaac, J.T., Wang, Y.T., 2004. Receptor trafficking and synaptic plasticity. Nat. Rev. Neurosci. 5, 952–962.

Collingridge, G.L., Peineau, S., Howland, J.G., Wang, Y.T., 2010. Long-term depression in the CNS. Nat. Rev. Neurosci. 11, 459–473.

Costa, R.O., et al., 2012. Endoplasmic reticulum stress occurs downstream of GluN2B subunit of N-methyl-D-aspartate receptor in mature hippocampal cultures treated with amyloid-beta oligomers. Aging Cell 11, 823–833.

Cramer, P.E., et al., 2012. ApoE-directed therapeutics rapidly clear beta-amyloid and reverse deficits in AD mouse models. Science 335, 1503–1506.

Cunnane, S.C., Chouinard-Watkins, R., Castellano, C.A., Barberger-Gateau, P., 2013. Docosahexaenoic acid homeostasis, brain aging and Alzheimer's disease: can we reconcile the evidence? Prostaglandins Leukot. Essent. Fatty Acids 88, 61–70.

daCosta, C.J., Dey, L., Therien, J.P., Baenziger, J.E., 2013. A distinct mechanism for activating uncoupled nicotinic acetylcholine receptors. Nat. Chem. Biol. 9, 701–707.

Dalskov, S.M., et al., 2005. Lipid raft localization of GABA A receptor and Na+, K+-ATPase in discrete microdomain clusters in rat cerebellar granule cells. Neurochem. Int. 46, 489–499.

Daviglus, M.L., et al., 2011. Risk factors and preventive interventions for Alzheimer disease: state of the science. Arch. Neurol. 68, 1185–1190.

Dawson, G., 2015. Measuring brain lipids. Biochim. Biophys. Acta 1851, 1026–1039.

de la Monte, S.M., Tong, M., 2014. Brain metabolic dysfunction at the core of Alzheimer's disease. Biochem. Pharmacol. 88, 548–559.

Decker, H., et al., 2010. N-methyl-D-aspartate receptors are required for synaptic targeting of Alzheimer's toxic amyloid-beta peptide oligomers. J. Neurochem. 115, 1520–1529.

del Toro, D., et al., 2010. Altered cholesterol homeostasis contributes to enhanced excitotoxicity in Huntington's disease. J. Neurochem. 115, 153–167.
Delint-Ramirez, I., Salcedo-Tello, P., Bermudez-Rattoni, F., 2008. Spatial memory formation induces recruitment of NMDA receptor and PSD-95 to synaptic lipid rafts. J. Neurochem. 106, 1658–1668.
Di Paolo, G., Kim, T.W., 2011. Linking lipids to Alzheimer's disease: cholesterol and beyond. Nat. Rev. Neurosci. 12, 284–296.
Djelti, F., et al., 2015. CYP46A1 inhibition, brain cholesterol accumulation and neurodegeneration pave the way for Alzheimer's disease. Brain 138, 2383–2398.
Do, C.B., et al., 2011. Web-based genome-wide association study identifies two novel loci and a substantial genetic component for Parkinson's disease. PLoS Genet. 7, e1002141.
Ehehalt, R., Keller, P., Haass, C., Thiele, C., Simons, K., 2003. Amyloidogenic processing of the Alzheimer beta-amyloid precursor protein depends on lipid rafts. J. Cell Biol. 160, 113–123.
Escriba, P.V., et al., 2015. Membrane lipid therapy: modulation of the cell membrane composition and structure as a molecular base for drug discovery and new disease treatment. Prog. Lipid Res. 59, 38–53.
Espenshade, P.J., Hughes, A.L., 2007. Regulation of sterol synthesis in eukaryotes. Annu. Rev. Genet. 41, 401–427.
Esposito, Z., et al., 2013. Amyloid beta, glutamate, excitotoxicity in Alzheimer's disease: are we on the right track? CNS Neurosci. Ther. 19, 549–555.
Fan, X., Jin, W.Y., Wang, Y.T., 2014. The NMDA receptor complex: a multifunctional machine at the glutamatergic synapse. Front Cell Neurosci. 8, 160.
Fang, C., et al., 2006. GODZ-mediated palmitoylation of GABA(A) receptors is required for normal assembly and function of GABAergic inhibitory synapses. J. Neurosci. 26, 12758–12768.
Fantini, J., Barrantes, F.J., 2009. Sphingolipid/cholesterol regulation of neurotransmitter receptor conformation and function. Biochim. Biophys. Acta 1788, 2345–2361.
Farooqui, A.A., Ong, W.Y., Horrocks, L.A., 2004. Biochemical aspects of neurodegeneration in human brain: involvement of neural membrane phospholipids and phospholipases A2. Neurochem. Res. 29, 1961–1977.
Ferreira, I.L., et al., 2012. Amyloid beta peptide 1-42 disturbs intracellular calcium homeostasis through activation of GluN2B-containing N-methyl-D-aspartate receptors in cortical cultures. Cell Calcium 51, 95–106.
Foley, P., 2010. Lipids in Alzheimer's disease: a century-old story. Biochim. Biophys. Acta 1801, 750–753.
Francesconi, A., Kumari, R., Zukin, R.S., 2009. Regulation of group I metabotropic glutamate receptor trafficking and signaling by the caveolar/lipid raft pathway. J. Neurosci. 29, 3590–3602.
Fukunaga, S., et al., 2012. GM1 cluster mediates formation of toxic Aβ fibrils by providing hydrophobic environments. Biochemistry 51, 8125–8131.
Gamba, P., et al., 2012. The link between altered cholesterol metabolism and Alzheimer's disease. Ann. N. Y Acad. Sci. 1259, 54–64.
Gamba, P., et al., 2015. Oxidized cholesterol as the driving force behind the development of Alzheimer's disease. Front Aging Neurosci. 7, 119.
Gaudreault, S.B., Chabot, C., Gratton, J.P., Poirier, J., 2004. The caveolin scaffolding domain modifies 2-amino-3-hydroxy-5-methyl-4-isoxazole propionate receptor binding properties by inhibiting phospholipase A2 activity. J. Biol. Chem. 279, 356–362.
Gentile, M.T., et al., 2012. Role of cytosolic calcium-dependent phospholipase A2 in Alzheimer's disease pathogenesis. Mol. Neurobiol. 45, 596–604.
Ghosh, S., Mukherjee, S., Basu, A., 2015. Chandipura virus perturbs cholesterol homeostasis leading to neuronal apoptosis. J. Neurochem. 135 (2), 368–380.
Gielen, E., et al., 2006. Rafts in oligodendrocytes: evidence and structure-function relationship. Glia 54, 499–512.
Gil, C., Soler-Jover, A., Blasi, J., Aguilera, J., 2005. Synaptic proteins and SNARE complexes are localized in lipid rafts from rat brain synaptosomes. Biochem. Biophys. Res. Commun. 329, 117–124.
Giovannoni, M.P., Piaz, V.D., Vergelli, C., Barlocco, D., 2003. Selective ACAT inhibitors as promising antihyperlipidemic, antiathero-sclerotic and anti-Alzheimer drugs. Mini Rev. Med. Chem. 3, 576–584.
Gladding, C.M., Raymond, L.A., 2011. Mechanisms underlying NMDA receptor synaptic/extrasynaptic distribution and function. Mol. Cell Neurosci. 48, 308–320.
Goedert, M., 2015. NEURODEGENERATION. Alzheimer's and Parkinson's diseases: the prion concept in relation to assembled Aβ, tau, and α-synuclein. Science 349, 1255555.
Gogas, K.R., 2006. Glutamate-based therapeutic approaches: NR2B receptor antagonists. Curr. Opin. Pharmacol. 6, 68–74.

Goldstein, J.L., DeBose-Boyd, R.A., Brown, M.S., 2006. Protein sensors for membrane sterols. Cell 124, 35–46.
Gong, Y., et al., 2006. Sterol-regulated ubiquitination and degradation of Insig-1 creates a convergent mechanism for feedback control of cholesterol synthesis and uptake. Cell Metab. 3, 15–24.
Goni, F.M., 2014. The basic structure and dynamics of cell membranes: an update of the Singer-Nicolson model. Biochim. Biophys. Acta 1838, 1467–1476.
Gonzalez, J., et al., 2015. NMDARs in neurological diseases: a potential therapeutic target. Int. J. Neurosci. 125, 315–327.
Gonzalez-Dominguez, R., Garcia-Barrera, T., Gomez-Ariza, J.L., 2014a. Metabolomic study of lipids in serum for biomarker discovery in Alzheimer's disease using direct infusion mass spectrometry. J. Pharm. Biomed. Anal. 98, 321–326.
Gonzalez-Dominguez, R., Garcia-Barrera, T., Vitorica, J., Gomez-Ariza, J.L., 2014b. Region-specific metabolic alterations in the brain of the APP/PS1 transgenic mice of Alzheimer's disease. Biochim. Biophys. Acta 1842, 2395–2402.
Gonzalez-Dominguez, R., Garcia-Barrera, T., Vitorica, J., Gomez-Ariza, J.L., 2015. Metabolomic screening of regional brain alterations in the APP/PS1 transgenic model of Alzheimer's disease by direct infusion mass spectrometry. J. Pharm. Biomed. Anal. 102, 425–435.
Grimm, M.O., Zimmer, V.C., Lehmann, J., Grimm, H.S., Hartmann, T., 2013. The impact of cholesterol, DHA, and sphingolipids on Alzheimer's disease. Biomed. Res. Int. 2013, 814390.
Grosgen, S., Grimm, M.O., Friess, P., Hartmann, T., 2010. Role of amyloid beta in lipid homeostasis. Biochim. Biophys. Acta 1801, 966–974.
Guijas, C., Rodriguez, J.P., Rubio, J.M., Balboa, M.A., Balsinde, J., 2014. Phospholipase A2 regulation of lipid droplet formation. Biochim. Biophys. Acta 1841, 1661–1671.
Guirland, C., Suzuki, S., Kojima, M., Lu, B., Zheng, J.Q., 2004. Lipid rafts mediate chemotropic guidance of nerve growth cones. Neuron 42, 51–62.
Haass, C., Selkoe, D.J., 2007. Soluble protein oligomers in neurodegeneration: lessons from the Alzheimer's amyloid beta-peptide. Nat. Rev. Mol. Cell Biol. 8, 101–112.
Halford, R.W., Russell, D.W., 2009. Reduction of cholesterol synthesis in the mouse brain does not affect amyloid formation in Alzheimer's disease, but does extend lifespan. Proc. Natl. Acad. Sci. U.S.A. 106, 3502–3506.
Hanson, J.E., et al., 2013. GluN2B antagonism affects interneurons and leads to immediate and persistent changes in synaptic plasticity, oscillations, and behavior. Neuropsychopharmacology 38, 1221–1233.
Hanson, J.E., Pare, J.F., Deng, L., Smith, Y., Zhou, Q., 2015. Altered GluN2B NMDA receptor function and synaptic plasticity during early pathology in the PS2APP mouse model of Alzheimer's disease. Neurobiol. Dis. 74, 254–262.
Hardingham, G.E., Bading, H., 2010. Synaptic versus extrasynaptic NMDA receptor signalling: implications for neurodegenerative disorders. Nat. Rev. Neurosci. 11, 682–696.
Hardingham, G.E., Fukunaga, Y., Bading, H., 2002. Extrasynaptic NMDARs oppose synaptic NMDARs by triggering CREB shut-off and cell death pathways. Nat. Neurosci. 5, 405–414.
Hardingham, G.E., 2009. Coupling of the NMDA receptor to neuroprotective and neurodestructive events. Biochem. Soc. Trans. 37, 1147–1160.
Harris, B., Pereira, I., Parkin, E., 2009. Targeting ADAM10 to lipid rafts in neuroblastoma SH-SY5Y cells impairs amyloidogenic processing of the amyloid precursor protein. Brain Res. 1296, 203–215.
Haughey, N.J., Bandaru, V.V., Bae, M., Mattson, M.P., 2010. Roles for dysfunctional sphingolipid metabolism in Alzheimer's disease neuropathogenesis. Biochim. Biophys. Acta 1801, 878–886.
Hayashi, H., et al., 2004. A seed for Alzheimer amyloid in the brain. J. Neurosci. 24, 4894–4902.
He, X., Jenner, A.M., Ong, W.Y., Farooqui, A.A., Patel, S.C., 2006. Lovastatin modulates increased cholesterol and oxysterol levels and has a neuroprotective effect on rat hippocampal neurons after kainate injury. J. Neuropathol. Exp. Neurol. 65, 652–663.
Head, B.P., et al., 2008. Caveolin-1 expression is essential for N-methyl-D-aspartate receptor-mediated Src and extracellular signal-regulated kinase 1/2 activation and protection of primary neurons from ischemic cell death. FASEB J. 22, 828–840.
Hering, H., Lin, C.C., Sheng, M., 2003. Lipid rafts in the maintenance of synapses, dendritic spines, and surface AMPA receptor stability. J. Neurosci. 23, 3262–3271.
Hibino, H., Kurachi, Y., 2007. Distinct detergent-resistant membrane microdomains (lipid rafts) respectively harvest K(+) and water transport systems in brain astroglia. Eur. J. Neurosci. 26, 2539–2555.
Hirsch, T.Z., Hernandez-Rapp, J., Martin-Lanneree, S., Launay, J.M., Mouillet-Richard, S., 2014. PrP(C) signalling in neurons: from basics to clinical challenges. Biochimie 104, 2–11.

Hoey, S.E., Williams, R.J., Perkinton, M.S., 2009. Synaptic NMDA receptor activation stimulates alpha-secretase amyloid precursor protein processing and inhibits amyloid-beta production. J. Neurosci. 29, 4442–4460.
Hong, Y.H., et al., 2009. Agonist-induced internalization of mGluR1alpha is mediated by caveolin. J. Neurochem. 111, 61–71.
Hong, C., Tontonoz, P., 2014. Liver X receptors in lipid metabolism: opportunities for drug discovery. Nat. Rev. Drug Discov. 13, 433–444.
Hoshino, T., Mahmood, M.I., Mori, K., Matsuzaki, K., 2013. Binding and aggregation mechanism of amyloid beta-peptides onto the GM1 ganglioside-containing lipid membrane. J. Phys. Chem. B 117, 8085–8094.
Hou, Q., et al., 2008. Regulation of AMPA receptor localization in lipid rafts. Mol. Cell Neurosci. 38, 213–223.
Hu, N.W., Ondrejcak, T., Rowan, M.J., 2012. Glutamate receptors in preclinical research on Alzheimer's disease: update on recent advances. Pharmacol. Biochem. Behav. 100, 855–862.
Hudry, E., et al., 2010. Adeno-associated virus gene therapy with cholesterol 24-hydroxylase reduces the amyloid pathology before or after the onset of amyloid plaques in mouse models of Alzheimer's disease. Mol. Ther. 18, 44–53.
Hulbert, A.J., Kelly, M.A., Abbott, S.K., 2013. Polyunsaturated fats, membrane lipids and animal longevity. J. Comp. Physiol. B 184, 149–166.
Huo, J.Z., Cortez, M.A., Snead 3rd, O.C., 2009. GABA receptor proteins within lipid rafts in the AY-9944 model of atypical absence seizures. Epilepsia 50, 776–788.
Hurtado, O., et al., 2008. Delayed post-ischemic administration of CDP-choline increases EAAT2 association to lipid rafts and affords neuroprotection in experimental stroke. Neurobiol. Dis. 29, 123–131.
Huttunen, H.J., Kovacs, D.M., 2008. ACAT as a drug target for Alzheimer's disease. Neurodegener Dis. 5, 212–214.
Ibarguren, M., Lopez, D.J., Escriba, P.V., 2014. The effect of natural and synthetic fatty acids on membrane structure, microdomain organization, cellular functions and human health. Biochim. Biophys. Acta 1838, 1518–1528.
Ikeda, Y., et al., 2009. Regulated endoplasmic reticulum-associated degradation of a polytopic protein: p97 recruits proteasomes to Insig-1 before extraction from membranes. J. Biol. Chem. 284, 34889–34900.
Jeon, T.I., Osborne, T.F., 2012. SREBPs: metabolic integrators in physiology and metabolism. Trends Endocrinol. Metab. 23, 65–72.
Jiang, T., Yu, J.T., Tan, L., 2012. Novel disease-modifying therapies for Alzheimer's disease. J. Alzheimers Dis. 31, 475–492.
Jin, H., et al., 2014. Ring finger protein 34 (RNF34) interacts with and promotes γ-aminobutyric acid type-A receptor degradation via ubiquitination of the γ2 subunit. J. Biol. Chem. 289, 29420–29436.
Jo, S., et al., 2014. GABA from reactive astrocytes impairs memory in mouse models of Alzheimer's disease. Nat. Med. 20, 886–896.
Jones, L., Harold, D., Williams, J., 2010. Genetic evidence for the involvement of lipid metabolism in Alzheimer's disease. Biochim. Biophys. Acta 1801, 754–761.
Kakio, A., Nishimoto, S., Kozutsumi, Y., Matsuzaki, K., 2003. Formation of a membrane-active form of amyloid beta-protein in raft-like model membranes. Biochem. Biophys. Res. Commun. 303, 514–518.
Kalia, L.V., Kalia, S.K., Salter, M.W., 2008. NMDA receptors in clinical neurology: excitatory times ahead. Lancet Neurol. 7, 742–755.
Kalmijn, S., et al., 1997. Dietary fat intake and the risk of incident dementia in the Rotterdam Study. Ann. Neurol. 42, 776–782.
Kalvodova, L., et al., 2005. Lipids as modulators of proteolytic activity of BACE: involvement of cholesterol, glycosphingolipids, and anionic phospholipids in vitro. J. Biol. Chem. 280, 36815–36823.
Kamenetz, F., et al., 2003. APP processing and synaptic function. Neuron 37, 925–937.
Karakas, E., Regan, M.C., Furukawa, H., 2015. Emerging structural insights into the function of ionotropic glutamate receptors. Trends Biochem. Sci. 40, 328–337.
Kawarabayashi, T., et al., 2004. Dimeric amyloid beta protein rapidly accumulates in lipid rafts followed by apolipoprotein E and phosphorylated tau accumulation in the Tg2576 mouse model of Alzheimer's disease. J. Neurosci. 24, 3801–3809.
Khmelinskaia, A., et al., 2014. Changes in membrane organization upon spontaneous insertion of 2-hydroxylated unsaturated fatty acids in the lipid bilayer. Langmuir 30, 2117–2128.
Kolsch, H., et al., 2002. Polymorphism in the cholesterol 24S-hydroxylase gene is associated with Alzheimer's disease. Mol. Psychiatry 7, 899–902.

Kolsch, H., Lutjohann, D., Tulke, A., Bjorkhem, I., Rao, M.L., 1999. The neurotoxic effect of 24-hydroxycholesterol on SH-SY5Y human neuroblastoma cells. Brain Res. 818, 171–175.

Korade, Z., Kenworthy, A.K., 2008. Lipid rafts, cholesterol, and the brain. Neuropharmacology 55, 1265–1273.

Kostylev, M.A., et al., 2015. Prion-Protein-interacting amyloid-beta oligomers of high molecular weight are tightly correlated with memory impairment in multiple Alzheimer mouse models. J. Biol. Chem. 290, 17415–17438.

Kotti, T.J., Ramirez, D.M., Pfeiffer, B.E., Huber, K.M., Russell, D.W., 2006. Brain cholesterol turnover required for geranylgeraniol production and learning in mice. Proc. Natl. Acad. Sci. U.S.A. 103, 3869–3874.

Kritis, A.A., Stamoula, E.G., Paniskaki, K.A., Vavilis, T.D., 2015. Researching glutamate – induced cytotoxicity in different cell lines: a comparative/collective analysis/study. Front Cell Neurosci. 9, 91.

Kubo, S., Hatano, T., Hattori, N., 2015. Lipid rafts involvement in the pathogenesis of Parkinson's disease. Front Biosci. (Landmark Ed.) 20, 263–279.

Lai, T.W., Shyu, W.C., Wang, Y.T., 2011. Stroke intervention pathways: NMDA receptors and beyond. Trends Mol. Med. 17, 266–275.

Lai, T.W., Zhang, S., Wang, Y.T., 2014. Excitotoxicity and stroke: identifying novel targets for neuroprotection. Prog. Neurobiol. 115, 157–188.

Lathe, R., Sapronova, A., Kotelevtsev, Y., 2014. Atherosclerosis and Alzheimer–diseases with a common cause? Inflammation, oxysterols, vasculature. BMC Geriatr. 14, 36.

Lauren, J., Gimbel, D.A., Nygaard, H.B., Gilbert, J.W., Strittmatter, S.M., 2009. Cellular prion protein mediates impairment of synaptic plasticity by amyloid-beta oligomers. Nature 457, 1128–1132.

Ledesma, M.D., Dotti, C.G., 2012. Peripheral cholesterol, metabolic disorders and Alzheimer's disease. Front Biosci. (Elite Ed.) 4, 181–194.

Lee, S.J., et al., 1998. A detergent-insoluble membrane compartment contains A beta in vivo. Nat. Med. 4, 730–734.

Lee, J.N., Ye, J., 2004. Proteolytic activation of sterol regulatory element-binding protein induced by cellular stress through depletion of Insig-1. J. Biol. Chem. 279, 45257–45265.

Lee, J.N., Gong, Y., Zhang, X., Ye, J., 2006a. Proteasomal degradation of ubiquitinated Insig proteins is determined by serine residues flanking ubiquitinated lysines. Proc. Natl. Acad. Sci. U.S.A. 103, 4958–4963.

Lee, J.N., Song, B., DeBose-Boyd, R.A., Ye, J., 2006b. Sterol-regulated degradation of Insig-1 mediated by the membrane-bound ubiquitin ligase gp78. J. Biol. Chem. 281, 39308–39315.

Lee, J.N., Zhang, X., Feramisco, J.D., Gong, Y., Ye, J., 2008. Unsaturated fatty acids inhibit proteasomal degradation of Insig-1 at a postubiquitination step. J. Biol. Chem. 283, 33772–33783.

Lemkul, J.A., Bevan, D.R., 2013. Aggregation of Alzheimer's amyloid beta-peptide in biological membranes: a molecular dynamics study. Biochemistry 52, 4971–4980.

Leoni, V., Caccia, C., 2013a. 24S-hydroxycholesterol in plasma: a marker of cholesterol turnover in neurodegenerative diseases. Biochimie 95, 595–612.

Leoni, V., Caccia, C., 2013b. Potential diagnostic applications of side chain oxysterols analysis in plasma and cerebrospinal fluid. Biochem. Pharmacol. 86, 26–36.

Lesne, S., et al., 2005. NMDA receptor activation inhibits alpha-secretase and promotes neuronal amyloid-beta production. J. Neurosci. 25, 9367–9377.

Leuba, G., et al., 2014. Pathological reorganization of NMDA receptors subunits and postsynaptic protein PSD-95 distribution in Alzheimer's disease. Curr. Alzheimer Res. 11, 86–96.

Levental, I., Grzybek, M., Simons, K., 2010. Greasing their way: lipid modifications determine protein association with membrane rafts. Biochemistry 49, 6305–6316.

Li, S., et al., 2011. Soluble Aβ oligomers inhibit long-term potentiation through a mechanism involving excessive activation of extrasynaptic NR2B-containing NMDA receptors. J. Neurosci. 31, 6627–6638.

Li, K., et al., 2012. Association study between two novel single nucleotide polymorphisms and sporadic Parkinson's disease in Chinese Han population. Neurosci. Lett. 517, 56–59.

Li, L., et al., 2014. Mass spectrometry methodology in lipid analysis. Int. J. Mol. Sci. 15, 10492–10507.

Li, X., Serwanski, D.R., Miralles, C.P., Bahr, B.A., De Blas, A.L., 2007. Two pools of Triton X-100-insoluble GABA(A) receptors are present in the brain, one associated to lipid rafts and another one to the post-synaptic GABAergic complex. J. Neurochem. 102, 1329–1345.

Liang, T., Li, R., Cheng, O., 2015. Statins for treating Alzheimer's disease: truly ineffective? Eur. Neurol. 73, 360–366.

Limon, A., Reyes-Ruiz, J.M., Miledi, R., 2012. Loss of functional GABA(A) receptors in the Alzheimer diseased brain. Proc. Natl. Acad. Sci. U.S.A. 109, 10071–10076.

Linetti, A., et al., 2010. Cholesterol reduction impairs exocytosis of synaptic vesicles. J. Cell Sci. 123, 595–605.

Lipton, S.A., 2006. Paradigm shift in neuroprotection by NMDA receptor blockade: memantine and beyond. Nat. Rev. Drug Discov. 5, 160–170.

Liu, Y., et al., 2007. NMDA receptor subunits have differential roles in mediating excitotoxic neuronal death both in vitro and in vivo. J. Neurosci. 27, 2846–2857.

Liu, Q., Xie, X., Emadi, S., Sierks, M.R., Wu, J., 2015. A novel nicotinic mechanism underlies beta-amyloid-induced neurotoxicity. Neuropharmacology 97, 457–463.

Lombardo, S., Maskos, U., 2015. Role of the nicotinic acetylcholine receptor in Alzheimer's disease pathology and treatment. Neuropharmacology 96, 255–262.

Lopes da Silva, S., et al., 2014. Plasma nutrient status of patients with Alzheimer's disease: systematic review and meta-analysis. Alzheimers Dement 10, 485–502.

Lourenco, M.V., Ferreira, S.T., De Felice, F.G., 2015. Neuronal stress signaling and eIF2alpha phosphorylation as molecular links between Alzheimer's disease and diabetes. Prog. Neurobiol. 129, 37–57.

Lucke-Wold, B.P., et al., 2015. Common mechanisms of Alzheimer's disease and ischemic stroke: the role of protein kinase C in the progression of age-related neurodegeneration. J. Alzheimers Dis. 43, 711–724.

Lund, E.G., Guileyardo, J.M., Russell, D.W., 1999. cDNA cloning of cholesterol 24-hydroxylase, a mediator of cholesterol homeostasis in the brain. Proc. Natl. Acad. Sci. U.S.A. 96, 7238–7243.

Luthi-Carter, R., et al., 2010. SIRT2 inhibition achieves neuroprotection by decreasing sterol biosynthesis. Proc. Natl. Acad. Sci. U.S.A. 107, 7927–7932.

Ma, L., Wang, J., Li, Y., 2015. Insulin resistance and cognitive dysfunction. Clin. Chim. Acta 444, 18–23.

Marcello, E., et al., 2007. Synapse-associated protein-97 mediates alpha-secretase ADAM10 trafficking and promotes its activity. J. Neurosci. 27, 1682–1691.

Marchand, S., Devillers-Thiery, A., Pons, S., Changeux, J.P., Cartaud, J., 2002. Rapsyn escorts the nicotinic acetylcholine receptor along the exocytic pathway via association with lipid rafts. J. Neurosci. 22, 8891–8901.

Marin, R., Rojo, J.A., Fabelo, N., Fernandez, C.E., Diaz, M., 2013. Lipid raft disarrangement as a result of neuropathological progresses: a novel strategy for early diagnosis? Neuroscience 245, 26–39.

Marques-da-Silva, D., Gutierrez-Merino, C., 2012. L-type voltage-operated calcium channels, N-methyl-D-aspartate receptors and neuronal nitric-oxide synthase form a calcium/redox nano-transducer within lipid rafts. Biochem. Biophys. Res. Commun. 420, 257–262.

Marques-da-Silva, D., Gutierrez-Merino, C., 2014. Caveolin-rich lipid rafts of the plasma membrane of mature cerebellar granule neurons are microcompartments for calcium/reactive oxygen and nitrogen species cross-talk signaling. Cell Calcium 56, 108–123.

Marques-da-Silva, D., Samhan-Arias, A.K., Tiago, T., Gutierrez-Merino, C., 2010. L-type calcium channels and cytochrome b5 reductase are components of protein complexes tightly associated with lipid rafts microdomains of the neuronal plasma membrane. J. Proteomics 73, 1502–1510.

Martin, V., et al., 2010. Lipid alterations in lipid rafts from Alzheimer's disease human brain cortex. J. Alzheimers Dis. 19, 489–502.

Mateos, M.V., Salvador, G.A., Giusto, N.M., 2010. Selective localization of phosphatidylcholine-derived signaling in detergent-resistant membranes from synaptic endings. Biochim. Biophys. Acta 1798, 624–636.

Matsuzaki, K., 2014. How do membranes initiate Alzheimer's disease? Formation of toxic amyloid fibrils by the amyloid beta-protein on ganglioside clusters. Acc. Chem. Res. 47, 2397–2404.

McGuinness, B., et al., 2010. Statins for the treatment of dementia. Cochrane Database Syst. Rev. CD007514.

McKay, B.E., Placzek, A.N., Dani, J.A., 2007. Regulation of synaptic transmission and plasticity by neuronal nicotinic acetylcholine receptors. Biochem. Pharmacol. 74, 1120–1133.

McPherson, R., Gauthier, A., 2004. Molecular regulation of SREBP function: the Insig-SCAP connection and isoform-specific modulation of lipid synthesis. Biochem. Cell Biol. 82, 201–211.

Mehta, A., Prabhakar, M., Kumar, P., Deshmukh, R., Sharma, P.L., 2013. Excitotoxicity: bridge to various triggers in neurodegenerative disorders. Eur. J. Pharmacol. 698, 6–18.

Meitzen, J., Mermelstein, P.G., 2011. Estrogen receptors stimulate brain region specific metabotropic glutamate receptors to rapidly initiate signal transduction pathways. J. Chem. Neuroanat. 42, 236–241.

Mendoza-Oliva, A., Zepeda, A., Arias, C., 2014. The complex actions of statins in brain and their relevance for Alzheimer's disease treatment: an analytical review. Curr. Alzheimer Res. 11, 817–833.

Mermelstein, P.G., 2009. Membrane-localised oestrogen receptor alpha and beta influence neuronal activity through activation of metabotropic glutamate receptors. J. Neuroendocrinol. 21, 257–262.

Michal, P., Rudajev, V., El-Fakahany, E.E., Dolezal, V., 2009. Membrane cholesterol content influences binding properties of muscarinic M2 receptors and differentially impacts activation of second messenger pathways. Eur. J. Pharmacol. 606, 50–60.

Michal, P., El-Fakahany, E.E., Dolezal, V., 2014. Changes in membrane cholesterol differentially influence preferential and non-preferential signaling of the M1 and M3 muscarinic acetylcholine receptors. Neurochem. Res. 40 (10), 2068–2077.

Milnerwood, A.J., et al., 2010. Early increase in extrasynaptic NMDA receptor signaling and expression contributes to phenotype onset in Huntington's disease mice. Neuron 65, 178–190.

Milnerwood, A.J., Raymond, L.A., 2010. Early synaptic pathophysiology in neurodegeneration: insights from Huntington's disease. Trends Neurosci. 33, 513–523.

Mohajeri, M.H., Troesch, B., Weber, P., 2015. Inadequate supply of vitamins and DHA in the elderly: implications for brain aging and Alzheimer-type dementia. Nutrition 31, 261–275.

Mohamed, A., Saavedra, L., Di Pardo, A., Sipione, S., Posse de Chaves, E., 2012. beta-amyloid inhibits protein prenylation and induces cholesterol sequestration by impairing SREBP-2 cleavage. J. Neurosci. 32, 6490–6500.

Molander-Melin, M., et al., 2005. Structural membrane alterations in Alzheimer brains found to be associated with regional disease development; increased density of gangliosides GM1 and GM2 and loss of cholesterol in detergent-resistant membrane domains. J. Neurochem. 92, 171–182.

Mony, L., Kew, J.N., Gunthorpe, M.J., Paoletti, P., 2009. Allosteric modulators of NR2B-containing NMDA receptors: molecular mechanisms and therapeutic potential. Br. J. Pharmacol. 157, 1301–1317.

Mota, S.I., Ferreira, I.L., Rego, A.C., 2014. Dysfunctional synapse in Alzheimer's disease – a focus on NMDA receptors. Neuropharmacology 76 (Pt A), 16–26.

Mucke, L., Selkoe, D.J., 2012. Neurotoxicity of amyloid beta-protein: synaptic and network dysfunction. Cold Spring Harb Perspect. Med. 2, a006338.

Muniz, M., Zurzolo, C., 2014. Sorting of GPI-anchored proteins from yeast to mammals—common pathways at different sites? J. Cell Sci. 127, 2793–2801.

Murphy, S.R., et al., 2013. Acat1 knockdown gene therapy decreases amyloid-beta in a mouse model of Alzheimer's disease. Mol. Ther. 21, 1497–1506.

Nicolas, M., Hassan, B.A., 2014. Amyloid precursor protein and neural development. Development 141, 2543–2548.

Nicolson, G.L., 2014. The Fluid-Mosaic Model of Membrane Structure: still relevant to understanding the structure, function and dynamics of biological membranes after more than 40 years. Biochim. Biophys. Acta 1838, 1451–1466.

Noguchi, N., Saito, Y., Urano, Y., 2014. Diverse functions of 24(S)-hydroxycholesterol in the brain. Biochem. Biophys. Res. Commun. 446, 692–696.

Noguchi, N., Urano, Y., Takabe, W., Saito, Y., 2015. New aspects of 24S-hydroxycholesterol in modulating neuronal cell death. Free Radic. Biol. Med. 87, 366–372.

Nothdurfter, C., et al., 2013. Lipid raft integrity affects GABAA receptor, but not NMDA receptor modulation by psychopharmacological compounds. Int. J. Neuropsychopharmacol. 16, 1361–1371.

Ohshiro, T., Tomoda, H., 2015. Acyltransferase inhibitors: a patent review (2010-present). Expert Opin. Ther. Pat. 25, 145–158.

Okamoto, K., et al., 2006. Sterol regulatory element binding protein (SREBP)-1 expression in brain is affected by age but not by hormones or metabolic changes. Brain Res. 1081, 19–27.

Olsen, K.M., Sheng, M., 2012. NMDA receptors and BAX are essential for Aβ impairment of LTP. Sci. Rep. 2, 225.

Ong, W.Y., Tanaka, K., Dawe, G.S., Ittner, L.M., Farooqui, A.A., 2013. Slow excitotoxicity in Alzheimer's disease. J. Alzheimers Dis. 35, 643–668.

Ong, W.Y., Farooqui, T., Kokotos, G., Farooqui, A.A., 2015. Synthetic and natural inhibitors of phospholipases A2: their importance for understanding and treatment of neurological disorders. ACS Chem. Neurosci. 6, 814–831.

Oshikawa, J., et al., 2003. Nicotinic acetylcholine receptor alpha 7 regulates cAMP signal within lipid rafts. Am. J. Physiol. Cell Physiol. 285, C567–C574.

Owens, D.F., Kriegstein, A.R., 2002. Is there more to GABA than synaptic inhibition? Nat. Rev. Neurosci. 3, 715–727.

Paoletti, P., Neyton, J., 2007. NMDA receptor subunits: function and pharmacology. Curr. Opin Pharmacol. 7, 39–47.

Paoletti, P., 2011. Molecular basis of NMDA receptor functional diversity. Eur. J. Neurosci. 33, 1351–1365.

Papassotiropoulos, A., et al., 2002. 24S-hydroxycholesterol in cerebrospinal fluid is elevated in early stages of dementia. J. Psychiatr. Res. 36, 27–32.

Papouin, T., et al., 2012. Synaptic and extrasynaptic NMDA receptors are gated by different endogenous coagonists. Cell 150, 633–646.

Parkin, E.T., Turner, A.J., Hooper, N.M., 1999. Amyloid precursor protein, although partially detergent-insoluble in mouse cerebral cortex, behaves as an atypical lipid raft protein. Biochem. J. 344 (Pt 1), 23–30.

Parsons, M.P., Raymond, L.A., 2014. Extrasynaptic NMDA receptor involvement in central nervous system disorders. Neuron 82, 279–293.

Paula-Lima, A.C., Brito-Moreira, J., Ferreira, S.T., 2013. Deregulation of excitatory neurotransmission underlying synapse failure in Alzheimer's disease. J. Neurochem. 126, 191–202.

Pena, V.B., Bonini, I.C., Antollini, S.S., Kobayashi, T., Barrantes, F.J., 2011. Alpha 7-type acetylcholine receptor localization and its modulation by nicotine and cholesterol in vascular endothelial cells. J. Cell Biochem. 112, 3276–3288.

Peters, C., Espinoza, M.P., Gallegos, S., Opazo, C., Aguayo, L.G., 2015. Alzheimer's Aβ interacts with cellular prion protein inducing neuronal membrane damage and synaptotoxicity. Neurobiol. Aging 36, 1369–1377.

Pierrot, N., et al., 2013. Amyloid precursor protein controls cholesterol turnover needed for neuronal activity. EMBO Mol. Med. 5, 608–625.

Pike, L.J., 2006. Rafts defined: a report on the keystone symposium on lipid rafts and cell function. J. Lipid Res. 47, 1597–1598.

Pol, A., Gross, S.P., Parton, R.G., 2014. Review: biogenesis of the multifunctional lipid droplet: lipids, proteins, and sites. J. Cell Biol. 204, 635–646.

Ponce, J., et al., 2008. Simvastatin reduces the association of NMDA receptors to lipid rafts: a cholesterol-mediated effect in neuroprotection. Stroke 39, 1269–1275.

Pouladi, M.A., Morton, A.J., Hayden, M.R., 2013. Choosing an animal model for the study of Huntington's disease. Nat. Rev. Neurosci. 14, 708–721.

Raina, A., Kaul, D., 2010. LXR-alpha genomics programmes neuronal death observed in Alzheimer's disease. Apoptosis 15, 1461–1469.

Ramirez, D.M., Andersson, S., Russell, D.W., 2008. Neuronal expression and subcellular localization of cholesterol 24-hydroxylase in the mouse brain. J. Comp. Neurol. 507, 1676–1693.

Rammes, G., Hasenjager, A., Sroka-Saidi, K., Deussing, J.M., Parsons, C.G., 2011. Therapeutic significance of NR2B-containing NMDA receptors and mGluR5 metabotropic glutamate receptors in mediating the synaptotoxic effects of beta-amyloid oligomers on long-term potentiation (LTP) in murine hippocampal slices. Neuropharmacology 60, 982–990.

Rathenberg, J., Kittler, J.T., Moss, S.J., 2004. Palmitoylation regulates the clustering and cell surface stability of GABAA receptors. Mol. Cell Neurosci. 26, 251–257.

Regan, M.C., Romero-Hernandez, A., Furukawa, H., 2015. A structural biology perspective on NMDA receptor pharmacology and function. Curr. Opin. Struct. Biol. 33, 68–75.

Reisberg, B., et al., 2003. Memantine in moderate-to-severe Alzheimer's disease. N. Engl. J. Med. 348, 1333–1341.

Richardson, K., et al., 2013. Statins and cognitive function: a systematic review. Ann. Intern. Med. 159, 688–697.

Ronicke, R., et al., 2011. Early neuronal dysfunction by amyloid beta oligomers depends on activation of NR2B-containing NMDA receptors. Neurobiol. Aging 32, 2219–2228.

Rudy, C.C., Hunsberger, H.C., Weitzner, D.S., Reed, M.N., 2015. The role of the tripartite glutamatergic synapse in the pathophysiology of Alzheimer's disease. Aging Dis. 6, 131–148.

Rush, T., Buisson, A., 2014. Reciprocal disruption of neuronal signaling and Aβ production mediated by extrasynaptic NMDA receptors: a downward spiral. Cell Tissue Res. 356, 279–286.

Saavedra, L., Mohamed, A., Ma, V., Kar, S., de Chaves, E.P., 2007. Internalization of beta-amyloid peptide by primary neurons in the absence of apolipoprotein E. J. Biol. Chem. 282, 35722–35732.

Salem Jr., N., Litman, B., Kim, H.Y., Gawrisch, K., 2001. Mechanisms of action of docosahexaenoic acid in the nervous system. Lipids 36, 945–959.

Sanchez-Mejia, R.O., et al., 2008. Phospholipase A2 reduction ameliorates cognitive deficits in a mouse model of Alzheimer's disease. Nat. Neurosci. 11, 1311–1318.

Santangelo, R.M., et al., 2012. Novel NMDA receptor modulators: an update. Expert Opin. Ther. Pat. 22, 1337–1352.

Saraceno, C., et al., 2014. SAP97-mediated ADAM10 trafficking from Golgi outposts depends on PKC phosphorylation. Cell Death Dis. 5, e1547.

Sasahara, K., Morigaki, K., Shinya, K., 2013. Effects of membrane interaction and aggregation of amyloid beta-peptide on lipid mobility and membrane domain structure. Phys. Chem. Chem. Phys. 15, 8929–8939.

Sasahara, K., Morigaki, K., Mori, Y., 2015. Uptake of raft components into amyloid beta-peptide aggregates and membrane damage. Anal. Biochem. 481, 18–26.
Schneider, A., et al., 2008. Flotillin-dependent clustering of the amyloid precursor protein regulates its endocytosis and amyloidogenic processing in neurons. J. Neurosci. 28, 2874–2882.
Sebastiao, A.M., Colino-Oliveira, M., Assaife-Lopes, N., Dias, R.B., Ribeiro, J.A., 2013. Lipid rafts, synaptic transmission and plasticity: impact in age-related neurodegenerative diseases. Neuropharmacology 64, 97–107.
Seeburg, P.H., et al., 1995. The NMDA receptor channel: molecular design of a coincidence detector. Recent Prog. Horm. Res. 50, 19–34.
Segatto, M., Di Giovanni, A., Marino, M., Pallottini, V., 2012. Analysis of the protein network of cholesterol homeostasis in different brain regions: an age and sex dependent perspective. J. Cell Physiol. 228, 1561–1567.
Segatto, M., Leboffe, L., Trapani, L., Pallottini, V., 2014. Cholesterol homeostasis failure in the brain: implications for synaptic dysfunction and cognitive decline. Curr. Med. Chem. 21, 2788–2802.
Shankar, G.M., et al., 2007. Natural oligomers of the Alzheimer amyloid-beta protein induce reversible synapse loss by modulating an NMDA-type glutamate receptor-dependent signaling pathway. J. Neurosci. 27, 2866–2875.
Shepardson, N.E., Shankar, G.M., Selkoe, D.J., 2011a. Cholesterol level and statin use in Alzheimer disease: I. Review of epidemiological and preclinical studies. Arch. Neurol. 68, 1239–1244.
Shepardson, N.E., Shankar, G.M., Selkoe, D.J., 2011b. Cholesterol level and statin use in Alzheimer disease: II. Review of human trials and recommendations. Arch. Neurol. 68, 1385–1392.
Shevchenko, A., Simons, K., 2010. Lipidomics: coming to grips with lipid diversity. Nat. Rev. Mol. Cell Biol. 11, 593–598.
Shibuya, Y., et al., 2015. Acyl-coenzyme A:cholesterol acyltransferase 1 blockage enhances autophagy in the neurons of triple transgenic Alzheimer's disease mouse and reduces human P301L-tau content at the presymptomatic stage. Neurobiol. Aging 36, 2248–2259.
Shibuya, Y., Chang, C.C., Huang, L.H., Bryleva, E.Y., Chang, T.Y., 2014. Inhibiting ACAT1/SOAT1 in microglia stimulates autophagy-mediated lysosomal proteolysis and increases Aβ1-42 clearance. J. Neurosci. 34, 14484–14501.
Shinohara, M., et al., 2014. Possible modification of Alzheimer's disease by statins in midlife: interactions with genetic and non-genetic risk factors. Front Aging Neurosci. 6, 71.
Simons, K., Ehehalt, R., 2002. Cholesterol, lipid rafts, and disease. J. Clin. Invest. 110, 597–603.
Simons, K., Gerl, M.J., 2010. Revitalizing membrane rafts: new tools and insights. Nat. Rev. Mol. Cell Biol. 11, 688–699.
Singer, S.J., Nicolson, G.L., 1972. The fluid mosaic model of the structure of cell membranes. Science 175, 720–731.
Singh, S., Kushwah, A.S., Singh, R., Farswan, M., Kaur, R., 2012. Current therapeutic strategy in Alzheimer's disease. Eur. Rev. Med. Pharmacol. Sci. 16, 1651–1664.
Smith, M.H., Ploegh, H.L., Weissman, J.S., 2011. Road to ruin: targeting proteins for degradation in the endoplasmic reticulum. Science 334, 1086–1090.
Snyder, E.M., et al., 2005. Regulation of NMDA receptor trafficking by amyloid-beta. Nat. Neurosci. 8, 1051–1058.
Sodero, A.O., et al., 2012. Cholesterol loss during glutamate-mediated excitotoxicity. EMBO J. 31, 1764–1773.
Sodero, A.O., Weissmann, C., Ledesma, M.D., Dotti, C.G., 2011. Cellular stress from excitatory neurotransmission contributes to cholesterol loss in hippocampal neurons aging in vitro. Neurobiol. Aging 32, 1043–1053.
Sonnino, S., et al., 2014. Lipid rafts in neurodegeneration and neuroprotection. Mol. Neurobiol 50, 130–148.
Spell, C., et al., 2004. SREBP-1a polymorphism influences the risk of Alzheimer's disease in carriers of the ApoE4 allele. Dement Geriatr. Cogn. Disord. 18, 245–249.
St Pierre, P., Nabi, I.R., 2012. The Gp78 ubiquitin ligase: probing endoplasmic reticulum complexity. Protoplasma 249 (Suppl. 1), S11–S18.
Stillwell, W., Shaikh, S.R., Zerouga, M., Siddiqui, R., Wassall, S.R., 2005. Docosahexaenoic acid affects cell signaling by altering lipid rafts. Reprod. Nutr. Dev. 45, 559–579.
Su, H.M., 2010. Mechanisms of n-3 fatty acid-mediated development and maintenance of learning memory performance. J. Nutr. Biochem. 21, 364–373.
Sun, M.K., Alkon, D.L., 2014. The "memory kinases": roles of PKC isoforms in signal processing and memory formation. Prog. Mol. Biol. Transl. Sci. 122, 31–59.
Suzuki, T., et al., 2011. Association of membrane rafts and postsynaptic density: proteomics, biochemical, and ultrastructural analyses. J. Neurochem. 119, 64–77.
Suzuki, T., 2002. Lipid rafts at postsynaptic sites: distribution, function and linkage to postsynaptic density. Neurosci. Res. 44, 1–9.

Swanwick, C.C., Shapiro, M.E., Yi, Z., Chang, K., Wenthold, R.J., 2009. NMDA receptors interact with flotillin-1 and -2, lipid raft-associated proteins. FEBS Lett. 583, 1226–1230.

Tackenberg, C., et al., 2013. NMDA receptor subunit composition determines beta-amyloid-induced neurodegeneration and synaptic loss. Cell Death Dis. 4, e608.

Taghibiglou, C., et al., 2009a. Essential role of SBP-1 activation in oxygen deprivation induced lipid accumulation and increase in body width/length ratio in *Caenorhabditis elegans*. FEBS Lett. 583, 831–834.

Taghibiglou, C., et al., 2009b. Mechanisms involved in cholesterol-induced neuronal insulin resistance. Neuropharmacology 57, 268–276.

Taghibiglou, C., et al., 2009c. Role of NMDA receptor-dependent activation of SREBP1 in excitotoxic and ischemic neuronal injuries. Nat. Med. 15, 1399–1406.

Taghibiglou, C., Lu, J., Mackenzie, I.R., Wang, Y.T., Cashman, N.R., 2011. Sterol regulatory element binding protein-1 (SREBP1) activation in motor neurons in excitotoxicity and amyotrophic lateral sclerosis (ALS): Indip, a potential therapeutic peptide. Biochem. Biophys. Res. Commun. 413, 159–163.

Taghibiglou, C., 2013. The sterol regulatory element binding transcription factor 1 (SREBP1): an attractive therapeutic target in CNS drug discoveries. J. Pharmacol. Biomed. Anal. 1, 1.

Tajima, Y., et al., 2013. Lipidomic analysis of brain tissues and plasma in a mouse model expressing mutated human amyloid precursor protein/tau for Alzheimer's disease. Lipids Health Dis. 12, 68.

Takayasu, Y., et al., 2010. Caveolin-1 knockout mice exhibit impaired induction of mGluR-dependent long-term depression at CA3-CA1 synapses. Proc. Natl. Acad. Sci. U.S.A. 107, 21778–21783.

Tanabe, F., Nakajima, T., Ito, M., 2012. Involvement of diacylglycerol produced by phospholipase D activation in Aβ-induced reduction of sAPPα secretion in SH-SY5Y neuroblastoma cells. Biochem. Biophys. Res. Commun. 446, 933–939.

Taverna, E., et al., 2007. Localization of synaptic proteins involved in neurosecretion in different membrane microdomains. J. Neurochem. 100, 664–677.

Teunissen, C.E., et al., 2007. 24S-hydroxycholesterol in relation to disease manifestations of acute experimental autoimmune encephalomyelitis. J. Neurosci. Res. 85, 1499–1505.

Thomas, G.M., Huganir, R.L., 2004. MAPK cascade signalling and synaptic plasticity. Nat. Rev. Neurosci. 5, 173–183.

Tian, G., Kong, Q., Lai, L., Ray-Chaudhury, A., Lin, C.L., 2010. Increased expression of cholesterol 24S-hydroxylase results in disruption of glial glutamate transporter EAAT2 association with lipid rafts: a potential role in Alzheimer's disease. J. Neurochem. 113, 978–989.

Torres, M., et al., 2014. Membrane lipid modifications and therapeutic effects mediated by hydroxydocosahexaenoic acid on Alzheimer's disease. Biochim. Biophys. Acta 1838, 1680–1692.

Torres, M., Marcilla-Etxenike, A., Fiol-deRoque, M.A., Escriba, P.V., Busquets, X., 2015. The unfolded protein response in the therapeutic effect of hydroxy-DHA against Alzheimer's disease. Apoptosis 20, 712–724.

Tsai, Y.H., Liu, X., Seeberger, P.H., 2012. Chemical biology of glycosylphosphatidylinositol anchors. Angew. Chem. Int. Ed. Engl. 51, 11438–11456.

Tu, W., et al., 2010. DAPK1 interaction with NMDA receptor NR2B subunits mediates brain damage in stroke. Cell 140, 222–234.

Ueno, H., et al., 2014. Comparison between the aggregation of human and rodent amyloid beta-proteins in GM1 ganglioside clusters. Biochemistry 53, 7523–7530.

Ulrich, D., 2015. Amyloid-beta impairs synaptic inhibition via GABAA receptor endocytosis. J. Neurosci. 35, 9205–9210.

Um, J.W., et al., 2012. Alzheimer amyloid-beta oligomer bound to postsynaptic prion protein activates Fyn to impair neurons. Nat. Neurosci. 15, 1227–1235.

Urano, Y., Ochiai, S., Noguchi, N., 2013. Suppression of amyloid-beta production by 24S-hydroxycholesterol via inhibition of intracellular amyloid precursor protein trafficking. FASEB J. 27, 4305–4315.

Uto, Y., 2015. Imidazo[1,2-a]pyridines as cholesterol 24-hydroxylase (CYP46A1) inhibitors: a patent evaluation (WO2014061676). Expert Opin. Ther. Pat. 25, 373–377.

Verdile, G., Fuller, S.J., Martins, R.N., 2015. The role of type 2 diabetes in neurodegeneration. Neurobiol. Dis. 84, 22–38.

Vignini, A., et al., 2013. Alzheimer's disease and diabetes: new insights and unifying therapies. Curr. Diabetes Rev. 9, 218–227.

Wada, S., et al., 2003. Gamma-secretase activity is present in rafts but is not cholesterol-dependent. Biochemistry 42, 13977–13986.

Wang, D.D., Kriegstein, A.R., 2009. Defining the role of GABA in cortical development. J. Physiol. 587, 1873–1879.
Wang, D., Jacobs, S.A., Tsien, J.Z., 2014. Targeting the NMDA receptor subunit NR2B for treating or preventing age-related memory decline. Expert Opin. Ther. Targets 18, 1121–1130.
Wang, C., Wang, M., Han, X., 2015. Applications of mass spectrometry for cellular lipid analysis. Mol. Biosyst. 11, 698–713.
Wassall, S.R., Stillwell, W., 2009. Polyunsaturated fatty acid-cholesterol interactions: domain formation in membranes. Biochim. Biophys. Acta 1788, 24–32.
Wenk, M.R., 2005. The emerging field of lipidomics. Nat. Rev. Drug Discov. 4, 594–610.
Williams, T.L., Serpell, L.C., 2011. Membrane and surface interactions of Alzheimer's Aβ peptide–insights into the mechanism of cytotoxicity. FEBS J. 278, 3905–3917.
Williamson, R., Sutherland, C., 2011. Neuronal membranes are key to the pathogenesis of Alzheimer's disease: the role of both raft and non-raft membrane domains. Curr. Alzheimer Res. 8, 213–221.
Willmann, R., et al., 2006. Cholesterol and lipid microdomains stabilize the postsynapse at the neuromuscular junction. EMBO J. 25, 4050–4060.
Wishart, D.S., et al., 2013. Hmdb 3.0—The human metabolome database in 2013. Nucleic Acids Res. 41, D801–D807.
Wood, W.G., Li, L., Muller, W.E., Eckert, G.P., 2014. Cholesterol as a causative factor in Alzheimer's disease: a debatable hypothesis. J. Neurochem. 129, 559–572.
Wyllie, D.J., Livesey, M.R., Hardingham, G.E., 2013. Influence of GluN2 subunit identity on NMDA receptor function. Neuropharmacology 74, 4–17.
Xia, P., Chen, H.S., Zhang, D., Lipton, S.A., 2010. Memantine preferentially blocks extrasynaptic over synaptic NMDA receptor currents in hippocampal autapses. J. Neurosci. 30, 11246–11250.
Yamamoto, N., et al., 2015. Midazolam inhibits the formation of amyloid fibrils and GM1 ganglioside-rich microdomains in presynaptic membranes through the gamma-aminobutyric acid A receptor. Biochem. Biophys. Res. Commun. 457, 547–553.
Yamamoto, N., Tanida, M., Kasahara, R., Sobue, K., Suzuki, K., 2014. Leptin inhibits amyloid beta-protein fibrillogenesis by decreasing GM1 gangliosides on the neuronal cell surface through PI3K/Akt/mTOR pathway. J. Neurochem. 131, 323–332.
Yamanaka, K., Saito, Y., Yamamori, T., Urano, Y., Noguchi, N., 2011. 24(S)-hydroxycholesterol induces neuronal cell death through necroptosis, a form of programmed necrosis. J. Biol. Chem. 286, 24666–24673.
Yamanaka, K., Urano, Y., Takabe, W., Saito, Y., Noguchi, N., 2014. Induction of apoptosis and necroptosis by 24(S)-hydroxycholesterol is dependent on activity of acyl-CoA:cholesterol acyltransferase 1. Cell Death Dis. 5, e990.
Yang, J.X., et al., 2015. Caveolin-1 in the anterior cingulate cortex modulates chronic neuropathic pain via regulation of NMDA receptor 2B subunit. J. Neurosci. 35, 36–52.
Yang, X., Sun, G.Y., Eckert, G.P., Lee, J.C., 2014. Cellular membrane fluidity in amyloid precursor protein processing. Mol. Neurobiol. 50, 119–129.
Yano, S., Tokumitsu, H., Soderling, T.R., 1998. Calcium promotes cell survival through CaM-K kinase activation of the protein-kinase-B pathway. Nature 396, 584–587.
Yu, W., et al., 1998. Co-compartmentalization of MAP kinases and cytosolic phospholipase A2 at cytoplasmic arachidonate-rich lipid bodies. Am. J. Pathol. 152, 759–769.
Zadori, D., et al., 2014. Glutamatergic dysfunctioning in Alzheimer's disease and related therapeutic targets. J. Alzheimers Dis. 42 (Suppl. 3), S177–S187.
Zha, Q., Ruan, Y., Hartmann, T., Beyreuther, K., Zhang, D., 2004. GM1 ganglioside regulates the proteolysis of amyloid precursor protein. Mol. Psychiatry 9, 946–952.
Zhang, S., et al., 2013. Critical role of increased PTEN nuclear translocation in excitotoxic and ischemic neuronal injuries. J. Neurosci. 33, 7997–8008.
Zhao, F.G., et al., 2005. Association between acyl-coenzyme A: cholesterol acyltransferase gene and risk for Alzheimer's disease in Chinese. Neurosci. Lett. 388, 17–20.
Zhou, X., et al., 2014. Lipid rafts participate in aberrant degradative autophagic-lysosomal pathway of amyloid-beta peptide in Alzheimer's disease. Neural Regen. Res. 9, 92–100.
Zhu, D., Xiong, W.C., Mei, L., 2006. Lipid rafts serve as a signaling platform for nicotinic acetylcholine receptor clustering. J. Neurosci. 26, 4841–4851.

CHAPTER

10

Mitochondria as a Therapeutic Target for the Treatment of Alzheimer's Disease

K.R. Valasani, E. Carlson, J.R. Vangavaragu, S.S. Yan

OUTLINE

INTRODUCTION

Alzheimer's disease (AD) is a progressive neurodegenerative disease that affects 44 million people worldwide and 5.4 million people in the United States. Over the past decade the death rate has increased by 68%, making this disease the sixth leading cause of death in the United States. It primarily affects the elderly and is characterized by severe memory loss and cognitive impairment (Andrade and Radhakrishnan, 2009; Possin, 2010; Hedden and Gabrieli, 2005; Chetelat et al., 2011). With no effective cure for AD and a constantly enlarging aging population, AD has become a major public health issue and places an ever-increasing burden

Drug Discovery Approaches for the Treatment of Neurodegenerative Disorders
http://dx.doi.org/10.1016/B978-0-12-802810-0.00010-6

on global economies. Only five drugs are currently approved by the Food and Drug Administration (FDA) to specifically treat AD. At best these drugs only alleviate the symptoms but show no effect on disease progression.

Since there are currently very limited drug targets for the treatment of AD, it is critical for researchers to explore and develop new therapeutic targets for halting and treating this disease. Clearly, new and more effective AD drugs are needed. Any approach that would decrease the rate of progression would represent a major contribution to both medical science and public health. Considerable effort toward this goal has already been expended within the scientific community with little success.

Despite progression in understanding its pathogenesis, the effective drug target remains unavailable. So far the therapeutic paradigm of one-compound-one-target has failed to produce an effective treatment for AD. Multiple pathogenic mechanisms appear to be involved in AD including amyloid-β (Aβ) aggregation to form amyloid plaques, tau hyperphosphorylation that disrupts microtubules to form neurofibrillary tangles, calcium imbalance, enhanced oxidative stress, impaired mitochondrial function, apoptotic neuronal death, and deterioration of synaptic transmission, particularly at cholinergic neurons (Godoy et al., 2014; Leon et al., 2013; Eckert et al., 2011a,b; Du et al., 2008, 2011; Du and Yan, 2010). This is consistent with an underlying complex network of factors that is most likely comprised of genetics, enzyme activities, receptor expression, protein interactions, alteration of metal concentrations, cell cycle survival disruption, ion homeostasis dysregulation, and protein misfolding (Du et al., 2008; Baines et al., 2005; Rosenstock et al., 2004; Ray et al., 2014; Streck et al., 2013; Pope et al., 2008; Mancuso et al., 2006; Schapira, 1996; Tritschler et al., 1994). Given that AD is a multifaceted disease; multitargeted approaches will probably be the most effective method for treatment.

CURRENT TREATMENT FOR ALZHEIMER'S DISEASE

Several different FDA-approved medications are currently used to treat memory loss, behavioral changes, sleep problems, and other symptoms of AD (Table 10.1). It has been known for some time that acetylcholine (ACh) deficiency is associated with AD. This gave rise to one of the oldest AD hypotheses, the cholinergic hypothesis, and associated therapies that inhibit the enzymatic activity of cholinesterases (ChEs) to increase ACh levels in the brain (Berman et al., 2000; Stasiak et al., 2014; Lane et al., 2006; Falugi and Aluigi,

TABLE 10.1 Food and Drug Administration (FDA)–Approved Alzheimer's Disease (AD) Drugs

Drug Name	Brand Name	Approved for	FDA Approved
1. Tacrine	Cognex	Mild-to-moderate AD	1993
2. Donepezil	Aricept	All stages of AD	1996
3. Rivastigmine	Exelon	Mild-to-moderate AD	2000
4. Galantamine	Razadyne	Mild-to-moderate AD	2001
5. Memantine	Namenda	Moderate-to-severe AD	2003

2012; Valasani et al., 2013a). Brain acetylcholinesterase (AChE) has been a main drug target and its inhibitors have demonstrated functionality in the symptomatic treatment of AD. AChE inhibitors are the most frequently prescribed drugs for AD, which promote memory function and delay the cognitive decline without altering the underlying pathology (Gotz et al., 2011; Bonda et al., 2010; Forstl, 2008; Dickey and Petrucelli, 2006; Arsland, 1998; Schenk et al., 1997).

The first four of the FDA-approved drugs are ChE inhibitors and three of these are used to treat mild-to-moderate stages of AD. Donepezil has been used to treat all stages of AD. The fifth FDA-approved AD drug, memantine, is not a ChE inhibitor and therefore works by a different mechanism than other Alzheimer's treatments. It is thought to play a protective role in the brain by regulating the activity of glutamate. Brain cells in patients with AD release more glutamate than normal leading to excitoneurotoxicity and neuronal cell death. Memantine helps regulate the synaptic release and activity of glutamate. Since memantine has a different mode of action, it may have an increased benefit in AD treatment, particularly when used in combination with the ChE inhibitors. Side effects for most of these medications are usually mild and include diarrhea, vomiting, nausea, fatigue, insomnia, loss of appetite, and weight loss. Tacrine, which was the first AD drug approved by the FDA, may cause liver damage so it is no longer used clinically.

A cure for AD is probably not on the horizon nor is a drug that will reverse the disease. But if AD was diagnosed early enough and an effective treatment was available to slow the progression of disease, people could carry out their daily activities and live independently for a much longer period time than at present. This is the approach that is presently being pursued since it would at least provide some relief for family members and the health care system. In addition to the FDA-approved AD drugs, health care providers also use other medicines to help manage symptoms of AD, including depression, sleeplessness, and behavioral problems such as agitation and aggression. Planning and medical/social management can help ease the burden on both patients and family members. Physical exercise, healthy nutrition, mental activities, and social interactions in a calm, structured environment also help people with AD to continue functioning as independently as possible.

MITOCHONDRIAL ENERGY METABOLISM AND OXIDATIVE STRESS

Mitochondria are complex organelles in the cell where cellular respiration or oxidation occurs. They are responsible for most of the energy used by eukaryotic cells and meet cellular energy and metabolic needs in response to physiological and environmental cues. Within the cell, adenosine triphosphate (ATP) is the major energy form produced in mitochondria. This energy source is generated through the collaboration of the tricarboxylic acid (TCA) cycle and the electron transport chain (ETC).

As shown in Fig. 10.1, TCA cycle-specific enzymes produce reduced nicotinamide adenine dinucleotide (NADH) (McCormack, 1985). Succinate dehydrogenase, a key enzyme associated with ETC complex II, oxidizes succinate and produces flavin adenine dinucleotide ($FADH_2$) in the TCA cycle (Yankovskaya et al., 2003). Subsequently, the reduced NADH and $FADH_2$ act as electron donors to the ETC complexes. The electrons are then transferred to complex III, which are integrated into cytochrome c and delivered to complex IV

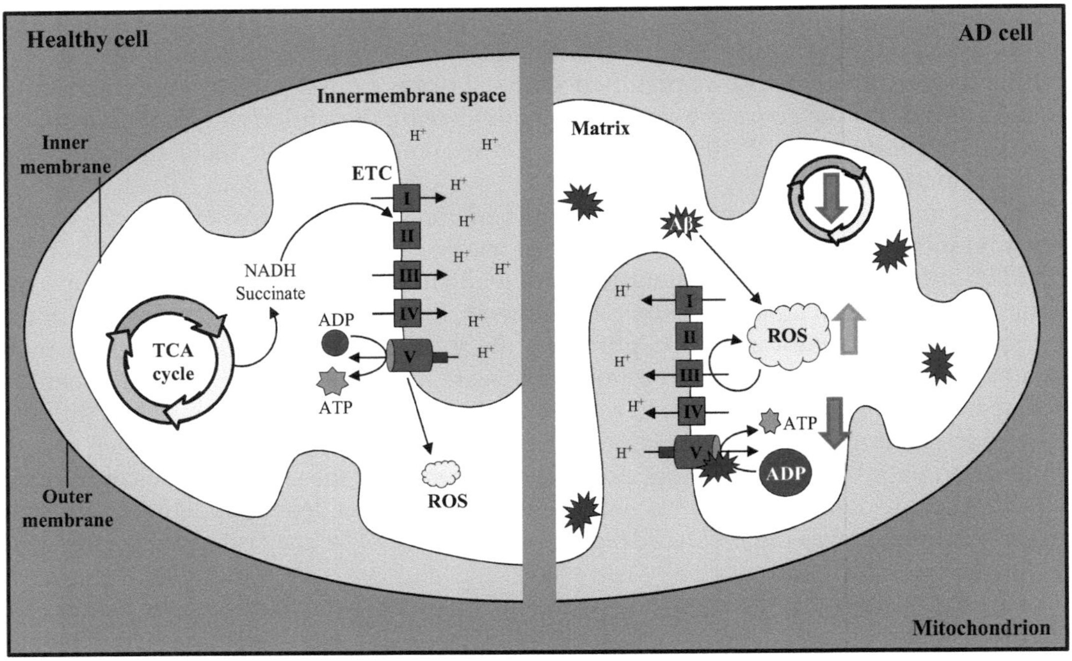

FIGURE 10.1 **Mitochondrial bioenergetics in healthy cells and Alzheimer's disease (AD)-affected cells.** Left: In healthy cells, the tricarboxylic acid (TCA) cycle works to reduce nicotinamide adenine dinucleotide (NADH) and oxidize succinate molecules, which are then used by the electron transport chain (ETC) to generate an electrochemical gradient between the inner membrane space and matrix. Complex V [adenosine triphosphate (ATP) synthase] uses the gradient to produce ATP molecules with manageable levels of reactive oxygen species (ROS) generation. Right: In AD-affected cells, TCA cycle enzyme activities are decreased (*blue arrow, very dark gray in print version*), leading to reduced ATP production (*blue arrow, very dark gray in print version*). Aβ molecules are also able to increase bioenergetic dysfunction by binding to complex V and limiting ATP levels, and enhance ROS production directly. Furthermore, ETC complex deficiencies lead to elevated ROS levels (*pink arrow, light gray in print version*).

(McCormack et al., 1990). Complex IV plays an essential role in ATP synthesis through the reduction of oxygen to water (Takehara et al., 1995).

During the respiratory process, proton gradients are produced across the mitochondrial inner membrane and then used by ATP synthase (complex V) for the synthesis of ATP from adenosine diphosphate and inorganic phosphate (Fig. 10.1) (Nalin and Cross, 1982). ATP is utilized for various essential cellular activities, such as calcium homeostasis, signal transduction, and DNA synthesis (LaNoue et al., 1972).

It has been recognized that the mechanism underlying Aβ toxicity involves loss of calcium homeostasis leading to reactive oxygen species (ROS) overproduction and energy metabolism reductions (Ferreira et al., 2010). There is considerable evidence that altered mitochondrial bioenergetics play a critical role in AD (Swerdlow, 2012). For instance, many TCA cycle enzymes exhibit decreased activity correlating with decreased ATP levels in AD (Sorbi et al., 1983; Gibson et al., 1998). Furthermore, Aβ has been observed to negatively regulate ATP generation by binding to the α-subunit of ATP synthase (Schmidt et al., 2008; Xing et al., 2012). Also reduced glucose metabolism has been reported (Fukuyama et al., 1994), indicating that both metabolic processes are affected during the progression of AD.

Many studies have shown that energy metabolism is diminished in AD brain in conjunction with oxidative stress from mitochondrial ROS overproduction (Markesbery, 1997). Data by Sun and associates, however, proposed that the decrease in energy metabolism seen in AD is in fact a protective response (Sun et al., 2012). In the AD microenvironment, cells reduce energy metabolism to adjust to lower levels of oxygen and nutrient demand. Thus AD-affected neuronal cells may adjust energy metabolism as a last effort to reestablish homeostatic condition.

Besides changes in energy metabolism, AD mitochondria also display impairments in the ETC complexes leading to an elevated ROS generation (Perry et al., 1998). Impairment has been observed in all complexes (Aksenov et al., 1999; Kim et al., 2000), though the most severe defects are seen in complex IV (Parker Jr. et al., 1994; Valla et al., 2001). Additionally, several groups have observed that Aβ aggregate formation can induce the production of ROS (Coraci et al., 2002; Tabner et al., 2001). Vast amounts of data support the oxidative stress hypothesis as a mechanism for AD development and progression.

MITOCHONDRIAL DYSFUNCTION IN AD

Much evidence indicates that mitochondrial dysfunction is connected with aging and age-related neurological diseases (Reddy, 2008; Lee et al., 2009; Kasiviswanathan et al., 2009; Taylor and Turnbull, 2005). Mitochondria are essential cellular organelles in producing efficient energy, detoxifying oxygen, maintaining the cellular redox potential, controlling calcium homeostasis, synthesizing heme and iron–sulfur clusters, and other key metabolites. Mitochondria are also implicated in the production of ROS, particularly under pathological conditions where a disparity in the ETC energy extracting mechanism occurs because of the dysfunction of a specific component such as selective decrease in complex IV activity (Lansbury and Lashuel, 2006). In the AD-affected brain, the biochemical and physiological composition of mitochondria appears abnormal. Dysfunctional mitochondria are presumed to influence neuronal plasticity and neuronal response to metabolic challenges, physiologic and environmental cues, and formation of new memory (Li et al., 2004; Atamna and Frey, 2007).

Increased mitochondrial production of ROS can further induce oxidative stress in neuronal cells; this event occurs in many pathological conditions where the respiratory chain is impaired (Albano, 2006; Wu and Cederbaum, 2003). For instance, increased ROS levels promote the formation and opening of the mitochondrial permeability transition pore (mPTP) that mediates apoptosis, leading to neuronal death (Du et al., 2008; Üttara et al., 2009; Paradies et al., 2014).

Aβ-INDUCED MITOCHONDRIAL DYSFUNCTION IN AD

Aβ, one of the main offending peptides involved in AD pathogenesis, has been linked to mitochondrial dysfunction. Aβ is a proteolytic product of amyloid precursor protein (APP) and AD neuropathology is characterized by abnormal metabolism of APP with excessive accumulation of Aβ peptides (Lustbader et al., 2004; Devi et al., 2006). Both proteins are known to accumulate within mitochondria in the brains of AD patients and AD mouse models. This accumulation in brain tissue causes the abnormality of mitochondrial enzymes including complex IV. It is particularly significant that Aβ is found in cells and mitochondria, especially in disease condition (Devi and Ohno, 2012; Pavlov et al., 2009).

AD pathology has been shown to be accompanied by mitochondrial dysfunction. Studies have shown a relationship between mitochondrial Aβ accumulation and synaptic mitochondrial dysfunction (Andrade and Radhakrishnan, 2009; Kulic et al., 2011; Eckert et al., 2011a,b).

Aβ-related mitochondrial dysfunction drastically impacts mitochondria and their host cells. For instance, irregular protein–protein interactions, reduced mitochondrial ATP manufacturing, impaired respiratory chain function leading to diminished energy metabolism, excessive ROS production promoting enhanced oxidative stress, DNA/RNA mutations that increase mitochondrial vulnerability to other toxicities, and disruption of calcium homeostasis leading to modification of mitochondrial membranes and eventual cell death can all occur because of Aβ-mediated mitochondrial dysfunction (Du et al., 2008, 2011; Lustbader et al., 2004).

Nevertheless, the pathogenic roles of these dysfunctions are poorly established as the synaptic and neuronal degeneration may be induced by Aβ in numerous ways. It is well known that Aβ is present within mitochondria and it interacts with many proteins. Below, we describe two such recently identified proteins of pharmacological significance (Du et al., 2008, 2011; Lustbader et al., 2004).

hPreP is a mitochondrial organellar metalloendopeptidase that functions as a peptide scavenger in the mitochondrial matrix to remove unstructured toxic peptides like Aβ, whose accumulation in the brain of AD patients and its binding to mitochondrial proteins such as CypD and Aβ-binding alcohol dehydrogenase (ABAD), also called 17β-hydroxysteroid dehydrogenase type 10, leads to the sequential events (such as increased oxidative stress, mPTP formation) that trigger mitochondrial damage and neuronal cell death (Fig. 10.2). Increasing hPreP activity enhances Aβ clearance in mitochondria and thereby halts its contribution to mitochondrial dysfunction and neuronal cell death (Alikhani et al., 2011; Yao et al., 2011). An effective AD treatment might result by identifying low-molecular weight compounds that may increase the activity of hPreP. One can use these compounds in combination with Aβ–CypD inhibitors and/or other AD treatments to more effectively protect mitochondrial dysfunction in AD brain.

Mitochondrial Aβ also interacts with CypD, which is a vital component of the mPTP that potentiates ROS production, causes synaptic failure, and promotes apoptosis induction via pore opening (Du and Yan, 2010; Rao et al., 2014). It was previously revealed that CypD can bind to Aβ within the mitochondria of cortical neurons from APP mutant mice, and that these complexes increased CypD translocation from the matrix to the inner membrane. Furthermore, CypD inhibition was able to diminish Aβ-mediated mitochondrial dysfunction in APP transgenic mice (Du et al., 2008). For instance, calcium-induced mitochondrial swelling, mitochondrial calcium uptake, and impaired mitochondrial respiratory function were restored.

These findings agree with the AD hypothesis of an intracellular Aβ toxicity cascade: the toxic Aβ species causes biochemical and molecular impairment as intracellular oligomeric aggregates, other than extracellular insoluble plaques (Fernandez-Vizarra et al., 2004; Lustbader et al., 2004). This hypothesis implies that preventing interactions between Aβ and hPreP and/or CypD could provide feasible ways to treat or prevent AD.

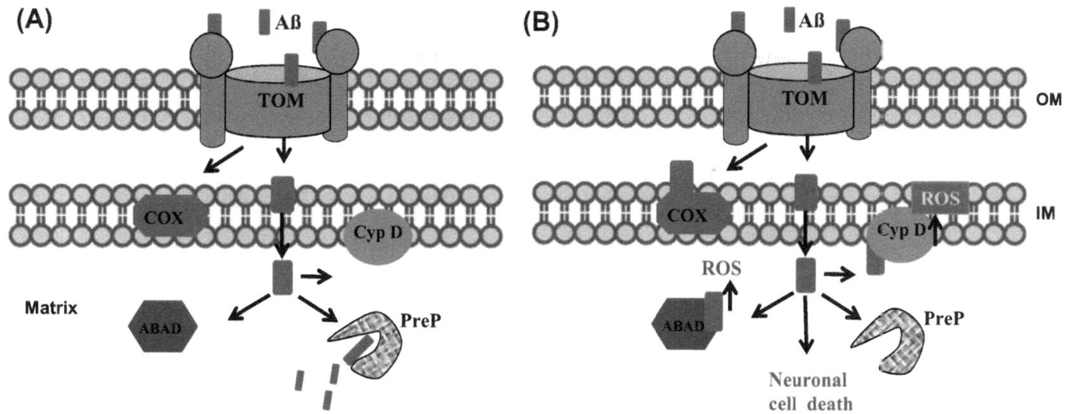

FIGURE 10.2 Role of human presequence protease (hPreP) that lies exclusively in the mitochondrial matrix. (A) This protease has a large active site that can clean mitochondria of unstructured peptides up to 65 amino acids in length and can totally digest Aβ40 and Aβ42. Aβ is imported into mitochondria through the translocase of the outer membrane (TOM) machinery and it resides preferentially in the inner membrane. The imported Aβ can reside in the inner membrane inhibiting the cytochrome c oxidase (COX). However, Aβ can also reach the matrix, where it can be degraded by the hPreP that lies exclusively in the mitochondrial matrix as shown in A. If Aβ is somehow not degraded by hPreP in the matrix, elevated Aβ and reactive oxygen species (ROS) levels exacerbate mitochondrial perturbation and neuronal cell death through Aβ targeting proteins such as Aβ-binding alcohol dehydrogenase (ABAD) and cyclophilin D (CypD)(B).

TARGETING PreP OR CypD FOR PREVENTING OR TREATING AD

PreP as a Potential AD Target

Many mitochondrial proteins are encoded by nuclear genes that are synthesized on cytosolic polyribosomes as precursor proteins each containing a presequence, which is a cleavable peptide extension on the N-terminus. The function of the presequence is to target specific proteins to the right organelles. The presequence is removed by the mitochondrial processing peptidase after it is imported into the mitochondrial matrix (Gabaldon and Huynen, 2004; Glaser and Dessi, 1999). However, free presequences inside mitochondria can be harmful as they can infiltrate the mitochondrial inner membrane to cause disruption of the membrane potential and uncoupling of oxidative phosphorylation (Alikhani et al., 2009; Ieva et al., 2013; King et al., 2014; Kmiec et al., 2014; Bonn et al., 2011). To prevent these events, presequence protease (PreP), located in the matrix, functions to degrade free presequences thereby completing the final step of the protein importation process (Teixeira and Glaser, 2013; Johnson et al., 2006).

PreP was originally identified in *Arabidopsis thaliana* (At) and was found to degrade targeting peptides of mitochondria and chloroplasts. Additionally, PreP is able to degrade a large assortment of unstructured peptides ranging from 10 to 65 amino acids in length (Johnson et al., 2006; Stahl et al., 2005; Ponpuak et al., 2007). This is demonstrated by the crystal structure of AtPreP1, which showed a large catalytic chamber roughly 10,000 $Å^3$ in size that could accommodate unstructured peptides up to 65 amino acids long (Johnson et al., 2006).

hPreP was originally identified as human zinc metalloprotease 1, because it is a member of the pitrilysin M16C family of peptidases containing an inverted zinc-binding motif. hPreP is an ATP-independent protease consisting of 1037 amino acids and is located within the mitochondrial matrix (Vangavaragu et al., 2014b; Teixeira et al., 2012; Chen et al., 2014). hPreP exhibits a 31% sequence similarity to AtPreP, and also performs similar functions in the degradation of presequences and other unstructured peptides. In addition, hPreP was found to be the only mitochondrial protease to degrade Aβ (Ponpuak et al., 2007; Alikhani et al., 2011). In vitro, hPreP can degrade Aβ1–40, Aβ1–42, and the Aβ arctic form (Aβ1–40 E22G), which is a peptide that promotes increased fibril formation and early onset of a familial variant of AD. Mass spectrometry analysis of the hPreP cleavage sites on Aβ revealed the production of several fragments unique for hPreP including cleavage sites in the very hydrophobic C-terminus portion of Aβ that is prone to aggregation. There was a minor preference for hydrophobic and small uncharged amino acids at the P1 and P′1 positions (Alikhani et al., 2011). Although Aβ peptides differ from presequences in terms of physicochemical properties and amino acid composition, the absence of stringent sequence specificity for cleavage allows hPreP to degrade numerous substrates (Vangavaragu et al., 2014).

As hPreP is able to degrade mitochondria-localized Aβ peptides, it is an important regulator of Aβ concentration within mitochondria; thus reduction of hPreP activity influences Aβ accumulation (Fig. 10.2) (Alikhani et al., 2011). hPreP activity has been analyzed in mitochondrial matrix fractions isolated from an area of the brain highly susceptible to Aβ accrual, the temporal lobe of AD patients, and age-matched controls using three different substrates (Aβ1–40, Aβ1–42, and F1β presequence) (Vangavaragu et al., 2014). When the activity was measured in mitochondria isolated from an area unaffected by AD, such as cerebellum, no differences in hPreP activity were observed between AD brains and age-matched controls. Similar experiments using mitochondria isolated from the brains of AD transgenic mouse models overexpressing APP or APP together with ABAD demonstrated lower hPreP activity compared with age-matched nontransgenic mice.

Additionally, the proteolytic activity of hPreP was reduced in an age-dependent manner demonstrating lower activity in 12-month-old mice compared to 5-month-old mice (Alikhani et al., 2011). From a functional point of view, reduced hPreP activity in AD brain mitochondria increases both Aβ and free presequence peptide accumulation (Alikhani et al., 2011). The possible toxic effects of presequence peptide accumulation in mitochondria when hPreP activity is low exacerbates mitochondrial dysfunction, but the specific relevance of this accrual remains to be clarified. Nevertheless, these data suggest that an effective AD treatment may be to increase hPreP activity in the AD-affected brain. Small molecule activators provide a possible therapeutic avenue. Developing small molecules that regulate the function of hPreP could lead to enhanced degradation and clearance of mitochondrial small unstructured peptides, including Aβ. A structure-based virtual screening was used to identify the ability of several compounds to enhance hPreP proteolytic activity. Compounds 3c and 4c of benzimidazole increased hPreP-mediated proteolysis of Aβ1–42, pF1β (2–54), and fluorogenic-substrate V (Vangavaragu et al., 2014b). These results imply that activation of hPreP using small benzimidazole derivatives may provide a promising option for AD treatment.

CypD as a Potential AD Target

CypD is a peptidyl prolyl isomerase F that resides in the mitochondrial matrix, associates with the inner mitochondrial membrane, and plays a central role in the opening of the mPTP during the mitochondrial membrane permeability transition (Rao et al., 2014; Du et al., 2008; Khaspekov et al., 1999; Valasani et al., 2014b). CypD levels are significantly elevated in neurons of AD-affected regions where CypD forms a complex with mitochondrial Aβ in the brains of AD patients and transgenic mice overexpressing a mutant form of human APP and Aβ (TgmAPP) (Du et al., 2008). Surface plasmon resonance has been used to show a high-affinity binding of recombinant CypD protein to Aβ. Aβ-mediated mitochondrial and synaptic dysfunction was reduced when CypD was absent. Blocking CypD protects against Aβ- and oxidative stress-induced mitochondrial and synaptic degeneration, and improves mitochondrial and cognitive function (Du et al., 2008). mPTP formation is usually associated with ROS generation, perturbed intracellular calcium regulation, mitochondrial morphology regulation, and release of proapoptotic factors. Calcium overload or oxidative stress in cells causes CypD translocation from the mitochondrial matrix to the inner membrane, leading to the opening of the mPTP (Du et al., 2008).

Two other channels have been considered as possible constituents of the mPTP: voltage-dependent anion channel (VDAC) along the outer mitochondrial membrane responsible for taking up ions into the organelle, and adenine nucleotide translocase (ANT). which catalyzes the ATP/ADP exchange through the inner mitochondrial membrane. Studies have shown that VDAC is not essential for mPTP formation (Baines et al., 2007) and neither is ANT (Baines et al., 2007; Kokoszka et al., 2004).

Calcium concentration has a dominant influence on mitochondrial function and integrity. If calcium concentration is increased, ROS concentrations are increased, whereas ATP levels are decreased, which lead to release of apoptotic factors and cell death. The absence of CypD protects against Aβ-mediated mitochondrial oxidative stress and rescues mitochondrial and synaptic dysfunction (Petrosillo et al., 2004; Paradies et al., 2004a,b; Rosenstock et al., 2004; Baines et al., 2005; Du and Yan, 2010). These studies have advanced our understanding of Aβ toxicity and its relation to AD pathogenesis. This suggests that blockade of CypD to prevent mPTP opening appears to be an excellent approach for the treatment of AD (Du et al., 2008, 2011; Du and Yan, 2010; Valasani et al., 2014a).

Cyclosporin A (CsA) is an FDA-approved hydrophobic undecapeptide that inhibits cyclophilins, a family of peptidyl prolyl *cis–trans* isomerases (PPIases) including CypD (Crompton et al., 1988; Tanveer et al., 1996; Griffiths and Halestrap, 1991). Although CsA is currently the most specific CypD inhibitor, it unfortunately lacks clinical significance because it also inhibits the calcineurin phosphatase pathway and is unable to easily pass through the blood–brain barrier (BBB). Other researchers have developed numerous CsA derivatives that include N-Me-Ala-6-cyclosporin A and N-Me-Val-4-cyclosporin (Griffiths and Halestrap, 1995; Nicolli et al., 1996; Khaspekov et al., 1999). However, both of them possess the same unfavorable immunosuppressive effects as CsA but are still potent inhibitors of the PPIase activity of CypD, thereby antagonizing mPTP opening and apoptosis induction.

CsA and its derivatives are high-molecular weight molecules with low cell permeability that have difficulty crossing the BBB. Smaller CypD inhibitors with much lower molecular weights and good drug-like properties provide a promising avenue for improving mitochondrial and neuronal function relevant to neurodegenerative diseases like AD (Vangavaragu et al., 2014a; Valasani et al., 2014b, 2013b; Valasani et al., 2014).

INSIGHTS AND FUTURE

There is little doubt that AD is associated with the aging process except in familial cases, which constitute only a small percentage. The costs associated with the care and treatments of AD patients are already enormous and will further increase with increasing life expectancy. Researchers around the world are expending enormous efforts to find a cure for AD or means to slow its progression. The present FDA-approved AD drugs only provide minimal relief for some of its symptoms. There are currently no approved drugs that offer a cure or reverse AD pathology. Since AD is almost certainly a multifaceted ailment, it makes sense to adopt a multifaceted approach for its treatment. We have described two specific places where small molecules can interact productively with proteins as potential drugs for treating AD: enhancing hPreP protease activity and inhibiting CypD-mediated mPTP. Several other targets have also been mentioned (CsA inhibitors of CypD, mPTP, and Ca^{2+} channel blockers) but each of these has serious shortcomings. Clearly, the search for new AD drugs that are both safe and effective must be intensified at both the experimental and clinical levels. Better diagnostic tools are also needed to identify the specific pathological changes as early as possible when preventive measures can be taken. People who develop healthy lifestyles, attain higher education, maintain nutritious food habits, and participate in physical activities may stand a much better chance of living longer and disease-free lives.

Since multiple pathogenic mechanisms, such as genetics, enzyme activities, receptor expression, protein interactions, alteration of metal concentrations, cell cycle survival disruption, ion homeostasis dysregulation, protein misfolding, etc. all appear to be involved in AD pathogenesis, efforts should be made to determine the relative impact each of these might have on the onset and progression of the disease. A successful cure or treatment for AD will therefore almost certainly require researchers from around the globe and from a diverse set of disciplines to share their respective expertise. There will probably not be a single bullet or a single target and this proposition clearly makes it desirable to pursue all promising avenues for a safe and effective treatment. Ultimately, an AD patient may take a drug "cocktail" for relief or cure.

ABBREVIATIONS

Aβ Amyloid-β
ABAD Aβ-binding alcohol dehydrogenase
ACh Acetylcholine
AChE Acetylcholinesterase
AD Alzheimer's disease
ANT Adenine nucleotide translocase
APP Amyloid precursor protein
At *Arabidopsis thaliana*
ATP Adenosine triphosphate
BBB Blood–brain barrier
ChEs Cholinesterases
CsA Cyclosporin A
CypD Cyclophilin D
ETC Electron transport chain

FDA Food and Drug Administration
h Human
M Mouse
mPTP Mitochondrial permeability transition pore
mtDNA Mitochondrial DNA
NADH or NAD+ Nicotinamide adenine dinucleotide
PPIases Peptidyl-prolyl *cis–trans* isomerases
PreP Presequence protease
ROS Reactive oxygen species
TCA Tricarboxylic acid
Tg Transgenic
VDAC Voltage-dependent anion channel

Funding

This work was supported by grant awards from the National Institute of Health.

References

Aksenov, M.Y., et al., 1999. The expression of several mitochondrial and nuclear genes encoding the subunits of electron transport chain enzyme complexes, cytochrome c oxidase, and NADH dehydrogenase, in different brain regions in Alzheimer's disease. Neurochem. Res. 24 (6), 767–774.

Albano, E., 2006. Alcohol, oxidative stress and free radical damage. Proc. Nutr. Soc. 65 (3), 278–290.

Alikhani, N., et al., 2011. Decreased proteolytic activity of the mitochondrial amyloid-β degrading enzyme, PreP peptidasome, in Alzheimer's disease brain mitochondria. J. Alzheimers Dis. 27 (1), 75–87.

Alikhani, N., Ankarcrona, M., Glaser, E., 2009. Mitochondria and Alzheimer's disease: amyloid-β peptide uptake and degradation by the presequence protease, hPreP. J. Bioenerg. Biomembr. 41 (5), 447–451.

Andrade, C., Radhakrishnan, R., 2009. The prevention and treatment of cognitive decline and dementia: an overview of recent research on experimental treatments. Indian J. Psychiatry 51 (1), 12–25.

Arsland, D., 1998. The cholinergic hypothesis of Alzheimer's disease: strategies for the treatment of cognitive and emotional dysfunction. Nordic J. Psychiatry 52, 57.

Atamna, H., Frey 2nd, W.H., 2007. Mechanisms of mitochondrial dysfunction and energy deficiency in Alzheimer's disease. Mitochondrion 7 (5), 297–310.

Baines, C.P., et al., 2005. Loss of cyclophilin D reveals a critical role for mitochondrial permeability transition in cell death. Nature 434 (7033), 658–662.

Baines, C.P., et al., 2007. Voltage-dependent anion channels are dispensable for mitochondrial-dependent cell death. Nat. Cell Biol. 9 (5), 550–555.

Berman, H.M., et al., 2000. The protein data bank and the challenge of structural genomics. Nat. Struct. Biol. 7 (Suppl.), 957–959.

Bonda, D.J., et al., 2010. Mitochondrial dynamics in Alzheimer's disease opportunities for future treatment strategies. Drugs Aging 27 (3), 181–192.

Bonn, F., et al., 2011. Presequence-dependent folding ensures MrpL32 processing by the m-AAA protease in mitochondria. EMBO J. 30 (13), 2545–2556.

Chen, J., et al., 2014. Mechanism of oxidative inactivation of human presequence protease by hydrogen peroxide. Free Radic. Biol. Med. 77, 57–63.

Chetelat, G., et al., 2011. Independent contribution of temporal β-amyloid deposition to memory decline in the pre-dementia phase of Alzheimer's disease. Brain 134 (Pt 3), 798–807.

Coraci, I.S., et al., 2002. CD36, a class B scavenger receptor, is expressed on microglia in Alzheimer's disease brains and can mediate production of reactive oxygen species in response to β-amyloid fibrils. Am. J. Pathol. 160 (1), 101–112.

Crompton, M., Ellinger, H., Costi, A., 1988. Inhibition by cyclosporin A of a Ca^{2+} dependent pore in heart-mitochondria activated by inorganic-phosphate and oxidative stress. Biochem. J. 255 (1), 357–360.

Devi, L., et al., 2006. Accumulation of amyloid precursor protein in the mitochondrial import channels of human Alzheimer's disease brain is associated with mitochondrial dysfunction. J. Neurosci. 26 (35), 9057–9068.

Devi, L., Ohno, M., 2012. Mitochondrial dysfunction and accumulation of the β-secretase-cleaved C-terminal fragment of APP in Alzheimer's disease transgenic mice. Neurobiol. Dis. 45 (1), 417–424.

Dickey, C.A., Petrucelli, L., 2006. Current strategies for the treatment of Alzheimer's disease and other tauopathies. Expert Opin. Ther. Targets 10 (5), 665–676.

Du, H., et al., 2008. Cyclophilin D deficiency attenuates mitochondrial and neuronal perturbation and ameliorates learning and memory in Alzheimer's disease. Nat. Med. 14 (10), 1097–1105.

Du, H., et al., 2011. Cyclophilin D deficiency improves mitochondrial function and learning/memory in aging Alzheimer disease mouse model. Neurobiol. Aging 32 (3), 398–406.

Du, H., Yan, S.S., 2010. Mitochondrial permeability transition pore in Alzheimer's disease: cyclophilin D and amyloid β. Biochim. Biophys. Acta 1802 (1), 198–204.

Eckert, A., Schmitt, K., Gotz, J., 2011a. Mitochondrial dysfunction – the beginning of the end in Alzheimer's disease? Separate and synergistic modes of tau and amyloid-β toxicity. Alzheimers Res. Ther. 3 (2), 15.

Eckert, A., Schmitt, K., Gotz, J., 2011b. Mitochondrial dysfunction – the beginning of the end in Alzheimer's disease? Separate and synergistic modes of tau and amyloid-β toxicity. Alzheimers Res. Ther. 3 (3).

Falugi, C., Aluigi, M.G., 2012. Early appearance and possible functions of non-neuromuscular cholinesterase activities. Front. Mol. Neurosci. 5.

Fernandez-Vizarra, P., et al., 2004. Intra- and extracellular AB and PHF in clinically evaluated cases of Alzheimer's disease. Histol. Histopathol. 19 (3), 823–844.

Ferreira, I.L., et al., 2010. Multiple defects in energy metabolism in Alzheimer's disease. Curr. Drug Targets 11 (10).

Forstl, H., 2008. Treatment and care strategies for Alzheimer's disease and related dementias. Nervenarzt 79 (5), 617–628.

Fukuyama, H., et al., 1994. Altered cerebral energy metabolism in Alzheimer's disease: a PET study. J. Nucl. Med. 35 (1), 1–6.

Gabaldon, T., Huynen, M.A., 2004. Shaping the mitochondrial proteome. Biochim. Biophys. Acta 1659 (2–3), 212–220.

Gibson, G.E., et al., 1998. Alpha-ketoglutarate dehydrogenase in Alzheimer brains bearing the APP670/671 mutation. Ann. Neurol. 44 (4), 676–681.

Glaser, E., Dessi, P., 1999. Integration of the mitochondrial-processing peptidase into the cytochrome bc(1) complex in plants. J. Bioenerg. Biomembr. 31 (3), 259–274.

Godoy, J.A., et al., 2014. Signaling pathway cross talk in Alzheimer's disease. Cell Commun. Signal 12, 23.

Gotz, J., Ittner, L.M., Matamales, M., 2011. Novel treatment strategies for Alzheimer's disease. Eur. Neuropsychopharmacol. 21, S187–S188.

Griffiths, E.J., Halestrap, A.P., 1991. Further evidence that cyclosporine-a protects mitochondria from calcium overload by inhibiting a matrix peptidyl-prolyl cis-trans isomerase – implications for the immunosuppressive and toxic effects of cyclosporine. Biochem. J. 274, 611–614.

Griffiths, E.J., Halestrap, A.P., 1995. Mitochondrial non-specific pores remain closed during cardiac ischaemia, but open upon reperfusion. Biochem. J. 307 (Pt 1), 93–98.

Hedden, T., Gabrieli, J.D., 2005. Healthy and pathological processes in adult development: new evidence from neuroimaging of the aging brain. Curr. Opin. Neurol. 18 (6), 740–747.

Ieva, R., et al., 2013. Mitochondrial inner membrane protease promotes assembly of presequence translocase by removing a carboxy-terminal targeting sequence. Nat. Commun. 4.

Johnson, K.A., et al., 2006. The closed structure of presequence protease PreP forms a unique 10,000 Å^3 chamber for proteolysis. EMBO J. 25 (9), 1977–1986.

Kasiviswanathan, R., et al., 2009. Disease mutations in the human mitochondrial DNA polymerase thumb subdomain impart severe defects in mitochondrial DNA replication. J. Biol. Chem. 284 (29), 19501–19510.

Khaspekov, L., et al., 1999. Cyclosporin A and its nonimmunosuppressive analogue N-Me-Val-4-cyclosporin A mitigate glucose/oxygen deprivation-induced damage to rat cultured hippocampal neurons. Eur. J. Neurosci. 11 (9), 3194–3198.

Kim, S.H., et al., 2000. Decreased levels of complex III core protein 1 and complex V beta chain in brains from patients with Alzheimer's disease and Down syndrome. Cell. Mol. Life Sci. 57 (12), 1810–1816.

King, J.V., et al., 2014. Molecular basis of substrate recognition and degradation by human presequence protease. Structure 22 (7), 996–1007.

Kmiec, B., Teixeira, P.F., Glaser, E., 2014. Phenotypical consequences of expressing the dually targeted presequence protease, AtPreP, exclusively in mitochondria. Biochimie 100C, 167–170.

Kokoszka, J.E., et al., 2004. The ADP/ATP translocator is not essential for the mitochondrial permeability transition pore. Nature 427 (6973), 461–465.

Kulic, L., et al., 2011. Combined expression of tau and the Harlequin mouse mutation leads to increased mitochondrial dysfunction, tau pathology and neurodegeneration. Neurobiol. Aging 32 (10), 1827–1838.

Lane, R.M., Potkin, S.G., Enz, A., 2006. Targeting acetylcholinesterase and butyrylcholinesterase in dementia. Int. J. Neuropsychopharmacol. 9 (1), 101–124.

LaNoue, K.F., Bryla, J., Williamson, J.R., 1972. Feedback interactions in the control of citric acid cycle activity in rat heart mitochondria. J. Biol. Chem. 247 (3), 667–679.

Lansbury, P.T., Lashuel, H.A., 2006. A century-old debate on protein aggregation and neurodegeneration enters the clinic. Nature 443 (7113), 774–779.

Lee, Y.S., Kennedy, W.D., Yin, Y.W., 2009. Structural insight into processive human mitochondrial DNA synthesis and disease-related polymerase mutations. Cell 139 (2), 312–324.

Leon, R., Garcia, A.G., Marco-Contelles, J., 2013. Recent advances in the multitarget-directed ligands approach for the treatment of Alzheimer's disease. Med. Res. Rev. 33 (1), 139–189.

Li, Z., et al., 2004. The importance of dendritic mitochondria in the morphogenesis and plasticity of spines and synapses. Cell 119 (6), 873–887.

Lustbader, J.W., et al., 2004. ABAD directly links A β to mitochondrial toxicity in Alzheimer's disease. Science 304 (5669), 448–452.

Mancuso, M., et al., 2006. Mitochondrial dysfunction, oxidative stress and neurodegeneration. J. Alzheimers Dis. 10 (1), 59–73.

Markesbery, W.R., 1997. Oxidative stress hypothesis in Alzheimer's disease. Free Radic. Biol. Med. 23 (1), 134–147.

McCormack, J.G., Halestrap, A.P., Denton, R.M., 1990. Role of calcium ions in regulation of mammalian intramitochondrial metabolism. Physiol. Rev. 70 (2), 391–425.

McCormack, J.G., 1985. Characterization of the effects of Ca^{2+} on the intramitochondrial Ca^{2+}-sensitive enzymes from rat liver and within intact rat liver mitochondria. Biochem. J. 231 (3), 581–595.

Nalin, C.M., Cross, R.L., 1982. Adenine nucleotide binding sites on beef heart F1-ATPase. Specificity of cooperative interactions between catalytic sites. J. Biol. Chem. 257 (14), 8055–8060.

Nicolli, A., et al., 1996. Interactions of cyclophilin with the mitochondrial inner membrane and regulation of the permeability transition pore, and cyclosporin A-sensitive channel. J. Biol. Chem. 271 (4), 2185–2192.

Paradies, G., et al., 2004a. Decrease in mitochondrial complex I activity in ischemic/reperfused rat heart – involvement of reactive oxygen species and cardiolipin. Circ. Res. 94 (1), 53–59.

Paradies, G., et al., 2004b. Mitochondrial dysfunction in ischemic/reperfused rat heart: role of ROS and cardiolipin. Biochim. Biophys. Acta 1658, 233.

Paradies, G., et al., 2014. Oxidative stress, cardiolipin and mitochondrial dysfunction in nonalcoholic fatty liver disease. World J. Gastroenterol. 20 (39), 14205–14218.

Parker Jr., W.D., et al., 1994. Electron transport chain defects in Alzheimer's disease brain. Neurology 44 (6), 1090–1096.

Pavlov, P.F., et al., 2009. Mitochondrial accumulation of APP and Aβ: significance for Alzheimer disease pathogenesis. J. Cell. Mol. Med. 13 (10), 4137–4145.

Perry, G., et al., 1998. Reactive oxygen species mediate cellular damage in Alzheimer disease. J. Alzheimers Dis. 1 (1), 45–55.

Petrosillo, G., et al., 2004. Ca^{2+}-induced reactive oxygen species production promotes cytochrome c release from rat liver mitochondria via mitochondrial permeability transition (MPT)-dependent and MPT-independent mechanisms – role of cardiolipin. J. Biol. Chem. 279 (51), 53103–53108.

Ponpuak, M., et al., 2007. A role for falcilysin in transit peptide degradation in the *Plasmodium falciparum* apicoplast. Mol. Microbiol. 63 (2), 314–334.

Pope, S., Land, J.M., Heales, S.J., 2008. Oxidative stress and mitochondrial dysfunction in neurodegeneration; cardiolipin a critical target? Biochim. Biophys. Acta 1777 (7–8), 794–799.

Possin, K.L., 2010. Visual spatial cognition in neurodegenerative disease. Neurocase 16 (6), 466–487.

Rao, V.K., Carlson, E.A., Yan, S.S., 2014. Mitochondrial permeability transition pore is a potential drug target for neurodegeneration. Biochim. Biophys. Acta 1842 (8), 1267–1272.

Ray, A., et al., 2014. Mitochondrial dysfunction, oxidative stress, and neurodegeneration elicited by a bacterial metabolite in a *C. elegans* Parkinson's model. Cell Death Dis. 5, e984.

Reddy, P.H., 2008. Mitochondrial medicine for aging and neurodegenerative diseases. Neuromolecular Med. 10 (4), 291–315.

Rosenstock, T.R., et al., 2004. Mitochondrial calcium, oxidative stress and apoptosis in a neurodegenerative disease model induced by 3-nitropropionic acid. J. Neurochem. 88 (5), 1220–1228.

Schapira, A.H., 1996. Oxidative stress and mitochondrial dysfunction in neurodegeneration. Curr. Opin. Neurol. 9 (4), 260–264.

Schenk, D., et al., 1997. Therapeutic strategies for treatment of Alzheimer's disease aimed at reduction of β-amyloid production. J. Neurochem. 69, S104.

Schmidt, C., et al., 2008. Amyloid precursor protein and amyloid β-peptide bind to ATP synthase and regulate its activity at the surface of neural cells. Mol. Psychiatry 13 (10), 953–969.

Sorbi, S., Bird, E.D., Blass, J.P., 1983. Decreased pyruvate dehydrogenase complex activity in Huntington and Alzheimer brain. Ann. Neurol. 13 (1), 72–78.

Stahl, A., et al., 2005. Two novel targeting peptide degrading proteases, PrePs, in mitochondria and chloroplasts, so similar and still different. J. Mol. Biol. 349 (4), 847–860.

Stasiak, A., et al., 2014. Effects of novel monoamine oxidases and cholinesterases targeting compounds on brain neurotransmitters and behavior in rat model of vascular dementia. Curr. Pharm. Des. 20 (2), 161–171.

Streck, E.L., Czapski, G.A., da Silva, C.G., 2013. Neurodegeneration, mitochondrial dysfunction, and oxidative stress. Oxid. Med. Cell. Longevity 826046.

Sun, J., et al., 2012. Down-regulation of energy metabolism in Alzheimer's disease is a protective response of neurons to the microenvironment. J. Alzheimers Dis. 28 (2), 389–402.

Swerdlow, R.H., 2012. Mitochondria and cell bioenergetics: increasingly recognized components and a possible etiologic cause of Alzheimer's disease. Antioxid. Redox Signal. 16 (12), 1434–1455.

Tabner, B.J., et al., 2001. Production of reactive oxygen species from aggregating proteins implicated in Alzheimer's disease, Parkinson's disease and other neurodegenerative diseases. Curr. Top. Med. Chem. 1 (6), 507–517.

Takehara, Y., et al., 1995. Oxygen-dependent regulation of mitochondrial energy metabolism by nitric oxide. Arch. Biochem. Biophys. 323 (1), 27–32.

Tanveer, A., et al., 1996. Involvement of cyclophilin D in the activation of a mitochondrial pore by Ca^{2+} and oxidant stress. Eur. J. Biochem. 238 (1), 166–172.

Taylor, R.W., Turnbull, D.M., 2005. Mitochondrial DNA mutations in human disease. Nat. Rev. Genet. 6 (5), 389–402.

Teixeira, P.F., et al., 2012. In vitro oxidative inactivation of human presequence protease (hPreP). Free Radic. Biol. Med. 53 (11), 2188–2195.

Teixeira, P.F., Glaser, E., 2013. Processing peptidases in mitochondria and chloroplasts. Biochim. Biophys. Acta 1833 (2), 360–370.

Tritschler, H.J., Packer, L., Medori, R., 1994. Oxidative stress and mitochondrial dysfunction in neurodegeneration. Biochem. Mol. Biol. Int. 34 (1), 169–181.

Uttara, B., et al., 2009. Oxidative stress and neurodegenerative diseases: a review of upstream and downstream antioxidant therapeutic options. Curr. Neuropharmacol. 7 (1), 65–74.

Valasani, K.R., et al., 2014. Identification of human ABAD inhibitors for rescuing Aβ-mediated mitochondrial dysfunction. Curr. Alzheimer Res. 11 (2), 128–136.

Valasani, K.R., et al., 2013a. Acetylcholinesterase inhibitors: structure based design, synthesis, pharmacophore modeling, and virtual screening. J. Chem. Inf. Model. 53 (8), 2033–2046.

Valasani, K.R., et al., 2013b. Structure-based design and synthesis of benzothiazole phosphonate analogues with inhibitors of human ABAD-Aβ for treatment of Alzheimer's disease. Chem. Biol. Drug Des. 81 (2), 238–249.

Valasani, K.R., et al., 2014a. High-resolution crystal structures of two crystal forms of human cyclophilin D in complex with PEG 400 molecules. Acta Crystallogr. F Struct. Biol. Commun. 70, 717–722.

Valasani, K.R., et al., 2014b. Structure based design, synthesis, pharmacophore modeling, virtual screening, and molecular docking studies for identification of novel cyclophilin D inhibitors. J. Chem. Inf. Model. 54 (3), 902–912.

Valla, J., Berndt, J.D., Gonzalez-Lima, F., 2001. Energy hypometabolism in posterior cingulate cortex of Alzheimer's patients: superficial laminar cytochrome oxidase associated with disease duration. J. Neurosci. 21 (13), 4923–4930.

Vangavaragu, J.R., et al., 2014a. Determination of small molecule ABAD inhibitors crossing blood–brain barrier and pharmacokinetics. J. Alzheimers Dis. 42 (1), 333–344.

Vangavaragu, J.R., et al., 2014b. Identification of human presequence protease (hPreP) agonists for the treatment of Alzheimer's disease. Eur. J. Med. Chem. 76, 506–516 2015. 93, 625.

Wu, D.F., Cederbaum, A.I., 2003. Alcohol, oxidative stress, and free radical damage. Alcohol Res. Health 27 (4), 277–284.

Xing, S.L., et al., 2012. β-amyloid peptide binds and regulates ectopic ATP synthase alpha-chain on neural surface. Int. J. Neurosci. 122 (6), 290–297.

Yankovskaya, V., et al., 2003. Architecture of succinate dehydrogenase and reactive oxygen species generation. Science 299 (5607), 700–704.

Yao, J., et al., 2011. Inhibition of amyloid-β (Aβ) peptide-binding alcohol dehydrogenase-Aβ interaction reduces Aβ accumulation and improves mitochondrial function in a mouse model of Alzheimer's disease. J. Neurosci. 31 (6), 2313–2320.

CHAPTER

11

Simple In Vivo Models of Alzheimer's Disease

S.W. Caito, J.L. Newell-Caito

OUTLINE

INTRODUCTION

The increasing diagnoses of neurodegenerative diseases, such as Alzheimer's disease (AD), combined with an aging population, warrants a better understanding of the pathological processes involved in the initiation and progression of these conditions in in vivo systems.

Drug Discovery Approaches for the Treatment of Neurodegenerative Disorders
http://dx.doi.org/10.1016/B978-0-12-802810-0.00011-8

However, modeling neurodegenerative diseases in vivo presents many challenges, including complexity of the model organism's nervous system, lifespan, available reagents, disease inducing reagents, and cost. There are no perfect models; however, each model has its own merits. While mammalian models of AD are common, there are disadvantages to their use, the major being cost and time needed to achieve an aged population. The use of nonmammalian genetic model organisms is an attractive alternative to rodent and primate models to investigate mechanisms involved in AD pathology and pharmacological intervention. Many of these organisms, such as *Caenorhabditis elegans* and *Drosophila melanogaster*, have been used for decades for neurological and developmental research, and are highly amenable to pharmacological and toxicity testing.

AD, along with Parkinson's disease (PD) and amyotrophic lateral sclerosis (ALS), is a complex multifactorial disease characterized by the loss of neurons as the primary pathological lesion, leading to cognitive, behavioral, and/or motor alterations. AD is characterized by synaptic damage and neural loss with the presence of senile plaques composed of β-amyloid (Aβ), produced by cleavage of β-amyloid precursor protein (APP) by β- and γ-secretases (Jacobsen and Iverfeldt, 2009), and hyperphosphorylated and aggregated microtubule-associated tau protein (Li et al., 2007). Neurodegenerative diseases appear with age, making it an important component for the generation of an in vivo model. Although there are familial genetic mutations that give rise to neurodegenerative diseases, the majority of AD, PD, and ALS cases are sporadic idiopathic in origin. Epidemiological studies have shown links between an individual's environment and the development of neurodegenerative diseases. Exposure to acrolein, heavy metals, and the pesticide DTT have been associated with the development of AD (Graham et al., 2014; Huang et al., 2013; Li et al., 2015). The contribution of heavy metal toxicity to AD has been the most studied. Copper (Cu), zinc (Zn), iron (Fe), and/or aluminum (Al) are present in senile plaques in AD brains (Bolognin et al., 2009), with enhanced Zn in the neuropil and Cu in the rims of the plaques (Lovell et al., 1998). The presence of heavy metals, such as Cu, Zn, and Fe, causes conformational changes in Aβ allowing for the stabilization of the oligomeric form and enhances oxidative stress (Faller, 2009; Faller and Hureau, 2009). With this complex interplay of age, genetics, and environment, one needs a model system where all three components can be easily integrated. Nonmammalian model organisms have well-characterized genomes allowing for the generation of numerous mutant strains and subsequent crossing of multiple mutant strains together. Simple in vivo model organisms are amenable to both treatments of environmental contaminants and pharmaceuticals, allowing one to make observations on the effects of selected compounds on wild-type and several mutant lines. Screening of numerous mutants with test compounds is highly amenable and has been performed for neurodegenerative endpoints.

The complexity of the mammalian brain and time to achieve an aged phenotype are major challenges for data interpretation. Investigating questions of age effects in rodents is a lengthy process, spanning the course of up to 2 years. This can produce significant cost of maintaining rodent colonies for such a prolonged period of time. Simple model organisms have short lifespans that allow for quicker observations and are inexpensive in their maintenance. *C. elegans* lives only 21 days and consumes a diet of *Escherichia coli* grown on agar plates, making its care inexpensive and aging studies quick. The mammalian brain contains numerous cell types and distinct brain regions, which complicate data acquisition and interpretation. Nonmammalian model organisms have smaller, less complex nervous systems, which perform similar functions. While the degree of complexity is smaller, the nervous systems of these organisms tend to be highly tractable. Cell fate is very well understood, from differentiation and migration patterns and connectivity of neurons in *C. elegans* and *D. melanogaster*. Additionally, zebrafish (*Danio rerio*) present an option of a less complex vertebrate brain.

In this chapter we give an overview of the most common nonmammalian model organisms used in neurodegenerative research, highlighting their advantages and caveats to their use. AD phenotypes will be described; both the available mutant strains will be described as well as the contribution of heavy metals to AD pathology. Additionally, pharmacological studies and screens will be examined, demonstrating the great utility of these organisms for drug discovery.

CAENORHABDITIS ELEGANS

C. elegans is a small soil-dwelling nematode that has been used in biomedical research for over 60 years. This worm species has a short lifespan (21 days), making it ideal for age-related studies. Worms are maintained on a lawn of *E. coli* grown on agar plates and are housed in 20°C incubators, making their upkeep inexpensive. These worms have made significant contributions in the fields of neuroscience, developmental biology, apoptosis, microRNAs, and RNA interference. The advantages of using *C. elegans* in neurodegeneration studies are summarized in Table 11.1.

The power behind the *C. elegans* model system arises from the organism's genetics. Worms share ~60–80% of human disease-related genes, making them a highly homologous species

TABLE 11.1 Advantages and Disadvantages of *Caenorhabditis elegans*, *Drosophila*, and Zebrafish for Studying Neurodegeneration

	C. elegans	*Drosophila*	Zebrafish
ADVANTAGES			
Short lifespan	✓	✓	
Easily genetically manipulable	✓	✓	✓
Fully sequenced and annotated genome	✓	✓	✓
Highly homologous to humans	✓	✓	✓
Conserved neural functions	✓	✓	✓
Multiple mutant strains available	✓	✓	✓
Inexpensive	✓	✓	✓
Transparent	✓		As embryos
Cryopreservation	✓		
DISADVANTAGES			
Significantly different anatomy	✓	✓	✓
Rudimentary immune system	✓	✓	
No myelin	✓	✓	

for research. The full sequence for the *C. elegans* genome was one of the first described (Waterston and Sulston, 1995), and has a high-density map of polymorphisms for the wild-type nematode. This allows for mapping of genetic mutations and linking of mechanisms to genetic susceptibility. The Caenorhabditis Genetics Center maintains a bank of available strains available for purchase. *C. elegans* is also highly genetically manipulable, with well-established protocols available for RNA interference, tagging proteins, and creation of knock-down, functionally null, and overexpressing strains. While the majority of a worm population is hermaphrodite, the rare males are beneficial in generating lines with multiple mutations, which become easily sustained by the self-fertilizing hermaphrodites.

C. elegans has one of the most well-characterized nervous systems available to study, partially because of its origin as a tool to study neurodevelopment (Brenner, 1974). There are a total of 302 neurons in the worm, which have been three dimensionally mapped (Hobert, 2005). The characterization of the worm's nervous system is meticulous, with resources available to follow individual cells from differentiation in the embryo and larval stages, as well as migration patterns elucidated and synaptic connections in the adult (Emmons, 2015; Sulston and Horvitz, 1977; Sulston et al., 1983). This allows for easy analysis of changes in nervous system in response to mutations, environmental insults, and pharmaceuticals. Along with the mapped-out nervous system, *C. elegans* has numerous defined behaviors that are directly linked to specific neural circuits, such as thrashing, chemotaxis, and pharyngeal pumping. Molecular mechanisms for neuronal functions are highly conserved in the worm. Neurotransmitter systems, synaptic release, and trafficking are also conserved.

Finally, *C. elegans* is completely transparent, allowing for in vivo visualization of fluorescently labeled proteins. A number of strains are available with individual neuronal populations fluorescently tagged (cholinergic, GABAergic, dopaminergic, serotonergic, glutaminergic, etc.). To visualize neurodegeneration in a mutant line, one can cross the mutant of interest with a fluorescently tagged strain and observe changes to neuronal morphology, such as discontinuous dendrites or axons, shrunken or lost cell bodies, or puncta and blebbing.

While there are multiple advantages to the *C. elegans* system, there are significant caveats one has to keep in mind. The simple anatomy of the worm includes a nervous system, digestive tract, reproductive system, and muscular system. There are no lungs, liver, kidney, pancreas, or vascular system in the worm. While there are cells in the digestive tract that perform similar functions as the liver and kidney, the lack of a vasculature makes their use in diseases that have a vascular component, such as AD, limited. Worms also have a rudimentary immune system that lacks an adaptive immunity. Many of the cytokines, chemokines, and inflammatory regulators, such as nuclear factor kappa B, are not present in the worm. Additionally, the neurons in *C. elegans* are not myelinated, making them a poor model for diseases such as multiple sclerosis.

Disease-Linked Mutations and Neurodegeneration

Amyloid Peptide Precursor Protein

Familial AD has been linked to several genetic mutations, many of which have been studied in *C. elegans* (Chartier-Harlin et al., 1991a,b; Goate et al., 1991). Amyloid peptide precursor protein (APP) and the presenilins, PS1 and PS2, were the first AD-associated proteins identified. APP is a membrane-bound protein that undergoes multiple cleavages around its transmembrane domain resulting in a secreted fragment (sAPP), the Aβ peptide, and the intracellular fragment APP-intracellular domain. The *C. elegans* homolog to the human APP gene is *apl-1*; however, the APL-1 protein lacks the Aβ peptide and the nematode genome does not encode a β-secretase (Daigle and Li, 1993; Jacobsen and Iverfeldt, 2009). The APL-1 protein is essential for worm viability as deletion of *apl-1* results in 100% larval lethality, and RNAi of *apl-1* reduces body size (Hornsten et al., 2007; Niwa et al., 2008). Worms expressing human Aβ42 are commonly used in research, with the most common strain expressing Aβ42 under the constitutive *unc-54* body-wall muscle promoter. These worms show progressive paralysis and intracellular cytoplasmic Aβ plaques (Link, 1995; Link et al., 2001). The role of the insulin-like signaling pathway has been examined in the *unc-54*/Aβ42 expressing strain. Knockdown of *daf-2* (insulin/IGF receptor ortholog) acting through *daf-16* (FOXO homolog) and *hsf-1* (heat shock factor ortholog) reduced Aβ42 toxicity; *daf-16* knockdown decreased the amount of Aβ aggregation whereas *hsf-1* knockdown increased aggregation (Cohen et al., 2010). Subsequently, DAF-16 expression to inhibit Aβ-induced paralysis was shown to require MDT-15 (ortholog of human mediator subunit MED15), which is involved in fat homeostasis (Zhang et al., 2013). Aβ-interacting proteins have been identified with mass spectrometry using the *unc-54*/Aβ42 strain, including HSP-70A and HSP-70C (HSP70 orthologs), HSP-16.1,16.2, and -16.48 (HSP16 orthologs) and the ortholog of the human SGT protein (Fonte et al., 2002; Liu and DeFranco, 1999). HSP-16 immunoprecipitates with intracellular Aβ; however, overexpression of HSP-16.2 has no effect on total Aβ accumulation (Fonte et al., 2002; 2008).

Worms expressing a temperature-inducible Aβ transcript driven by the *myo-3* muscle-specific promoter and regulated by an incorporated long 3′ untranslated region display a paralysis phenotype arising from stable Aβ42 mRNA and protein expression (Link, 2006; Link et al., 2003). DNA microarray study using these worms identified 67 upregulated and 240 downregulated genes associated with the intracellular accumulation of Aβ (Link et al., 2003). Of the upregulated genes, αB-crystallin and tumor necrosis factor-induced protein 1 were shown to be increased in AD brains (Link et al., 2003). An intraneuronal deposition model of Aβ toxicity shows hypersensitivity to serotonin and defects in chemotaxis (Link, 2006). Additionally, an inducible Aβ model with muscle-specific expression (driven by the *myo-3* promoter) leads to an accumulation of autophagic vesicles, dependent upon *asp-1*, *asp-4*, *asp-5*, and *asp-6* (aspartyl proteases), *lmp-1* and *lmp-2* (lysosomal-associated membrane proteins), and *vha-15* (vacuolar proton-translocating ATPase) (Florez-McClure et al., 2007).

Presenilins

Presenilins are the enzymatic units of γ-secretase that cleave APP into Aβ. Mutations in presenilins are associated with familial AD (Nunan and Small, 2000). *C. elegans* contains three presenilin orthologs: *sel-12*, *hop-1*, and *spe-4* (Baumeister et al., 1997; Levitan and Greenwald, 1995; Li and Greenwald, 1997). Mutations in the worm orthologs of presenilins display axonal abnormalities in acetylcholine-producing AIY neurons (Wittenburg et al., 2000). The presenilin mutant worms have deficits in memory as measured by the thermotaxis assay. In this assay, young adult worms incubated overnight at 20°C on nematode growth medium (NGM) plates with bacteria are washed off the plate and transferred to an unseeded plate at 20°C for 2 min. Individual animals are placed on new unseeded NGM plate for an incubation period between 0 and 18 h before a frozen vial of acetic acid is placed in the center of the plate at 26°C for 90 min to create a temperature gradient ranging from 17°C to 25°C. Worms associate food with a given growth temperature during the conditioning period and will isothermal track on the unseeded plates to the growth temperature to find food. The percentage of worms that track to the growth temperature reflects the ability of the worms to learn and by varying the initial incubation time one can evaluate memory. Studies using the presenilin mutant lines have also identified interactions of presenilin and apoptotic and Notch signaling pathways (Berezovska et al., 1998; Kitagawa et al., 2003).

Tau

The major component of neurofibrillary tangles is phosphorylated microtubule-associated protein tau (MAPT). In *C. elegans* the MAPT ortholog is *ptl-1*; however, because of differential posttranslational mutations, transgenic worm strains expressing human tau are better models (Goedert et al., 1996). There are worms that either express wild-type human tau or overexpress a pseudohyperphosphorylated tau protein (PTP), which is highly phosphorylated in the nematode similar to AD patients (Brandt et al., 2009). In the PTP strain, tau aggregates in worms and causes axonal abnormalities in inhibitory motor neurons associated with age-dependent uncoordinated movement (Brandt et al., 2009). Both of the strains expressing either wild-type human tau or PTP models show neurodegeneration and locomotor defects as a result of failed neurotransmission and other age-dependent motor neuron dysfunctions (Kraemer et al., 2003). Tau is involved in several neurodegenerative diseases, collectively referred to as tauopathies. Mutations in tau that are similar to those observed in frontotemporal dementia with parkinsonism chromosome 17 type (FTDP-17) are also available in *C. elegans*.

Metal-Induced Neurodegeneration

Studies in *C. elegans* on heavy metal toxicity and AD have centered on Cu. Cu exposure enhances the paralysis by human Aβ expression in *C. elegans* (Luo et al., 2011). Luo et al. have also reported that Cu exposure in the human Aβ expressing worms alters levels of Zn, manganese (Mn), and Fe (Luo et al., 2011). However, human Aβ-expressing worms alone have altered Fe content (Wan et al., 2011), which suggests that the presence human Aβ in worms may alter metal homeostasis. Mammalian APP contains a Cu-binding domain (CuBD) in its N-terminus, which not only binds Cu, but also reduces Cu(II) to Cu(I), producing reactive oxygen species (ROS) (Hesse et al., 1994; Multhaup et al., 1996). Overexpression of the Aβ fragment significantly alters metal homeostasis, causing decreased Cu and Fe levels and increased Mn level (Maynard et al., 2002), suggesting that Aβ aggregations potentially disrupt proper metal levels in AD. The CuBD of *C. elegans* is highly reactive to Cu^{2+}; injection of APL-1 into rat dorsal hippocampus confers protection against Cu^{2+} toxicity in vivo by enhancing Cu^{2+} uptake (Cerpa et al., 2004). The vertebrate CuBD contains essential histidine residues at positions 147 and 151. *C. elegans*' CuBD, however, contains a tyrosine residue at position 147 and a lysine residue at 151, which confer neuroprotection from Cu^{2+} exposure (White et al., 2002).

The expression of human Aβ in *C. elegans* muscle cells is altered upon exposure to Cu^{2+}. Instead of expressing the full-length Aβ product (residues 1–42), a truncated (residues 3–42) Aβ was formed, which aggregates faster in vitro than full-length Aβ (McColl et al., 2009).

C. elegans-expressing point mutations (V18A, E22G) in Aβ have decreased intracellular amyloid aggregation compared to worms expressing wild-type Aβ. The Aβ mutant worms show decreased sensitivity to Cu^{2+} exposure compared to control worms, in which Cu^{2+} enhances Aβ aggregation (Minniti et al., 2009). These data suggest that there are Cu responsive sites in Aβ that lie outside of the CuBD of APP.

Pharmaceutical Testing

C. elegans strains expressing AD mutations have been used to screen both pharmaceutical compounds and natural products for potential to alleviate Aβ toxicity and improve lifespan. Reserpine, a Food and Drug Administration (FDA)-approved antihypertensive drug and vesicular monoamine transporter inhibitor, showed increased longevity and decreased signs of aging in wild-type worms (Srivastava et al., 2008), and when tested in the *unc-54*/Aβ42 strain it also delayed paralysis and enhanced stress tolerance (Arya et al., 2009). These effects were found to be dependent on acetylcholinergic signaling, as cholinergic loss of function mutants showed no beneficial effects of reserpine (Saharia et al., 2012). The use of reserpine to treat AD, however, is a delicate issue, because both studies in rodents and *C. elegans* have shown dopaminergic neurotoxicity of reserpine, resembling a Parkinsonian syndrome (Leao et al., 2015; Reckziegel et al., 2015). Modulation of the acetylcholinergic system in AD was also examined using the acetylcholinesterase (AChE) inhibitor aldicarb. Sensitivity to aldicarb was dependent on APL-1; RNAi knockdown of *apl-1* increased sensitivity to aldicarb, which could be rescued by expressing full-length APL-1 in the mutant (Wiese et al., 2010). Benzofuran-chalcone hybrids similarly protect against Aβ toxicity in worms, through decreasing AChE levels, oxidative stress, and lipid content (Sashidhara et al., 2014). The choline analog JAY2-22-33 significantly reduced Aβ toxicity by delaying paralysis in the Aβ constitutive muscle-expression strain (Keowkase et al., 2010). These effects require the insulin signaling pathway and nicotinic acetylcholine receptors (Keowkase et al., 2010). NT219, an insulin/IGF signaling cascade inhibitor, decreased paralysis in the *unc-54*/Aβ42 strain with no effect on lifespan (El-Ami et al., 2014), suggesting that pathways independent of insulin signaling regulate lifespan in the *unc-54*/Aβ42 strain. The effects of the antidepressant fluoxetine, tetracyclines, and Cu chelators have also been examined. These compounds were found to protect against Aβ toxicity in worms, with increased lifespan and thermal stress resistance and decreased oxidative stress (Diomede et al., 2010; Keowkase et al., 2010). A donepezil–huprine hybrid has been tested in the *unc-54*/Aβ42 strain, showing decreased paralysis but no effect on reducing Aβ (Sola et al., 2015). In a screen of 140,000 chemicals, clioquinol was identified as able to attenuate Aβ toxicity in vitro in yeast and in worms (Matlack et al., 2014).

C. elegans has been useful in screening natural products for their protective effects on Aβ toxicity. *Ginkgo biloba* extract Egb 761, soy isoflavone glycitein, and ginkgolides increase lifespan, alleviate paralysis, serotonin hypersensitivity, and chemotaxis, and decrease toxic ROS levels in the *unc-54*/Aβ42 strain (Gutierrez-Zepeda et al., 2005; Wu and Luo, 2005; Wu et al., 2006). Polyphenolic compounds from apples (procyanidins) and quercetin decreased the amount of aggregated proteins in the *unc-54*/Aβ42 strain (Regitz et al., 2014; Toda et al., 2011). It was found that the protective effects of quercetin were caused by an activation of the unfolded protein response, because RNAi against these proteins diminished quercetin's effects (Regitz et al., 2014). Extracts from tea (tea seed pomace and aromatic fractions), oleuropein aglycone from extra virgin olive oil, and 13L, a peptide from cocoa, decrease Aβ deposits and oxidative stress in worms (Diomede et al., 2013; Martorell et al., 2013; Takahashi et al., 2014; Wei et al., 2014). Galantamine and hemanthidine are two alkaloids derived from *Lycoris radiate* that are AChE inhibitors. These compounds increase lifespan and decrease paralysis in Aβ-expressing worms (Xin et al., 2013).

DROSOPHILA MELANOGASTER

Drosophila fruit flies have been used in biomedical research for over 100 years, particularly in genetic research (Castle, 1906). They have a short lifespan of 120 days, which can vary depending on diet and stress conditions. *Drosophila* are grown in vials using yeast as a food source and are maintained at 21°C, making them an inexpensive model organism. The advantages of using flies in neurodegeneration studies are numerous and summarized in Table 11.1.

Drosophila was one of the first organisms with a fully sequenced genome (Adams et al., 2000; Myers et al., 2000), and as such has a multitude of genetic reagents available. Fruit flies have a small, minimally redundant genome containing approximately 13,600 protein-coding genes organized in only four chromosomes. Transgenic flies for overexpression, knockdowns, and functional null mutants are available from the Bloomington Drosophila Stock Center. Like *C. elegans*, *Drosophila* is highly genetically manipulable. Additionally, phenotyping of mutations under a dissecting microscope is easy. Body structures are easily observed, allowing for characterization of body color and size, position and integrity of wings, eye color, and bristle patterns. Importantly, flies share close to 70% of disease-causing genes with humans (Iijima et al., 2004).

The fly brain and nervous system are well studied and homologous to humans. *Drosophila* has a tripartite brain composed of several brain centers, including the antennal lobes, the mushroom bodies (thought to be involved in learning and memory), the central body complex, the protocerebrum, the posterior slope and lateral deutocerebrum, and the optic lobes. There are roughly 135,000 neurons in the fly brain, which have been three dimensionally mapped (Chiang et al., 2011). Similar to *C. elegans*, molecular mechanisms for neurotransmitter release, vesicle trafficking, and neuronal functions are highly conserved in humans. Unlike the worm, visual and olfactory sensations can be investigated in the fly. Finally, *Drosophila* has well characterized behaviors that can be used to probe for neurodegeneration. These include simple avoidance and flight ability measurements, to more sophisticated learning, memory, and cogitative assays.

Disease-Linked Mutations and Neurodegeneration

Amyloid Peptide Precursor Protein

The *Drosophila* homolog of the APP is *Appl*, which is expressed in the nervous system. *Appl* expression has been linked to nervous system development, circadian rhythms, synaptic organization, and the axonal injury response in flies (Blake et al., 2015; Leyssen et al., 2005; Merdes et al., 2004; Wentzell et al., 2012). Similar to mammals, the fly has all components of the γ-secretase complex, although the β-secretase-like enzyme has very low β-secretase activity (Periz and Fortini, 2004). The homology of APP and Appl is variable. Studies investigating the secreted extracellular fragments of APP (sAPP) investigating its role in synaptic remodeling and neuroprotection have shown similar results in both *Drosophila* and humans (Ashley et al., 2005; Wentzell et al., 2012). This is in contrast to the region of Appl that corresponds to Aβ, which lacks homology to APP (Luo et al., 1992). Interestingly, overexpression of the β-secretase-like protein allowing for the production of the Aβ-like peptide results in Aβ-like aggregation and age-dependent behavioral deficits and neurodegeneration (Carmine-Simmen et al., 2009). To examine human Aβ42-induced toxicity and neurodegeneration in *Drosophila*, transgenic flies have been constructed harboring a variety of inserted human proteins. Finelli et al. created a fly line expressing fully processed, secreted Aβ40 and Aβ42 peptides expressed solely in the nervous system (Finelli et al., 2004). Only the Aβ42-expressing flies showed age-dependent and dose-dependent neurodegeneration. Aβ42-expressing flies have impaired short-term memory, reduced lifespan, and age-related locomotor deficits (Iijima et al., 2008). Neuronal expression of an inducible Aβ42 causes intra- and extracellular accumulation of Aβ42 peptides, leading to neurotoxicity, locomotor defects, and reduced lifespan (Crowther et al., 2005). These effects are exacerbated in flies expressing Aβ42(E22G), a point mutation known to increase the rate of Aβ42 aggregation (Crowther et al., 2005; Nilsberth et al., 2001). Additionally, neuronal expression of Aβ42 in flies affects axonal transport of mitochondria, leading to depletion of mitochondria from the presynaptic active zone (Zhao et al., 2010). A more complex mutant line has been generated containing human APP, human β-secretase, and *Drosophila* γ-secretase presenilin with point mutations corresponding to familial AD mutations N141I, L235P, and E280A (Greeve et al., 2004; Ye and Fortini, 1999). This model allowed for the processing of human APP in *Drosophila* resulting in expression of human Aβ40 and Aβ42 peptides. The Aβ peptides formed plaques, and the flies developed age-dependent neurodegeneration as measured by photoreceptor cell loss (Greeve et al., 2004). This unique mutant demonstrates the similarities in the physiology and biochemistry of flies and humans in Aβ42-induced neurodegeneration.

Presenilins

Flies have a single homolog, *PSN*, compared to the two mammalian presenilin genes involved in familial AD. While ubiquitous knockdown of *PSN* is lethal, knockdown of *PSN* in the midgut produces viable flies that have reduced Cu levels and are more tolerant to excess dietary Cu. These flies have increased oxidative stress, because there is an inhibition of Cu, Zn superoxide dismutase and they are sensitive to oxidants (Southon et al., 2013). Flies expressing human mutant presenilins have reduced synaptic plasticity and impaired memory (Lu et al., 2007). Genetic screens have been performed to identify presenilin-interacting genes, which included members of the Notch signaling pathway and genes involved in intracellular calcium homeostasis (Mahoney et al., 2006; van de Hoef et al., 2009).

Tau

Flies contain an endogenous homolog to the tau protein. However, flies expressing Aβ42 do not show fibrillary structures composed of hyperphosphorylated tau by either biochemical or histological methods (Iijima et al., 2004). This observation has led to the development of fly lines expressing human tau or mutant tau proteins. Overexpression of human wild-type or mutant tau in the *Drosophila* nervous system causes vacuolization of the brain, leading to age-dependent neurodegeneration and decreased lifespan. Concomitant expression of both Aβ42 and tau in flies demonstrated exacerbated neuronal dysfunction, axonal transport defects, and decreased lifespan (Folwell et al., 2010). In the coexpression line, Aβ42 was shown to increase tau phosphorylation by downregulating the wingless signaling (Wnt) pathway (Folwell et al., 2010). Similar to the endogenous *Drosophila* tau, overexpressed human tau does not form large filamentous aggregates in the fly brain despite levels of hyperphosphorylation (Wittmann et al., 2001). Several mutant lines have been generated to examine the effects of tau phosphorylation in flies. Point mutations in tau include TauS2A, TauS11A, and TauS262A (Chatterjee et al., 2009; Iijima-Ando et al., 2010). These mutants were used in the rough eye phenotype (REP) assay. Retinal expression of genes that can cause neurodegeneration, such as tau, cause the fly's eye to have a rough appearance, which correlates to the loss of retinal cells and photoreceptors (Chatterjee et al., 2009; Jackson et al., 2002; Wittmann et al., 2001). Retinal expression of human tau causes degeneration of photoreceptor axons, evident by the appearance of vacuoles in the medulla, the projection target of photoreceptor axons (Wittmann et al., 2001). Examining transgenic lines crossed to the tau-expressing lines allows for genetic screening of modifiers of tau toxicity. For example, the fly ortholog of glycogen synthase kinase 3β (GSK3β) when overexpressed enhanced the REP, while crossing with a GSK3β-deficient line suppressed the REP (Jackson et al., 2002). Genetic screens using the TauS2A, TauS11A, and TauS262A lines identified kinases involved in tau phosphorylation, including protease-activated receptor 1 at ser2, GSK3β at ser11, and DNA damage-activated checkpoint kinase 2 at ser262 (Chatterjee et al., 2009; Iijima-Ando et al., 2010). Another phosphorylation-resistant mutant line was created in which all serine–proline/threonine–proline sites were mutated to alanines (TauAP), making the tau protein resistant to proline-directed kinases (Steinhilb et al., 2007). Additionally, these sites were also mutated to glutamines (TauE14) to mimic a hyperphosphorylated status of tau (Steinhilb et al., 2007). Flies expressing TauE14 flies showed characteristic tau toxicity, which was inhibited by expression of TauAP (Steinhilb et al., 2007). Finally, there are fly strains that express disease-related mutations associated with FTDP-17 (Ali et al., 2012; Feuillette et al., 2010).

Apolipoprotein E4

Drosophila has been used to investigate interactions between Aβ and apolipoprotein E, ApoE4, an allele variant that confers the largest known genetic risk factor for late-onset sporadic AD (Corder et al., 1993; Holtzman et al., 2012). It has been shown that ApoE binds Aβ and is a regulator of Aβ trafficking in the brain (Holtzman et al., 2012), and that ApoE null mouse models have reduced deposition of Aβ peptides (Kim et al., 2011). As discussed earlier, in *Drosophila* production of Aβ peptides from the either the endogenous *Appl* or from the expression of human Aβ peptides induces brain neurodegeneration; however, flies do not contain an ApoE4 homolog. Interestingly, flies contain Dementin, homolog of TMCC2, a protein that interacts with both ApoE and APP in mammals (Hopkins et al., 2011). Null mutants of Dementin display neurodegeneration and accumulation of Appl proteolytic products (Hopkins, 2013). ApoE mimetics examined in *Drosophila* inhibited neurodegeneration and improved learning and memory in flies expressing human APP (Sarantseva et al., 2009), suggesting further investigation is needed to characterize neuroprotective mechanisms of these compounds.

Metal-Induced Neurodegeneration

Drosophila models have been used to examine the contribution of Cu, Zn, Fe, and Al to the development of AD. Treatment of flies with either Cu or Zn enhances Aβ42-induced phenotypes, such as REP, decreased survival, and locomotor defects (Hua et al., 2011). This enhanced toxicity could be prevented by chelators, inhibition of Cu or Zn importers, or by expression of MTF-1, a conserved metal-responsive transcription factor that induces expression of metal ion scavenger proteins (Hua et al., 2011; Lang et al., 2012, 2013). Knockdown of the Zn importer dZIP1 also decreased the accumulation of Aβ fibrils in *Drosophila* brains (Lang et al., 2012). Similarly, Fe has been shown to enhance Aβ42-induced toxicity, which can be blocked by Fe-specific chelating agents and the overexpression of the Fe-binding protein ferritin (Liu et al., 2011). Overexpression of two subunits of ferritin prolonged the lifespan of Aβ42-expressing flies and decreased measures of oxidative damage to the fly's brain (Rival et al., 2009). The presence of Fe was found to alter the structure of Aβ fibrils delaying the formation of mature aggregates (Liu et al., 2011). These studies demonstrate that modulation of Aβ by heavy metals is important for the toxicity of Aβ42 peptides.

Feeding *Drosophila* Al, produces neurotoxicity similar to AD. Al exposure decreases lifespan and causes locomotor deficits, olfactory learning abnormalities, and vacuolization of the brain (Wu et al., 2012). Al increased levels of Fe in the flies and generated ROS (Wu et al., 2012). Chelation of Fe and expression of ferritin decreased Al toxicity (Wu et al., 2012), suggesting a role for altered Fe homeostasis in Al neurotoxicity. Interestingly, Al did not modulate neurotoxicity associated with expression of Aβ peptides or tau (Wu et al., 2012). This observation suggests that the three factors work independently of each other in producing an AD-like phenotype in *Drosophila*.

Pharmaceutical Testing

Drosophila has been used as a simple in vivo model to test the efficacy of several compounds identified in large pharmacological screens. In a study examining the effect of 65,000 small molecules on the ability to inhibit Aβ42 aggregation, eight compounds were identified, one of which, D737, was the most efficacious in both cell culture and *Drosophila* (McKoy et al., 2012). In flies, D737 not only reduced Aβ42 aggregation, but also decreased ROS generation and increased both lifespan and locomotive ability (McKoy et al., 2012). In a study, McKoy et al. (2014) examined structure–activity relationships of 11 analogs of D737, finding that fluorine substitutions on an aromatic ring greatly increased the inhibition of Aβ42 aggregation and increased the longevity of the transgenic Aβ42-expressing *Drosophila* as compared to the parent compound D737. It will be interesting to compare the effects of D737 in mammalian in vivo models to continue to examine its potential as a therapeutic. The effect of several porphyrins were examined in *Drosophila* for inhibition of the AChE enzyme, because it has been observed that in AD patients AChE inhibitors can increase regional cerebral blood flow (Hai et al., 2013). The most stable complex found between the fly AChE was with 5, 10, 15, 20-Tetrakis (4-sulfonatophenyl) porphyrinato iron(III) chloride (Hai et al., 2013), suggesting that the molecule may be a new specific AChE inhibitor. A similar screen was performed on flavonoid derivatives, identifying 2-(4′-benzyloxyphenyl)-3-hydroxy-chromen-4-one as protective against neurodegeneration (measured by REP), decreased amyloid plaques, and increased locomotor activity and lifespan (Singh et al., 2014). In flies expressing human tau, the microtubule-stabilizing peptide NAPVSIPQ (NAP) reversed microtubule destabilization, axonal transport disruption, synaptic defects, and behavioral impairments (Quraishe et al., 2013). NAP accomplished this without altering the abnormal tau levels (Quraishe et al., 2013), suggesting that the drug microtubule stabilization is independent of tau.

Testing FDA-approved drugs for AD therapeutic potential has been performed in *Drosophila* as a quick and inexpensive way to screen. Lithium decreased Aβ42 production by slowing protein synthesis in *Drosophila* (Sofola-Adesakin et al., 2014). The effects of lithium were dose dependent, where both low and high doses rescued the locomotory defects induced by Aβ42, but it rescued lifespan only at lower doses (Sofola-Adesakin et al., 2014). Gefitinib and erlotinib, epidermal growth factor receptor inhibitors that are currently used in cancer therapy, are able to prevent Aβ42-induced memory loss in flies (Wang et al., 2012). The combination of the AChE donepezil (Aricept) with smart soup, a traditional Chinese medicine formula composed of three herbaceous plants, increased both longevity and locomotive activity of Aβ42-expressing flies (Wang et al., 2015). There was also less Aβ deposition and neurodegeneration following the combined drug treatment (Wang et al., 2015). This combination therapy showed potential for use in human studies. A small retrospective cohort study was performed, demonstrating that AD patients receiving both Aricept and smart soup had better cognitive measures than those who did not receive the treatment (Wang et al., 2015). Further studies are needed to confirm these findings in humans and to determine whether there are beneficial effects on Aβ42 aggregation and neurodegeneration in mammals as was observed in flies.

DANIO RERIO

Zebrafish (*D. rerio*) are small freshwater fish native to India that have been used in developmental biology research for over 60 years. Zebrafish are extremely hardy and inexpensive compared to other vertebrate models. These fish are usually kept in a circulating tank system that continuously filters and aerates the water to maintain the water quality required for a healthy aquatic environment (Avdesh et al., 2012). Zebrafish are fed brine shrimp, which are equally easy to grow and maintain as a colony (Avdesh et al., 2012). Of the model organisms described in this chapter, zebrafish have the longest lifespan, with a mean of 3.5 years and a maximum of 5.5 years (Gerhard et al., 2002). While fish physiology is significantly different than mammalian, the presence of muscoskeletal system and vascular system gives zebrafish an advantage over both *Drosophila* and *C. elegans* in modeling human biology. Zebrafish develop rapidly ex utero from transparent embryos, of which greater than 100 embryos are produced per spawning. This allows for a high reproductive capacity and quick collection of numerous samples. A summary of advantages of the zebrafish system is presented in Table 11.1.

Zebrafish are an advantageous model for genetic analyses. The zebrafish genome is extensively annotated. However, human genes do have identifiable zebrafish orthologs, despite the genome duplication characteristic of teleost-bony fish (Catchen et al., 2011). Duplicated genes often have overlapping functions, which makes analysis of gene function difficult unless the function of both duplicate genes is altered. Zebrafish embryos are highly genetically manipulable through injection of morpholino antisense oligonucleotides, sense mRNA, transgenes, or genome engineering systems (Hisano et al., 2014; Hwang et al., 2013; Schmid and Haass, 2013). Morpholinos are designed to bind to particular sites in transcripts from a gene of interest. Injection of morpholino and mRNA are transient, with effects observed during embryogenesis (2–3 days postfertilization). Transgenic zebrafish can be generated by the Tol2 transposase system to insert genes under tissue-specific promoters (Kawakami et al., 2000) or the Cre/loxP (Hans et al., 2009) and GAL4-UAS (Halpern et al., 2008) systems for conditionally expressed transgenics. Zinc finger nucleases, transcription activator-like effector nucleases, and the type II prokaryotic clustered regularly interspaced short palindromic repeats/Cas systems are utilized for generation of point mutations and targeted modification of gene sequences (Hwang et al., 2013; Schmid and Haass, 2013).

The utility of zebrafish in neuroscience research is on the rise. Researchers are using zebrafish for a number of neuro-related applications, for studying sleep cycles, pain, fear, anxiety, learning, vision, and social interactions. Additionally, fish are being used to study neurological disorders such as autism, sleep disorders, epilepsy, depression, addiction, and neurodegeneration (reviewed nicely in Kalueff et al., 2014; Stewart et al., 2014). The zebrafish nervous system contains around 1 million neurons and has analogous functions in mammals. The brain is well characterized and has an online atlas available as a resource for neuroanatomy (www.zebrafishbrain.org). While there are similar brain regions in the fish as in mammals, not all brain regions are as developed in the fish, such as the cortex. Additionally, there are regions of the fish brain that do not clearly map to a mammalian counterpoint. There are many options available for imaging of the zebrafish brain. As transparent embryos, functional imaging is possible to measure changes in metabolism, blood flow, and chemical composition (Stewart et al., 2014). As nontransparent adults, zebrafish brains have been examined using magnetic resonance imaging or histology (Stewart et al., 2014). Finally, there are several behavioral assays that have been developed in zebrafish, many of which have similar mammalian protocols. For example, the novel tank test in fish is similar to the open field and elevated plus maze tests in rodents (Blaser et al., 2010; Stewart et al., 2012).

Disease-Linked Mutations and Neurodegeneration

Amyloid Peptide Precursor Protein

Zebrafish orthologs of APP are *appa* and *appb*, which have widespread and overlapping expression in the forebrain and vasculature, with *appb* expressed additionally in the spinal cord (Lee and Cole, 2007; Liao et al., 2012; Musa et al., 2001). Using gene traps, Liao et al. (2012) found that the mRNA transcripts for *appa* were contained solely in neuronal cells and not in endothelial cells of the vasculature, suggesting that the Appa protein is synthesized in neurons and then accumulates in the vasculature. The function of the two orthologs in zebrafish has been investigated using translation blocking morpholinos. Inhibition of *appa* showed minimal effects on the developing embryo; in contrast inhibition of *appb* resulted in developmental defects, such as decreased body length, deformed tail, defective convergent extension cellular movements, decreased motor axon outgrowth, and defective axonal outgrowth patterning and synapse formation (Abramsson et al., 2013; Joshi et al., 2009; Song and Pimplikar, 2012). Interestingly, injection of human wild-type APP into *appb* embryos can prevent these developmental defects (Abramsson et al., 2013), suggesting conserved functions between human and zebrafish APP. Injection of mutations associated with familial AD, however, are less effective in preventing the defects.

Because Appa and Appb proteins are acted upon by β- and γ-secretases, it is possible to examine the role of Aβ in zebrafish. To increase Aβ levels, zebrafish are exposed as embryos to Aβ in their aqueous environment. Treatment of embryos with Aβ40 caused defective vascular development and accelerated cell senescence (Donnini et al., 2010). In particular, high levels of Aβ increased cerebrovascular branching in the developing zebrafish hindbrain (Cameron et al., 2012). Diminishing Aβ levels by targeted APP morpholino injection and β-secretase inhibitor treatment also induced cerebrovascular defects (Luna et al., 2013). Injection of human Aβ42 could rescue the phenotype (Luna et al., 2013), further suggesting that Aβ may play a role in maintaining normal cerebrovascular function. Expression of human Aβ42 in zebrafish has been performed using the *mitfa* (nacre) gene, which drives expression in melanocytes (Newman et al., 2010). Unfortunately, no visible phenotype was produced until the fish were 16 months old (Newman et al., 2010), at which point the fish are old and infertile to set up genetic crosses to identify modifiers of Aβ42 toxicity. While this system could theoretically allow for drug screening for Aβ42 modifiers, the requirement of such old fish makes it inefficient for drug testing. As such, treatment with recombinant Aβ protein is the standard for increasing Aβ levels in fish.

Presenilins

The zebrafish orthologs of human presenilins are *psen1* and *psen2*, which are ubiquitously expressed in zebrafish embryos (Groth et al., 2002; Leimer et al., 1999). The presenilin orthologs in zebrafish interact with *bace1*, the zebrafish ortholog to beta-site Aβ A4 precursor protein-cleaving enzyme 1 to constitute a functional γ-secretase (Moussavi et al., 2012). Hypoxia that occurs during AD resulting from hypoperfusion of the vasculature leads to an increased expression of psen1, *psen2* and *bace1* (Moussavi Nik et al., 2012).

Zebrafish embryos injected with a psen1 translation-blocking morpholino have similar phenotypes to conditional Psen1 knockout mice, such as aberrant somite formation and Notch signaling defects (Nornes et al., 2003, 2008; Shen et al., 1997; Wong et al., 1997). A transgenic zebrafish mutant that lacks Psen1 activity has altered histaminergic neuronal function, showing decreased histaminergic neuronal numbers in embryonic fish and an increase in histaminergic neurons by 1 year (Sundvik et al., 2013). This implies that psen1 may be involved in neuronal plasticity or stem cell differentiation. Morpholinos against Psen2 translation affect the production of dorsal longitudinal ascending interneurons in the developing spinal cord of zebrafish larvae (Nornes et al., 2009). Blockage of Psen1 does not affect the dorsal longitudinal ascending interneurons, making this phenotype a possible marker to distinguish modifiers of Psen1 and Psen2 function. Currently, there are no transgenic zebrafish that express any of the mutations associated with familial AD. However, zebrafish engineered to exclude exon 8 or 9 from zebrafish psen1 transcripts to mimic the effects of the human PSEN1 L271V and Δ9 mutations have premature truncation of the open reading frame after exons 6 and 7, respectively (Nornes et al., 2008). The truncated transcripts evaded nonsense-mediated decay and produced Psen1 proteins with dominant negative activity and could suppress Psen2 activity (Nornes et al., 2008). Truncation of Psen1 led to activation of Notch signaling and suppressed APP cleavage (Newman et al., 2014). A naturally truncated Psen1 isoform in zebrafish, called PS1IV, has been identified that resembles a PSEN2 isoform in humans called PS2V (Moussavi Nik et al., 2015). PS2V is expressed in familial late-onset AD and is induced by hypoxia. Both the human PS2V and fish PS1IV stimulate γ-secretase activity, increasing Aβ formation, and suppress the unfolded protein response under hypoxic conditions (Moussavi Nik et al., 2015).

Tau

The zebrafish orthologs of the human MAPT gene are *mapta* and *maptb*, which have similar patterns of expression in developing embryos (Chen et al., 2009). The *mapt* gene transcript is alternatively spliced, giving rise to several protein isoforms, which can be classified based on the number of tubulin-binding motifs, either 3R or 4R. A ratio of 1:1 of 3R:4R promotes for normal functioning of the MAPT protein in the brain, while alterations of the ratio exist in AD (Conrad et al., 2007; Goedert and Spillantini, 2006). In zebrafish, *mapta* is spliced into 4R and 6R isoforms while *maptb* is spliced predominantly into 3R isoforms (Chen et al., 2009). This contrast in isoform composition makes the endogenous MAPT in zebrafish less attractive to model human MAPT. Alterations of *mapta* and *maptb* levels are altered by hypoxia, particularly the 6R and 4R isoforms of *mapta* and *maptb*, respectively (Moussavi Nik et al., 2014). Transgenic zebrafish expressing human MAPT 4R in zebrafish CNS neurons express MAPT at levels eightfold higher than in human brains, resulting in accumulations of tau in the fish brain that resembled neurofibrillary tangles (Bai et al., 2007). Additionally, there are transgenic zebrafish that express a mutant form of human MAPT associated with FTDP-17, TAU-P301L (Paquet et al., 2009). These transgenic fish lines may be useful tools in examining tau as a pharmaceutical target.

Fluorescent probes have been developed to visualize neurofibrillary tangles in brain tissue from AD patients. These probes are rhodanine-3-acetic acid derivatives that preferentially bind to the tangles over amyloid plaques. In zebrafish, these probes bind neurofibrillary tangles and show negligible cytotoxicity (Anumala et al., 2013), suggesting that there is potential for use in in vivo diagnostic testing.

Apolipoprotein E4

The zebrafish homologs to APOE4 are *apoea* and *apoeb*; however, very little is known about their functions. Both *apoea* and *apoeb* are expressed in the developing retina and yolk syncytial layer (Pujic et al., 2006; Raymond et al., 2006). Only *apoeb*, but not *apoea*, is expressed in macrophages and microglial cells, developing and regenerating fin tissue, epidermis, liver, intestine, and ovary (Levi et al., 2012; Lien et al., 2006; Monnot et al., 1999; Tingaud-Sequeira et al., 2006). Currently, more information is needed about this protein in vivo to be able to use zebrafish transgenics in AD-related studies.

Pharmaceutical Testing

Zebrafish have been underutilized in regards to pharmaceutical testing for AD. Testing of any compound in zebrafish requires water solubility, which may be a hurdle to overcome for certain compounds. Direct injection of Aβ42 into the hindbrain ventricle of zebrafish embryos results in cognitive deficits and increased tau phosphorylation by GSK3β in 5-day postfertilization larvae (Nery et al., 2014). These effects were reversed by lithium treatment, similar to what was observed in *Drosophila* (Nery et al., 2014; Sofola-Adesakin et al., 2014). Treatment of zebrafish with recombinant Aβ40 peptides causes a reduction of vessel branching in fish expressing GFP in endothelial cells, induced nicotinamide adenine dinucleotide phosphate oxidase-derived ROS, and impaired vascular endothelial growth factor (VEGF)-dependent angiogenesis (Lu et al., 2014). Pretreatment with puerarin, an isoflavone found in the roots of the *Pueraria* plant genus, attenuated Aβ40-induced vessel reduction and impairment to angiogenesis (Lu et al., 2014). Additionally, Aβ40 treatment decreased VEGF-dependent phosphorylation of Akt and endothelial nitric oxide synthase, which was attenuated by puerarin (Lu et al., 2014). This study suggests that puerarin treatment may be protective for Aβ40-induced vascular injury associated with AD.

CONCLUSIONS

The genetic model organisms *C. elegans*, *Drosophila*, and zebrafish offer an attractive alternative to rodent in vivo models. Research using these species can be performed quickly and inexpensively because of the organisms' high fertility rate and ease of maintenance. While many of the transgenics described express human proteins in nonmammalian systems, conservation of protein–protein interactions is high, allowing for results that are translatable to mammalian biology. While there are many uses for simple in vivo systems, their short lifespans, small body size, and care requirements allow for effective screening of genetic modifiers to disease, but also for potential neurotoxic compounds or effective pharmaceutical agents. It is important to understand the limitations to their use and the need to verify results in mammalian systems.

References

Abramsson, A., Kettunen, P., Banote, R.K., Lott, E., Li, M., Arner, A., et al., 2013. The zebrafish amyloid precursor protein-b is required for motor neuron guidance and synapse formation. Dev. Biol. 381 (2), 377–388.

Adams, M.D., Celniker, S.E., Holt, R.A., Evans, C.A., Gocayne, J.D., Amanatides, P.G., et al., 2000. The genome sequence of *Drosophila melanogaster*. Science 287 (5461), 2185–2195.

Ali, Y.O., Ruan, K., Zhai, R.G., 2012. NMNAT suppresses tau-induced neurodegeneration by promoting clearance of hyperphosphorylated tau oligomers in a *Drosophila* model of tauopathy. Hum. Mol. Genet. 21 (2), 237–250.

Anumala, U.R., Gu, J., Lo Monte, F., Kramer, T., Heyny-von Haussen, R., Holzer, J., et al., 2013. Fluorescent rhodanine-3-acetic acids visualize neurofibrillary tangles in Alzheimer's disease brains. Bioorg. Med. Chem. 21 (17), 5139–5144.

Arya, U., Dwivedi, H., Subramaniam, J.R., 2009. Reserpine ameliorates Abeta toxicity in the Alzheimer's disease model in *Caenorhabditis elegans*. Exp. Gerontol. 44 (6–7), 462–466.

Ashley, J., Packard, M., Ataman, B., Budnik, V., 2005. Fasciclin II signals new synapse formation through amyloid precursor protein and the scaffolding protein dX11/Mint. J. Neurosci. 25 (25), 5943–5955.

Avdesh, A., Chen, M., Martin-Iverson, M.T., Mondal, A., Ong, D., Rainey-Smith, S., et al., 2012. Regular care and maintenance of a zebrafish (*Danio rerio*) laboratory: an introduction. J. Vis. Exp. (69), e4196.

Bai, F., Xi, J.H., Andley, U.P., 2007. Up-regulation of tau, a brain microtubule-associated protein, in lens cortical fractions of aged alphaA-, alphaB-, and alphaA/B-crystallin knockout mice. Mol. Vis. 13, 1589–1600.

Baumeister, R., Leimer, U., Zweckbronner, I., Jakubek, C., Grunberg, J., Haass, C., 1997. Human presenilin-1, but not familial Alzheimer's disease (FAD) mutants, facilitate *Caenorhabditis elegans* Notch signalling independently of proteolytic processing. Genes Funct. 1 (2), 149–159.

Berezovska, O., Xia, M.Q., Hyman, B.T., 1998. Notch is expressed in adult brain, is coexpressed with presenilin-1, and is altered in Alzheimer disease. J. Neuropathol. Exp. Neurol. 57 (8), 738–745.

Blake, M.R., Holbrook, S.D., Kotwica-Rolinska, J., Chow, E.S., Kretzschmar, D., Giebultowicz, J.M., 2015. Manipulations of amyloid precursor protein cleavage disrupt the circadian clock in aging *Drosophila*. Neurobiol. Dis. 77, 117–126.

Blaser, R.E., Chadwick, L., McGinnis, G.C., 2010. Behavioral measures of anxiety in zebrafish (*Danio rerio*). Behav. Brain Res. 208 (1), 56–62.

Bolognin, S., Messori, L., Zatta, P., 2009. Metal ion physiopathology in neurodegenerative disorders. Neuromol. Med. 11 (4), 223–238.

Brandt, R., Gergou, A., Wacker, I., Fath, T., Hutter, H., 2009. A *Caenorhabditis elegans* model of tau hyperphosphorylation: induction of developmental defects by transgenic overexpression of Alzheimer's disease-like modified tau. Neurobiol. Aging 30 (1), 22–33.

Brenner, S., 1974. The genetics of *Caenorhabditis elegans*. Genetics 77 (1), 71–94.

Cameron, D.J., Galvin, C., Alkam, T., Sidhu, H., Ellison, J., Luna, S., et al., 2012. Alzheimer's-related peptide amyloid-beta plays a conserved role in angiogenesis. PLoS One 7 (7), e39598.

Carmine-Simmen, K., Proctor, T., Tschape, J., Poeck, B., Triphan, T., Strauss, R., et al., 2009. Neurotoxic effects induced by the *Drosophila* amyloid-beta peptide suggest a conserved toxic function. Neurobiol. Dis. 33 (2), 274–281.

Castle, W.E., 1906. Inbreeding, cross-breeding and sterility in *Drosophila*. Science 23 (578), 153.

Catchen, J.M., Braasch, I., Postlethwait, J.H., 2011. Conserved synteny and the zebrafish genome. Methods Cell Biol. 104, 259–285.

Cerpa, W.F., Barria, M.I., Chacon, M.A., Suazo, M., Gonzalez, M., Opazo, C., et al., 2004. The N-terminal copper-binding domain of the amyloid precursor protein protects against Cu^{2+} neurotoxicity in vivo. FASEB J. 18 (14), 1701–1703.

Chartier-Harlin, M.C., Crawford, F., Hamandi, K., Mullan, M., Goate, A., Hardy, J., et al., 1991a. Screening for the beta-amyloid precursor protein mutation (APP717: Val---Ile) in extended pedigrees with early onset Alzheimer's disease. Neurosci. Lett. 129 (1), 134–135.

Chartier-Harlin, M.C., Crawford, F., Houlden, H., Warren, A., Hughes, D., Fidani, L., et al., 1991b. Early-onset Alzheimer's disease caused by mutations at codon 717 of the beta-amyloid precursor protein gene. Nature 353 (6347), 844–846.

Chatterjee, S., Sang, T.K., Lawless, G.M., Jackson, G.R., 2009. Dissociation of tau toxicity and phosphorylation: role of GSK-3beta, MARK and Cdk5 in a *Drosophila* model. Hum. Mol. Genet. 18 (1), 164–177.

Chen, M., Martins, R.N., Lardelli, M., 2009. Complex splicing and neural expression of duplicated tau genes in zebrafish embryos. J. Alzheimers Dis. 18 (2), 305–317.

Chiang, A.S., Lin, C.Y., Chuang, C.C., Chang, H.M., Hsieh, C.H., Yeh, C.W., et al., 2011. Three-dimensional reconstruction of brain-wide wiring networks in *Drosophila* at single-cell resolution. Curr. Biol. 21 (1), 1–11.

Cohen, E., Du, D., Joyce, D., Kapernick, E.A., Volovik, Y., Kelly, J.W., et al., 2010. Temporal requirements of insulin/IGF-1 signaling for proteotoxicity protection. Aging Cell 9 (2), 126–134.

Conrad, C., Zhu, J., Schoenfeld, D., Fang, Z., Ingelsson, M., Stamm, S., et al., 2007. Single molecule profiling of tau gene expression in Alzheimer's disease. J. Neurochem. 103 (3), 1228–1236.

Corder, E.H., Saunders, A.M., Strittmatter, W.J., Schmechel, D.E., Gaskell, P.C., Small, G.W., et al., 1993. Gene dose of apolipoprotein E type 4 allele and the risk of Alzheimer's disease in late onset families. Science 261 (5123), 921–923.

Crowther, D.C., Kinghorn, K.J., Miranda, E., Page, R., Curry, J.A., Duthie, F.A., et al., 2005. Intraneuronal Abeta, non-amyloid aggregates and neurodegeneration in a *Drosophila* model of Alzheimer's disease. Neuroscience 132 (1), 123–135.

Daigle, I., Li, C., 1993. apl-1, a *Caenorhabditis elegans* gene encoding a protein related to the human beta-amyloid protein precursor. Proc. Natl. Acad. Sci. U.S.A. 90 (24), 12045–12049.

Diomede, L., Cassata, G., Fiordaliso, F., Salio, M., Ami, D., Natalello, A., et al., 2010. Tetracycline and its analogues protect *Caenorhabditis elegans* from beta amyloid-induced toxicity by targeting oligomers. Neurobiol. Dis. 40 (2), 424–431.

Diomede, L., Rigacci, S., Romeo, M., Stefani, M., Salmona, M., 2013. Oleuropein aglycone protects transgenic *C. elegans* strains expressing Aβ42 by reducing plaque load and motor deficit. PLoS One 8 (3), e58893.

Donnini, S., Solito, R., Cetti, E., Corti, F., Giachetti, A., Carra, S., et al., 2010. Abeta peptides accelerate the senescence of endothelial cells in vitro and in vivo, impairing angiogenesis. FASEB J. 24 (7), 2385–2395.

El-Ami, T., Moll, L., Carvalhal Marques, F., Volovik, Y., Reuveni, H., Cohen, E., 2014. A novel inhibitor of the insulin/IGF signaling pathway protects from age-onset, neurodegeneration-linked proteotoxicity. Aging Cell 13 (1), 165–174.

Emmons, S.W., 2015. The beginning of connectomics: a commentary on White et al. (1986) 'The structure of the nervous system of the nematode *Caenorhabditis elegans*'. Philos. Trans. R. Soc. Lond. B Biol. Sci. 370 (1666).

Faller, P., 2009. Copper and zinc binding to amyloid-beta: coordination, dynamics, aggregation, reactivity and metal-ion transfer. Chembiochem 10 (18), 2837–2845.

Faller, P., Hureau, C., 2009. Bioinorganic chemistry of copper and zinc ions coordinated to amyloid-beta peptide. [Review] Dalton Trans. (7), 1080–1094.

Feuillette, S., Deramecourt, V., Laquerriere, A., Duyckaerts, C., Delisle, M.B., Maurage, C.A., et al., 2010. Filamin-A and Myosin VI colocalize with fibrillary Tau protein in Alzheimer's disease and FTDP-17 brains. Brain Res. 1345, 182–189.

Finelli, A., Kelkar, A., Song, H.J., Yang, H., Konsolaki, M., 2004. A model for studying Alzheimer's Aβ42-induced toxicity in *Drosophila melanogaster*. Mol. Cell. Neurosci. 26 (3), 365–375.

Florez-McClure, M.L., Hohsfield, L.A., Fonte, G., Bealor, M.T., Link, C.D., 2007. Decreased insulin-receptor signaling promotes the autophagic degradation of beta-amyloid peptide in *C. elegans*. Autophagy 3 (6), 569–580.

Folwell, J., Cowan, C.M., Ubhi, K.K., Shiabh, H., Newman, T.A., Shepherd, D., et al., 2010. Abeta exacerbates the neuronal dysfunction caused by human tau expression in a *Drosophila* model of Alzheimer's disease. Exp. Neurol. 223 (2), 401–409.

Fonte, V., Kapulkin, W.J., Taft, A., Fluet, A., Friedman, D., Link, C.D., 2002. Interaction of intracellular beta amyloid peptide with chaperone proteins. Proc. Natl. Acad. Sci. U.S.A. 99 (14), 9439–9444.

Fonte, V., Kipp, D.R., Yerg 3rd, J., Merin, D., Forrestal, M., Wagner, E., et al., 2008. Suppression of in vivo beta-amyloid peptide toxicity by overexpression of the HSP-16.2 small chaperone protein. J. Biol. Chem. 283 (2), 784–791.

Gerhard, G.S., Kauffman, E.J., Wang, X., Stewart, R., Moore, J.L., Kasales, C.J., et al., 2002. Life spans and senescent phenotypes in two strains of Zebrafish (*Danio rerio*). Exp. Gerontol. 37 (8–9), 1055–1068.

Goate, A., Chartier-Harlin, M.C., Mullan, M., Brown, J., Crawford, F., Fidani, L., et al., 1991. Segregation of a missense mutation in the amyloid precursor protein gene with familial Alzheimer's disease. Nature 349 (6311), 704–706.

Goedert, M., Baur, C.P., Ahringer, J., Jakes, R., Hasegawa, M., Spillantini, M.G., et al., 1996. PTL-1, a microtubule-associated protein with tau-like repeats from the nematode *Caenorhabditis elegans*. J. Cell Sci. 109 (Pt 11), 2661–2672.

Goedert, M., Spillantini, M.G., 2006. A century of Alzheimer's disease. Science 314 (5800), 777–781.

Graham, S.F., Nasaruddin, M.B., Carey, M., Holscher, C., McGuinness, B., Kehoe, P.G., et al., 2014. Age-associated changes of brain copper, iron, and zinc in Alzheimer's disease and dementia with lewy bodies. J. Alzheimers Dis. 42 (4), 1407–1413.

Greeve, I., Kretzschmar, D., Tschape, J.A., Beyn, A., Brellinger, C., Schweizer, M., et al., 2004. Age-dependent neurodegeneration and Alzheimer-amyloid plaque formation in transgenic *Drosophila*. J. Neurosci. 24 (16), 3899–3906.

Groth, C., Nornes, S., McCarty, R., Tamme, R., Lardelli, M., 2002. Identification of a second presenilin gene in zebrafish with similarity to the human Alzheimer's disease gene presenilin2. Dev. Genes Evol. 212 (10), 486–490.

Gutierrez-Zepeda, A., Santell, R., Wu, Z., Brown, M., Wu, Y., Khan, I., et al., 2005. Soy isoflavone glycitein protects against beta amyloid-induced toxicity and oxidative stress in transgenic *Caenorhabditis elegans*. BMC Neurosci. 6, 54.

Hai, A., Kizilbash, N.A., Zaidi, S.H., Alruwaili, J., 2013. Porphyrin derivatives as inhibitors for acetylcholinesterase from *Drosophila melanogaster*. Bioinformation 9 (12), 645–649.

Halpern, M.E., Rhee, J., Goll, M.G., Akitake, C.M., Parsons, M., Leach, S.D., 2008. Gal4/UAS transgenic tools and their application to zebrafish. Zebrafish 5 (2), 97–110.

Hans, S., Kaslin, J., Freudenreich, D., Brand, M., 2009. Temporally-controlled site-specific recombination in zebrafish. PLoS One 4 (2), e4640.

Hesse, L., Beher, D., Masters, C.L., Multhaup, G., 1994. The beta A4 amyloid precursor protein binding to copper. FEBS Lett. 349 (1), 109–116.

Hisano, Y., Ota, S., Kawahara, A., 2014. Genome editing using artificial site-specific nucleases in zebrafish. Dev. Growth Differ. 56 (1), 26–33.

Hobert, O., 2005. Specification of the Nervous System. WormBook: the Online Review of *C. elegans* Biology, pp. 1–19.

Holtzman, D.M., Herz, J., Bu, G., 2012. Apolipoprotein E and apolipoprotein E receptors: normal biology and roles in Alzheimer disease. [Review] Cold Spring Harb. Perspect. Med. 2 (3), a006312.

Hopkins, P.C., 2013. Neurodegeneration in a *Drosophila* model for the function of TMCC2, an amyloid protein precursor-interacting and apolipoprotein E-binding protein. PLoS One 8 (2), e55810.

Hopkins, P.C., Sainz-Fuertes, R., Lovestone, S., 2011. The impact of a novel apolipoprotein E and amyloid-beta protein precursor-interacting protein on the production of amyloid-beta. J. Alzheimers Dis. 26 (2), 239–253.

Hornsten, A., Lieberthal, J., Fadia, S., Malins, R., Ha, L., Xu, X., et al., 2007. APL-1, a *Caenorhabditis elegans* protein related to the human beta-amyloid precursor protein, is essential for viability. Proc. Natl. Acad. Sci. U.S.A. 104 (6), 1971–1976.

Hua, H., Munter, L., Harmeier, A., Georgiev, O., Multhaup, G., Schaffner, W., 2011. Toxicity of Alzheimer's disease-associated Aβ peptide is ameliorated in a *Drosophila* model by tight control of zinc and copper availability. Biol. Chem. 392 (10), 919–926.

Huang, Y.J., Jin, M.H., Pi, R.B., Zhang, J.J., Ouyang, Y., Chao, X.J., et al., 2013. Acrolein induces Alzheimer's disease-like pathologies in vitro and in vivo. Toxicol. Lett. 217 (3), 184–191.

Hwang, W.Y., Fu, Y., Reyon, D., Maeder, M.L., Tsai, S.Q., Sander, J.D., et al., 2013. Efficient genome editing in zebrafish using a CRISPR-Cas system. Nat. Biotechnol. 31 (3), 227–229.

Iijima-Ando, K., Zhao, L., Gatt, A., Shenton, C., Iijima, K., 2010. A DNA damage-activated checkpoint kinase phosphorylates tau and enhances tau-induced neurodegeneration. Hum. Mol. Genet. 19 (10), 1930–1938.

Iijima, K., Chiang, H.C., Hearn, S.A., Hakker, I., Gatt, A., Shenton, C., et al., 2008. Aβ42 mutants with different aggregation profiles induce distinct pathologies in *Drosophila*. PLoS One 3 (2), e1703.

Iijima, K., Liu, H.P., Chiang, A.S., Hearn, S.A., Konsolaki, M., Zhong, Y., 2004. Dissecting the pathological effects of human Aβ40 and Aβ42 in *Drosophila*: a potential model for Alzheimer's disease. Proc. Natl. Acad. Sci. U.S.A. 101 (17), 6623–6628.

Jackson, G.R., Wiedau-Pazos, M., Sang, T.K., Wagle, N., Brown, C.A., Massachi, S., et al., 2002. Human wild-type tau interacts with wingless pathway components and produces neurofibrillary pathology in *Drosophila*. Neuron 34 (4), 509–519.

Jacobsen, K.T., Iverfeldt, K., 2009. Amyloid precursor protein and its homologues: a family of proteolysis-dependent receptors. [Review] Cell. Mol. Life Sci. 66 (14), 2299–2318.

Joshi, P., Liang, J.O., DiMonte, K., Sullivan, J., Pimplikar, S.W., 2009. Amyloid precursor protein is required for convergent-extension movements during Zebrafish development. Dev. Biol. 335 (1), 1–11.

Kalueff, A.V., Stewart, A.M., Gerlai, R., 2014. Zebrafish as an emerging model for studying complex brain disorders. Trends Pharmacol. Sci. 35 (2), 63–75.

Kawakami, K., Shima, A., Kawakami, N., 2000. Identification of a functional transposase of the Tol2 element, an Ac-like element from the Japanese medaka fish, and its transposition in the zebrafish germ lineage. Proc. Natl. Acad. Sci. U.S.A. 97 (21), 11403–11408.

Keowkase, R., Aboukhatwa, M., Adam, B.L., Beach, J.W., Terry Jr., A.V., Buccafussco, J.J., et al., 2010. Neuroprotective effects and mechanism of cognitive-enhancing choline analogs JWB 1-84-1 and JAY 2-22-33 in neuronal culture and *Caenorhabditis elegans*. Mol. Neurodegener. 5, 59.

Kim, J., Jiang, H., Park, S., Eltorai, A.E., Stewart, F.R., Yoon, H., et al., 2011. Haploinsufficiency of human APOE reduces amyloid deposition in a mouse model of amyloid-beta amyloidosis. J. Neurosci. 31 (49), 18007–18012.

Kitagawa, N., Shimohama, S., Oeda, T., Uemura, K., Kohno, R., Kuzuya, A., et al., 2003. The role of the presenilin-1 homologue gene sel-12 of *Caenorhabditis elegans* in apoptotic activities. J. Biol. Chem. 278 (14), 12130–12134.

Kraemer, B.C., Zhang, B., Leverenz, J.B., Thomas, J.H., Trojanowski, J.Q., Schellenberg, G.D., 2003. Neurodegeneration and defective neurotransmission in a *Caenorhabditis elegans* model of tauopathy. Proc. Natl. Acad. Sci. U.S.A. 100 (17), 9980–9985.

Lang, M., Fan, Q., Wang, L., Zheng, Y., Xiao, G., Wang, X., et al., 2013. Inhibition of human high-affinity copper importer Ctr1 orthologous in the nervous system of *Drosophila* ameliorates Aβ42-induced Alzheimer's disease-like symptoms. Neurobiol. Aging 34 (11), 2604–2612.

Lang, M., Wang, L., Fan, Q., Xiao, G., Wang, X., Zhong, Y., et al., 2012. Genetic inhibition of solute-linked carrier 39 family transporter 1 ameliorates aβ pathology in a *Drosophila* model of Alzheimer's disease. PLoS Genet. 8 (4), e1002683.

Leao, A.H., Sarmento-Silva, A.J., Santos, J.R., Ribeiro, A.M., Silva, R.H., 2015. Molecular, neurochemical, and behavioral hallmarks of reserpine as a model for Parkinson's disease: new perspectives to a long-standing model. Brain Pathol. 25 (4).

Lee, J.A., Cole, G.J., 2007. Generation of transgenic zebrafish expressing green fluorescent protein under control of zebrafish amyloid precursor protein gene regulatory elements. Zebrafish 4 (4), 277–286.

Leimer, U., Lun, K., Romig, H., Walter, J., Grunberg, J., Brand, M., et al., 1999. Zebrafish (*Danio rerio*) presenilin promotes aberrant amyloid beta-peptide production and requires a critical aspartate residue for its function in amyloidogenesis. Biochemistry 38 (41), 13602–13609.

Levi, L., Ziv, T., Admon, A., Levavi-Sivan, B., Lubzens, E., 2012. Insight into molecular pathways of retinal metabolism, associated with vitellogenesis in zebrafish. Am. J. Physiol. Endocrinol. Metabol. 302 (5), E626–E644.

Levitan, D., Greenwald, I., 1995. Facilitation of lin-12-mediated signalling by sel-12, a *Caenorhabditis elegans* S182 Alzheimer's disease gene. Nature 377 (6547), 351–354.

Leyssen, M., Ayaz, D., Hebert, S.S., Reeve, S., De Strooper, B., Hassan, B.A., 2005. Amyloid precursor protein promotes post-developmental neurite arborization in the *Drosophila* brain. EMBO J. 24 (16), 2944–2955.

Li, B., Chohan, M.O., Grundke-Iqbal, I., Iqbal, K., 2007. Disruption of microtubule network by Alzheimer abnormally hyperphosphorylated tau. Acta Neuropathol. 113 (5), 501–511.

Li, G., Kim, C., Kim, J., Yoon, H., Zhou, H., 2015. Common pesticide, dichlorodiphenyltrichloroethane (DDT), increases amyloid-beta levels by impairing the function of ABCA1 and IDE: implication for Alzheimer's disease. J. Alzheimers Dis. 46 (1).

Li, X., Greenwald, I., 1997. HOP-1, a *Caenorhabditis elegans* presenilin, appears to be functionally redundant with SEL-12 presenilin and to facilitate LIN-12 and GLP-1 signaling. Proc. Natl. Acad. Sci. U.S.A. 94 (22), 12204–12209.

Liao, H.K., Wang, Y., Noack Watt, K.E., Wen, Q., Breitbach, J., Kemmet, C.K., et al., 2012. Tol2 gene trap integrations in the zebrafish amyloid precursor protein genes appa and aplp2 reveal accumulation of secreted APP at the embryonic veins. Dev. Dyn. 241 (2), 415–425.

Lien, C.L., Schebesta, M., Makino, S., Weber, G.J., Keating, M.T., 2006. Gene expression analysis of zebrafish heart regeneration. PLoS Biol. 4 (8), e260.

Link, C.D., 1995. Expression of human beta-amyloid peptide in transgenic *Caenorhabditis elegans*. Proc. Natl. Acad. Sci. U.S.A. 92 (20), 9368–9372.

Link, C.D., 2006. *C. elegans* models of age-associated neurodegenerative diseases: lessons from transgenic worm models of Alzheimer's disease. Exp. Gerontol. 41 (10), 1007–1013.

Link, C.D., Johnson, C.J., Fonte, V., Paupard, M., Hall, D.H., Styren, S., et al., 2001. Visualization of fibrillar amyloid deposits in living, transgenic *Caenorhabditis elegans* animals using the sensitive amyloid dye, X-34. Neurobiol. Aging 22 (2), 217–226.

Link, C.D., Taft, A., Kapulkin, V., Duke, K., Kim, S., Fei, Q., et al., 2003. Gene expression analysis in a transgenic *Caenorhabditis elegans* Alzheimer's disease model. Neurobiol. Aging 24 (3), 397–413.

Liu, B., Moloney, A., Meehan, S., Morris, K., Thomas, S.E., Serpell, L.C., et al., 2011. Iron promotes the toxicity of amyloid beta peptide by impeding its ordered aggregation. J. Biol. Chem. 286 (6), 4248–4256.

Liu, J., DeFranco, D.B., 1999. Chromatin recycling of glucocorticoid receptors: implications for multiple roles of heat shock protein 90. Mol. Endocrinol. 13 (3), 355–365.

Lovell, M.A., Robertson, J.D., Teesdale, W.J., Campbell, J.L., Markesbery, W.R., 1998. Copper, iron and zinc in Alzheimer's disease senile plaques. J. Neurol. Sci. 158 (1), 47–52.

Lu, X.L., Liu, J.X., Wu, Q., Long, S.M., Zheng, M.Y., Yao, X.L., et al., 2014. Protective effects of puerarin against Aβ40-induced vascular dysfunction in zebrafish and human endothelial cells. Eur. J. Pharmacol. 732, 76–85.

Lu, Y., Lv, Y., Ye, Y., Wang, Y., Hong, Y., Fortini, M.E., et al., 2007. A role for presenilin in post-stress regulation: effects of presenilin mutations on Ca^{2+} currents in *Drosophila*. FASEB J. 21 (10), 2368–2378.

Luna, S., Cameron, D.J., Ethell, D.W., 2013. Amyloid-beta and APP deficiencies cause severe cerebrovascular defects: important work for an old villain. PLoS One 8 (9), e75052.

Luo, L., Tully, T., White, K., 1992. Human amyloid precursor protein ameliorates behavioral deficit of flies deleted for Appl gene. Neuron 9 (4), 595–605.

Luo, Y., Zhang, J., Liu, N., Zhao, B., 2011. Copper ions influence the toxicity of β-amyloid(1-42) in a concentration-dependent manner in a *Caenorhabditis elegans* model of Alzheimer's disease. Sci. China Life Sci. 54 (6), 527–534.

Mahoney, M.B., Parks, A.L., Ruddy, D.A., Tiong, S.Y., Esengil, H., Phan, A.C., et al., 2006. Presenilin-based genetic screens in *Drosophila melanogaster* identify novel notch pathway modifiers. Genetics 172 (4), 2309–2324.

Martorell, P., Bataller, E., Llopis, S., Gonzalez, N., Alvarez, B., Monton, F., et al., 2013. A cocoa peptide protects *Caenorhabditis elegans* from oxidative stress and beta-amyloid peptide toxicity. PLoS One 8 (5), e63283.

Matlack, K.E., Tardiff, D.F., Narayan, P., Hamamichi, S., Caldwell, K.A., Caldwell, G.A., et al., 2014. Clioquinol promotes the degradation of metal-dependent amyloid-beta (Aβ) oligomers to restore endocytosis and ameliorate Aβ toxicity. Proc. Natl. Acad. Sci. U.S.A. 111 (11), 4013–4018.

Maynard, C.J., Cappai, R., Volitakis, I., Cherny, R.A., White, A.R., Beyreuther, K., et al., 2002. Overexpression of Alzheimer's disease amyloid-beta opposes the age-dependent elevations of brain copper and iron. J. Biol. Chem. 277 (47), 44670–44676.

McColl, G., Roberts, B.R., Gunn, A.P., Perez, K.A., Tew, D.J., Masters, C.L., et al., 2009. The *Caenorhabditis elegans* A beta 1-42 model of Alzheimer disease predominantly expresses A beta 3-42. J. Biol. Chem. 284 (34), 22697–22702.

McKoy, A.F., Chen, J., Schupbach, T., Hecht, M.H., 2012. A novel inhibitor of amyloid β (Aβ) peptide aggregation: from high throughput screening to efficacy in an animal model of Alzheimer disease. J. Biol. Chem. 287 (46), 38992–39000.

McKoy, A.F., Chen, J., Schupbach, T., Hecht, M.H., 2014. Structure-activity relationships for a series of compounds that inhibit aggregation of the Alzheimer's peptide, Aβ42. Chem. Biol. Drug Des. 84 (5), 505–512.

Merdes, G., Soba, P., Loewer, A., Bilic, M.V., Beyreuther, K., Paro, R., 2004. Interference of human and *Drosophila* APP and APP-like proteins with PNS development in *Drosophila*. EMBO J. 23 (20), 4082–4095.

Minniti, A.N., Rebolledo, D.L., Grez, P.M., Fadic, R., Aldunate, R., Volitakis, I., et al., 2009. Intracellular amyloid formation in muscle cells of Aβ-transgenic *Caenorhabditis elegans*: determinants and physiological role in copper detoxification. Mol. Neurodegener. 4, 2.

Monnot, M.J., Babin, P.J., Poleo, G., Andre, M., Laforest, L., Ballagny, C., et al., 1999. Epidermal expression of apolipoprotein E gene during fin and scale development and fin regeneration in zebrafish. Dev. Dyn. 214 (3), 207–215.

Moussavi, N., Chen, M., Martins, R., Verdile, G., et al., 2014. Hypoxia alters expression of Zebrafish Microtubule-associated protein Tau (mapta, maptb) gene transcripts. BMC Res. Notes 7, 767.

Moussavi Nik, S.H., Newman, M., Wilson, L., Ebrahimie, E., Wells, S., Musgrave, I., et al., 2015. Alzheimer's disease-related peptide PS2V plays ancient, conserved roles in suppression of the unfolded protein response under hypoxia and stimulation of gamma-secretase activity. Hum. Mol. Genet. 24 (13).

Moussavi Nik, S.H., Wilson, L., Newman, M., Croft, K., Mori, T.A., Musgrave, I., et al., 2012. The BACE1-PSEN-AβPP regulatory axis has an ancient role in response to low oxygen/oxidative stress. J. Alzheimers Dis. 28 (3), 515–530.

Multhaup, G., Schlicksupp, A., Hesse, L., Beher, D., Ruppert, T., Masters, C.L., et al., 1996. The amyloid precursor protein of Alzheimer's disease in the reduction of copper(II) to copper(I). Science 271 (5254), 1406–1409.

Musa, A., Lehrach, H., Russo, V.A., 2001. Distinct expression patterns of two zebrafish homologues of the human APP gene during embryonic development. Dev. Genes Evol. 211 (11), 563–567.

Myers, E.W., Sutton, G.G., Delcher, A.L., Dew, I.M., Fasulo, D.P., Flanigan, M.J., et al., 2000. A whole-genome assembly of *Drosophila*. Science 287 (5461), 2196–2204.

Nery, L.R., Eltz, N.S., Hackman, C., Fonseca, R., Altenhofen, S., Guerra, H.N., et al., 2014. Brain intraventricular injection of amyloid-beta in zebrafish embryo impairs cognition and increases tau phosphorylation, effects reversed by lithium. PLoS One 9 (9), e105862.

Newman, M., Wilson, L., Camp, E., Verdile, G., Martins, R., Lardelli, M., 2010. A zebrafish melanophore model of amyloid beta toxicity. Zebrafish 7 (2), 155–159.

Newman, M., Wilson, L., Verdile, G., Lim, A., Khan, I., Moussavi Nik, S.H., et al., 2014. Differential, dominant activation and inhibition of Notch signalling and APP cleavage by truncations of PSEN1 in human disease. Hum. Mol. Genet. 23 (3), 602–617.

Nilsberth, C., Westlind-Danielsson, A., Eckman, C.B., Condron, M.M., Axelman, K., Forsell, C., et al., 2001. The 'Arctic' APP mutation (E693G) causes Alzheimer's disease by enhanced Abeta protofibril formation. Nat. Neurosci. 4 (9), 887–893.

Niwa, R., Zhou, F., Li, C., Slack, F.J., 2008. The expression of the Alzheimer's amyloid precursor protein-like gene is regulated by developmental timing microRNAs and their targets in *Caenorhabditis elegans*. Dev. Biol. 315 (2), 418–425.

Nornes, S., Groth, C., Camp, E., Ey, P., Lardelli, M., 2003. Developmental control of Presenilin1 expression, endoproteolysis, and interaction in zebrafish embryos. Exp. Cell Res. 289 (1), 124–132.

Nornes, S., Newman, M., Verdile, G., Wells, S., Stoick-Cooper, C.L., Tucker, B., et al., 2008. Interference with splicing of Presenilin transcripts has potent dominant negative effects on Presenilin activity. Hum. Mol. Genet. 17 (3), 402–412.

Nornes, S., Newman, M., Wells, S., Verdile, G., Martins, R.N., Lardelli, M., 2009. Independent and cooperative action of Psen2 with Psen1 in zebrafish embryos. Exp. Cell Res. 315 (16), 2791–2801.

Nunan, J., Small, D.H., 2000. Regulation of APP cleavage by alpha-, beta- and gamma-secretases. [Review] FEBS Lett. 483 (1), 6–10.

Paquet, D., Bhat, R., Sydow, A., Mandelkow, E.M., Berg, S., Hellberg, S., et al., 2009. A zebrafish model of tauopathy allows in vivo imaging of neuronal cell death and drug evaluation. J. Clin. Invest. 119 (5), 1382–1395.

Periz, G., Fortini, M.E., 2004. Functional reconstitution of gamma-secretase through coordinated expression of presenilin, nicastrin, Aph-1, and Pen-2. J. Neurosci. Res. 77 (3), 309–322.

Pujic, Z., Omori, Y., Tsujikawa, M., Thisse, B., Thisse, C., Malicki, J., 2006. Reverse genetic analysis of neurogenesis in the zebrafish retina. Dev. Biol. 293 (2), 330–347.

Quraishe, S., Cowan, C.M., Mudher, A., 2013. NAP (davunetide) rescues neuronal dysfunction in a *Drosophila* model of tauopathy. Mol. Psychiatry 18 (7), 834–842.

Raymond, P.A., Barthel, L.K., Bernardos, R.L., Perkowski, J.J., 2006. Molecular characterization of retinal stem cells and their niches in adult zebrafish. BMC Dev. Biol. 6, 36.

Reckziegel, P., Chen, P., Caito, S., Gubert, P., Soares, F.A., Fachinetto, R., et al., 2015. Extracellular dopamine and alterations on dopamine transporter are related to reserpine toxicity in *Caenorhabditis elegans*. Arch. Toxicol. 90 (3).

Regitz, C., Dussling, L.M., Wenzel, U., 2014. Amyloid-beta ($A\beta_{1-42}$)-induced paralysis in *Caenorhabditis elegans* is inhibited by the polyphenol quercetin through activation of protein degradation pathways. Mol. Nutr. Food Res. 58 (10), 1931–1940.

Rival, T., Page, R.M., Chandraratna, D.S., Sendall, T.J., Ryder, E., Liu, B., et al., 2009. Fenton chemistry and oxidative stress mediate the toxicity of the beta-amyloid peptide in a *Drosophila* model of Alzheimer's disease. Eur. J. Neurosci. 29 (7), 1335–1347.

Saharia, K., Arya, U., Kumar, R., Sahu, R., Das, C.K., Gupta, K., et al., 2012. Reserpine modulates neurotransmitter release to extend lifespan and alleviate age-dependent Abeta proteotoxicity in *Caenorhabditis elegans*. Exp. Gerontol. 47 (2), 188–197.

Sarantseva, S., Timoshenko, S., Bolshakova, O., Karaseva, E., Rodin, D., Schwarzman, A.L., et al., 2009. Apolipoprotein E-mimetics inhibit neurodegeneration and restore cognitive functions in a transgenic *Drosophila* model of Alzheimer's disease. PLoS One 4 (12), e8191.

Sashidhara, K.V., Modukuri, R.K., Jadiya, P., Dodda, R.P., Kumar, M., Sridhar, B., et al., 2014. Benzofuran-chalcone hybrids as potential multifunctional agents against Alzheimer's disease: synthesis and in vivo studies with transgenic *Caenorhabditis elegans*. ChemMedChem 9 (12), 2671–2684.

Schmid, B., Haass, C., 2013. Genomic editing opens new avenues for zebrafish as a model for neurodegeneration. J. Neurochem. 127 (4), 461–470.

Shen, J., Bronson, R.T., Chen, D.F., Xia, W., Selkoe, D.J., Tonegawa, S., 1997. Skeletal and CNS defects in Presenilin-1-deficient mice. Cell 89 (4), 629–639.

Singh, S.K., Gaur, R., Kumar, A., Fatima, R., Mishra, L., Srikrishna, S., 2014. The flavonoid derivative 2-(4′ Benzyloxyphenyl)-3-hydroxy-chromen-4-one protects against Aβ42-induced neurodegeneration in transgenic *Drosophila*: insights from in silico and in vivo studies. Neurotox. Res. 26 (4), 331–350.

Sofola-Adesakin, O., Castillo-Quan, J.I., Rallis, C., Tain, L.S., Bjedov, I., Rogers, I., et al., 2014. Lithium suppresses Aβ pathology by inhibiting translation in an adult *Drosophila* model of Alzheimer's disease. Front. Aging Neurosci. 6, 190.

Sola, I., Viayna, E., Gomez, T., Galdeano, C., Cassina, M., Camps, P., et al., 2015. Multigram synthesis and in vivo efficacy studies of a novel multitarget anti-Alzheimer's compound. Molecules 20 (3), 4492–4515.

Song, P., Pimplikar, S.W., 2012. Knockdown of amyloid precursor protein in zebrafish causes defects in motor axon outgrowth. PLoS One 7 (4), e34209.

Southon, A., Greenough, M.A., Ganio, G., Bush, A.I., Burke, R., Camakaris, J., 2013. Presenilin promotes dietary copper uptake. PLoS One 8 (5), e62811.

Srivastava, D., Arya, U., SoundaraRajan, T., Dwivedi, H., Kumar, S., Subramaniam, J.R., 2008. Reserpine can confer stress tolerance and lifespan extension in the nematode *C. elegans*. Biogerontology 9 (5), 309–316.

Steinhilb, M.L., Dias-Santagata, D., Mulkearns, E.E., Shulman, J.M., Biernat, J., Mandelkow, E.M., et al., 2007. S/P and T/P phosphorylation is critical for tau neurotoxicity in *Drosophila*. J. Neurosci. Res. 85 (6), 1271–1278.

Stewart, A., Gaikwad, S., Kyzar, E., Green, J., Roth, A., Kalueff, A.V., 2012. Modeling anxiety using adult zebrafish: a conceptual review. Neuropharmacology 62 (1), 135–143.

Stewart, A.M., Braubach, O., Spitsbergen, J., Gerlai, R., Kalueff, A.V., 2014. Zebrafish models for translational neuroscience research: from tank to bedside. Trends Neurosci. 37 (5), 264–278.

Sulston, J.E., Horvitz, H.R., 1977. Post-embryonic cell lineages of the nematode, *Caenorhabditis elegans*. Dev. Biol. 56 (1), 110–156.

Sulston, J.E., Schierenberg, E., White, J.G., Thomson, J.N., 1983. The embryonic cell lineage of the nematode *Caenorhabditis elegans*. Dev. Biol. 100 (1), 64–119.

Sundvik, M., Chen, Y.C., Panula, P., 2013. Presenilin1 regulates histamine neuron development and behavior in zebrafish, danio rerio. J. Neurosci. 33 (4), 1589–1597.

Takahashi, A., Watanabe, T., Fujita, T., Hasegawa, T., Saito, M., Suganuma, M., 2014. Green tea aroma fraction reduces beta-amyloid peptide-induced toxicity in *Caenorhabditis elegans* transfected with human beta-amyloid minigene. Biosci. Biotechnol. Biochem. 78 (7), 1206–1211.

Tingaud-Sequeira, A., Forgue, J., Andre, M., Babin, P.J., 2006. Epidermal transient down-regulation of retinol-binding protein 4 and mirror expression of apolipoprotein Eb and estrogen receptor 2a during zebrafish fin and scale development. Dev. Dyn. 235 (11), 3071–3079.

Toda, T., Sunagawa, T., Kanda, T., Tagashira, M., Shirasawa, T., Shimizu, T., 2011. Apple procyanidins suppress amyloid beta-protein aggregation. Biochem. Res. Int. 2011, 784698.
van de Hoef, D.L., Hughes, J., Livne-Bar, I., Garza, D., Konsolaki, M., Boulianne, G.L., 2009. Identifying genes that interact with *Drosophila presenilin* and amyloid precursor protein. Genesis 47 (4), 246–260.
Wan, L., Nie, G., Zhang, J., Luo, Y., Zhang, P., Zhang, Z., et al., 2011. β-Amyloid peptide increases levels of iron content and oxidative stress in human cell and *Caenorhabditis elegans* models of Alzheimer disease. Free Radic. Biol. Med. 50 (1), 122–129.
Wang, L., Chiang, H.C., Wu, W., Liang, B., Xie, Z., Yao, X., et al., 2012. Epidermal growth factor receptor is a preferred target for treating amyloid-beta-induced memory loss. Proc. Natl. Acad. Sci. U.S.A. 109 (41), 16743–16748.
Wang, Y., Sui, Y., Yu, H., Shen, X., Chen, S., Pei, G., et al., 2015. The combination of aricept with a traditional Chinese medicine formula, smart soup, may be a novel way to treat Alzheimer's disease. J. Alzheimers Dis. 45 (4).
Waterston, R., Sulston, J., 1995. The genome of *Caenorhabditis elegans*. Proc. Natl. Acad. Sci. U.S.A. 92 (24), 10836–10840.
Wei, C.C., Yu, C.W., Yen, P.L., Lin, H.Y., Chang, S.T., Hsu, F.L., et al., 2014. Antioxidant activity, delayed aging, and reduced amyloid-beta toxicity of methanol extracts of tea seed pomace from *Camellia tenuifolia*. J. Agric. Food Chem. 62 (44), 10701–10707.
Wentzell, J.S., Bolkan, B.J., Carmine-Simmen, K., Swanson, T.L., Musashe, D.T., Kretzschmar, D., 2012. Amyloid precursor proteins are protective in *Drosophila* models of progressive neurodegeneration. Neurobiol. Dis. 46 (1), 78–87.
White, A.R., Multhaup, G., Galatis, D., McKinstry, W.J., Parker, M.W., Pipkorn, R., et al., 2002. Contrasting, species-dependent modulation of copper-mediated neurotoxicity by the Alzheimer's disease amyloid precursor protein. J. Neurosci. 22 (2), 365–376.
Wiese, M., Antebi, A., Zheng, H., 2010. Intracellular trafficking and synaptic function of APL-1 in *Caenorhabditis elegans*. PLoS One 5 (9).
Wittenburg, N., Eimer, S., Lakowski, B., Rohrig, S., Rudolph, C., Baumeister, R., 2000. Presenilin is required for proper morphology and function of neurons in *C. elegans*. Nature 406 (6793), 306–309.
Wittmann, C.W., Wszolek, M.F., Shulman, J.M., Salvaterra, P.M., Lewis, J., Hutton, M., et al., 2001. Tauopathy in *Drosophila*: neurodegeneration without neurofibrillary tangles. Science 293 (5530), 711–714.
Wong, P.C., Zheng, H., Chen, H., Becher, M.W., Sirinathsinghji, D.J., Trumbauer, M.E., et al., 1997. Presenilin 1 is required for Notch1 and DII1 expression in the paraxial mesoderm. Nature 387 (6630), 288–292.
Wu, Y., Luo, Y., 2005. Transgenic *C. elegans* as a model in Alzheimer's research. Curr. Alzheimer Res. 2 (1), 37–45.
Wu, Y., Wu, Z., Butko, P., Christen, Y., Lambert, M.P., Klein, W.L., et al., 2006. Amyloid-beta-induced pathological behaviors are suppressed by Ginkgo biloba extract EGb 761 and ginkgolides in transgenic *Caenorhabditis elegans*. J. Neurosci. 26 (50), 13102–13113.
Wu, Z., Du, Y., Xue, H., Wu, Y., Zhou, B., 2012. Aluminum induces neurodegeneration and its toxicity arises from increased iron accumulation and reactive oxygen species (ROS) production. Neurobiol. Aging 33 (1) 199; e1–e12.
Xin, L., Yamujala, R., Wang, Y., Wang, H., Wu, W.H., Lawton, M.A., et al., 2013. Acetylcholineestarase-inhibiting alkaloids from *Lycoris radiata* delay paralysis of amyloid beta-expressing transgenic *C. elegans* CL4176. PLoS One 8 (5), e63874.
Ye, Y., Fortini, M.E., 1999. Apoptotic activities of wild-type and Alzheimer's disease-related mutant presenilins in *Drosophila melanogaster*. J. Cell Biol. 146 (6), 1351–1364.
Zhang, P., Judy, M., Lee, S.J., Kenyon, C., 2013. Direct and indirect gene regulation by a life-extending FOXO protein in *C. elegans*: roles for GATA factors and lipid gene regulators. Cell Metab. 17 (1), 85–100.
Zhao, X.L., Wang, W.A., Tan, J.X., Huang, J.K., Zhang, X., Zhang, B.Z., et al., 2010. Expression of beta-amyloid induced age-dependent presynaptic and axonal changes in *Drosophila*. J. Neurosci. 30 (4), 1512–1522.

CHAPTER

12

Rodent Models for Alzheimer's Disease in Drug Discovery

J.E. Barrett, P. McGonigle

OUTLINE

INTRODUCTION

Alzheimer's disease (AD) is a progressive and, currently, irreversible neurodegenerative condition that has several distinctive histopathological features in the CNS as well as a number of behavioral manifestations, the most prominent of which is cognitive impairment. The histopathological hallmarks of AD in the brain are extracellular deposits of amyloid-β (Aβ) plaques and tau proteins in intracellular neurofibrillary tangles. The accumulation of Aβ and tau begins approximately 15–20 years before the onset of AD dementia (Ising et al., 2015). The development of these pathological changes is associated with neuronal loss and synaptic pruning, along with marked changes in neurotransmitter systems in different brain regions. The behavioral manifestations of these neuropathological developments in the CNS include several features that, in addition to cognitive impairment, may consist of paranoid ideation,

Drug Discovery Approaches for the Treatment of Neurodegenerative Disorders
http://dx.doi.org/10.1016/B978-0-12-802810-0.00012-X

hallucinations, and disruptions in diurnal rhythms, as well as disturbances in anxiety and obsessive compulsive behaviors. The most common form of AD is referred to as sporadic AD, accounting for approximately 99% of cases. To date, no genetic mutations have been directly linked to this form of the disorder; however, expression of the apolipoprotein E4 allele has been established as a significant risk factor. Less than 1% of cases are characterized as familial AD, which has been directly linked to different mutations in the genes for amyloid precursor protein (APP) or presenilin 1 or 2 (PS1, PS2). The familial form exhibits all of the behavioral and pathological hallmarks of sporadic AD and these mutations have been incorporated into transgenic rodents in an effort to create animal models of this disorder. The heterogeneity of this complex disorder, together with its progressive debilitation, pose significant challenges for the development of appropriate animal models, which, in turn, pose significant barriers to the development of effective therapeutics to treat and, more importantly, to eventually prevent AD. This chapter will focus on the use of rodent models of AD in drug discovery, highlighting the diversity of these models and their utility in the preclinical assessment of potential pharmacotherapeutic treatments.

AD is generally a disease of aging, with the incidence highest in individuals over the age of 65. The number of individuals in this category is predicted to grow by over 62% in the next 15 years to approximately 1 billion worldwide (Masters et al., 2015; Qian et al., 2015). In the United States, an estimated 5.1 million people aged 65 or older have AD, with this number projected to increase to nearly 13.8 million by 2050 (Alzheimer's Association, 2015; Qian et al., 2015). Approximately 200,000 individuals under age 65 have early-onset AD. By 2050 it is estimated that every 33 s someone will develop AD, amounting to an increase of over 1 million new cases per year (Alzheimer's Association, 2015). The magnitude of these developments, left unaddressed, represents a significant burden on individuals affected by the disease, the family, caregivers, and society, with a major, potentially catastrophic impact on the health care system. This realization has led to a major effort to discover and develop new therapeutics to treat the symptoms and slow or prevent the progression of the disease.

Unfortunately, over the past two decades the failure rate in clinical trials for drugs to treat AD has been approximately 99.6% (Cummings et al., 2014). Over 200 AD drug candidates evaluated in over 1200 clinical trials have failed to reach approval to treat either the deterioration of the disease or to modify the course of its progression (Becker and Greig, 2012; Cavanaugh et al., 2014). The drugs currently approved to treat AD (donepezil, rivastigmine, galantamine, memantine, and a combination of memantine plus donepezil) are only modestly effective and do not alter the progression of the disease. Of particular relevance to this chapter, many of the drugs introduced into clinical development within the last decade demonstrated efficacy in preclinical animal models but were either not efficacious or had unacceptable side effects in humans. The striking failure rate of potential AD therapeutics raises inevitable questions about the predictive utility of both genetic and behavioral models and whether these approaches are sufficiently sensitive to detect clinical efficacy. It is widely acknowledged that the issues surrounding the validity and predictive utility of animal models are complex, ranging from publication bias to a lack of reproducibility and to whether the clinical trials reflect preclinical assessment (Hackam, 2007; Hackam and Redelmeier, 2006; McGonigle and Ruggeri, 2014; Pound and Bracken, 2014; Van der Worp et al., 2010). The sources of potential variability are extensive and a number of suggestions have been made to address and control some of these variables (eg, Bales, 2012; Justice and Dhillon, 2016; Zeiss, 2015).

This chapter will review the principal approaches using rodent models that have been developed to examine drugs to treat AD and will attempt to highlight the major issues confronting the field with a view toward providing a basis for approaching the many challenges that face this important area of research.

OVERVIEW OF ANIMAL MODELS OF ALZHEIMER'S DISEASE

The vexing issue of developing valid translational approaches based on robust and predictive preclinical rodent models, whether for AD or other neurodegenerative and neuropsychiatric disorders, has captured significant attention and concern for which, at the present time, no definitive solutions are available (McGonigle and Ruggeri, 2014). Some have suggested that, in light of the complex issues that are faced by these challenges, animal disease models should be skipped altogether and replaced with mechanism-based biomarkers in nondisease models (Tsukamoto, 2016). These biomarkers would include drug exposure at the target site of action necessary to elicit a pharmacological effect and binding to the pharmacological target together with the expression of pharmacological activity (see Morgan et al., 2012 for the "three pillars of survival" to phase II clinical development)—all directed at developing an integrated understanding of the fundamental pharmacokinetic/pharmacodynamic principles of drug exposure and target engagement that can be related to pharmacological activity. Although these approaches may be of value, it is undeniably important also to examine critically and in greater detail the use of animal models in the drug discovery process before abandoning their use.

A large number of approaches have been undertaken to mimic AD-like cognitive deficits in rodent models. The nongenetic methods employed have included lesions in specific regions of the brain believed to play a role in cognition, pharmacological models, and neurotoxins, with many of these approaches directed mainly toward manipulations of the cholinergic system. The cholinergic hypothesis of AD, in which acetylcholine was linked to AD because of the loss of cholinergic neurons in the basal ganglia (Davies and Maloney, 1976), was a significant influence in driving the majority of the early pharmacological efforts to examine the role of the cholinergic system in AD. Scopolamine-induced deficits in cognitive tasks were commonly used to examine the effects of various compounds to attenuate those deficits (Bartus et al., 1982; Craig et al., 2011; Van Dam and De Deyn, 2011). Although these various approaches provided insight into the involvement of the cholinergic system in cognitive dysfunction, there are several recognized shortcomings of these approaches. Among the most prominent have been concerns that, unlike AD, these models were relatively static and nonprogressive. Additionally, these approaches could not reproduce the fact that multiple systems are involved in AD and do not reproduce the full pathology of the disease. Despite these limitations, the majority of the drugs currently approved to treat AD (see earlier) work through the acetylcholinergic system. It has been known that there are interactions between the cholinergic system and Aβ, as has been demonstrated in a few studies where it has been found that, following cholinergic denervation and degeneration of this system in APP/PS1 or in APPswe/PS1dE9 transgenic mouse models of AD, there is an enhanced deposition of Aβ and amyloid plaques that is followed by cognitive impairment (Laursen et al., 2013; Ramos-Rodriguez et al., 2013).

In addition to the use of pharmacological models that focus on the role of the cholinergic system in AD, a number of studies have examined the effects of Aβ infusion models to mimic more closely the histopathological sequelae, toxic insults, and cognitive impairment associated with AD. These studies have used direct intracerebral injections of Aβ into different brain regions and, although generally producing cognitive dysfunction and some AD pathology, there are wide inconsistencies in the outcomes. Some of the variables contributing to the variability of results include the species of peptide used (eg, $A\beta_{1-40}$, $A\beta_{1-42}$, or $A\beta_{25-35}$), the aggregation state of the peptide, site of the infusion, as well as the interval between administration of the peptide and the behavioral assessment. Additionally, the concentrations of administered Aβ are typically much higher than those found in the brain or spinal fluid of AD patients, rendering the results of some of the studies difficult to interpret (Van Dam and De Deyn, 2011). Importantly, when attempting to challenge these models pharmacologically, as would be performed in preclinical studies focusing on compounds in development, it may be difficult to translate the results to the clinic because of the differences in these levels and the concentrations of the test compound required to produce meaningful effects. The rodent Aβ infusion models do, however, provide some advantages over transgenic rodent models. First, they induce some of the changes associated with Aβ deposition in humans, such as inflammation and microglial activation. Second, they do not require the lengthy time intervals to await plaque development that are associated with transgenic approaches, nor do they induce other changes in APP fragments that can occur following APP overexpression where APP overexpression may have neuroprotective or neurotoxic effects that can influence the outcome assessments.

GENETICALLY MODIFIED RODENT MODELS OF ALZHEIMER'S DISEASE

It is well known that aging rodents do not spontaneously develop histopathological hallmarks of AD. Although these animals may be of use to study cognitive decline associated with aging, they are of little use with regard to pharmacological studies directed toward preventing or attenuating the signature histopathological hallmarks of the disease. The discovery in the 1990s that specific gene mutations contributed to the development of familial forms of AD, coupled to the advances in molecular genetics, led to several efforts to develop a wide variety of transgenic mice to model this disease. Some of these transgenic models produce excess Aβ or promote the development of neurofibrillary tangles while others develop both forms of pathological changes in the CNS (see reviews by Gidyk et al., 2015; Webster et al., 2014). There are a wide variety of transgenic rodent models that have been developed to study AD that are based on the expression of one or more proteins carrying one or more mutations directly linked to familial AD (Table 12.1). The ability to develop transgenic models of AD was first reported by Games et al. (1995) with the PDAPP model that was followed by the Tg2576 (Hsiao et al., 1996) and the APP23 mouse models (Stürchler-Pierrat et al.,1997). The PDAPP model expresses human APP carrying the Indiana familial AD mutation (V717F) that is driven by the platelet-derived growth factor-β promoter. The Tg2576 and APP23 models also express human APP but with the Swedish mutation (K670N/M671L) that is driven by the hamster prion protein and the murine Thy-1 promoter, respectively (Van Dam and

TABLE 12.1 Notable Rodent Models of Alzheimer's

Model	Transgene	Pathology	Behavior	References
MOUSE				
PDAPP	hAPP Ind	Formation of Aβ plaques at 6–9 months	Learning and memory deficits apparent at 6 months	Games et al. (1995)
Tg2576	hAPP Swe	Formation of Aβ plaques at 9 months, activated microglia, decreased cholinergic and adrenergic neurons	Deficits in working and spatial memory, contextual and cued conditioning at 10 months	Holcomb et al. (1998)
APP/PS1	hAPP Swe hPS1dE9	Formation of Aβ plaques at 6 months, activated microglia, decrease in adrenergic neurons, females develop plaques before males	Deficits in working and spatial memory at 6 months	Jankowsky et al. (2004)
3xTg	hAPP Swe hMapt (P301L) hPsen1 (M146V)	Formation of Aβ plaques at 6 months, activated microglia, hyperphosphorylated tau, neurofibrillary tangles	Deficits in working and spatial memory at 4.5 months	Oddo et al. (2003)
5xFAD	hAPP Swe, Fl, Lon hPsen1 (M146L, L286V)	Formation of Aβ in 2 months, activated microglia, loss of cholinergic and adrenergic neurons	Deficits in working and spatial memory at 6 months	Oakley et al. (2006)
RAT				
PSAPP	hAPP695 Swe, Lon hPSEN1 (M146V)	Formation of Aβ, activated microglia, hyperphosphorylated tau	Deficits in long-term potentiation as well as spatial and working memory	Flood et al. (2009)
McGill-R-Thy1-APP	hAPP751 Swe, Ind	Formation of Aβ at 6–9 months	Deficits in spatial and working memory	Leon et al. (2010)
Tgf344-AD	hAPP695 Swe hPsen1dEp	Formation of Aβ, activated microglia, hyperphosphorylated tau, neurofibrillary tangle, neuronal loss, brain shrinkage	Deficits in working and spatial memory	Cohen et al. (2013)

De Deyn, 2011). All three of these models have provided support for the amyloid hypothesis insofar as they each display progressive diffuse and neuritic Aβ deposition as well as synaptic and neurotransmitter alterations along with cognitive deficits. Although these features represent several of the conditions paralleling human AD, a serious limitation of these models is that they lack the neurofibrillary tangles that are characteristic of AD.

These initial developments have been followed by several other transgenic models including the introduction of early-onset mutations in the presenilin (PSEN) genes but these models (PSEN1 and PSEN2) also have not demonstrated the presence of neurofibrillary tangles nor have they shown robust cognitive impairment or significant plaque pathology. In combination, as a double transgenic with APP, however, this double transgenic APP/PSEN has demonstrated accelerated Aβ pathology that includes neuronal loss, inflammation, and cognitive decline (McGowan et al., 2006; Van Dam and De Deyn, 2006); however, these models also do not develop neurofibrillary tangles, a shortcoming that was partially overcome by the development of mice with mutated human tau that were crossed with the APP model. Although these mice showed enhanced amyloid deposition along with tau phosphorylation, the formation of neurofibrillary-like tangles, and neuronal loss, these mice lacked the colocalization of plaques and neurofibrillary tangles in the relevant brain regions, including the hippocampus and the cortex (Van Dam and De Deyn, 2011). These issues were addressed by the subsequent development of a triple-transgenic mouse model (3xTg) harboring $PS1_{M146V}$, APP_{Swe}, and tau_{P301L} transgenic (Dodo et al., 2003). Rather than crossing independent lines, this model was derived by directly introducing two additional transgenes into single-cell embryos from homozygous $PS1_{M146V}$ knockin mice. This approach generated mice with the same genetic background as the 3xTg mice, progressively developing extracellular Aβ deposits prior to the formation of neurofibrillary tangles, a result consistent with the amyloid cascade hypothesis. These mice also had deficits in synaptic plasticity that included those of long-term potentiation while also demonstrating the neuropathological lesions in the hippocampus, amygdala, and cerebral cortex, those structures most affected in AD.

According to the Alzheimer's Forum (http://www.alzforum.org/research-models) there are over 118 models of AD. Although it is not possible to provide a comprehensive review of all these models, and many are not extensively characterized, it does seem worthwhile elucidating the distinctive characteristics of some of the more salient models. The various models differ in a number of dimensions that include the temporal progression of the disease as well as in the development of associated CNS pathology and cognitive symptoms (see reviews by Cavanaugh et al., 2014; Onos et al., 2016; Puzzo et al., 2015; Webster et al., 2014). For instance, Oakley et al. (2006) have developed a transgenic mouse based on five familial mutations with this mouse developing cerebral amyloid plaques and gliosis at 2 months of age, much faster development of this pathology than most other transgenic models. The differences in transgenic models have been elucidated most clearly in a very comprehensive review by Webster et al. (2014), who provide a detailed analysis of the progression of memory deficits in several different mouse strains of AD and in a number of different procedures to assess cognitive function. This analysis provides a number of very interesting differences in the various mouse strains that have been most frequently employed to examine the cognitive deficits. For example, one of the most consistent findings in cognitive impairment has been seen in procedures using fear conditioning where 4 of the 5 mouse strains that were examined with this procedure all demonstrated impairment. However, the age at which these impairments were manifested ranged from 1–2 months of age in the APP+PS1 strain, 3–5 months in the 5Xfad strain, to 6–8 months in the APP/PS1 and 3xtgADD strains. Thus there is considerable variability in this single measure of cognitive impairment among the different genetic strains of mice. It is also worth noting that these deficits in cognition followed the development of diffuse amyloid plaques for most of the strains by approximately 1 month with the exception of the APP/PS1 strain. In this strain, the onset of cognitive impairment in the fear-conditioning procedure occurred at 1–2 months of age, preceding the development of plaques that did not develop until 6–8 months of age. For the Tg2576 strain, the impairment in fear conditioning occurred at 3–5 months with the appearance of plaques occurring between 9 and 11 months of age. Thus there exists a wide degree of variability between the onset of neuronal pathology and the impairment in some cognitive tasks.

These authors also compared memory deficits in the Morris water maze (MWM) procedure where there was much more variability in cognitive impairment (Webster et al., 2014). For instance, the APP/PS1 demonstrated impairment in MWM at the same age as impairments occurred in the fear-conditioning procedure. By comparison, the APP+PS1 mice, although showing deficits in the fear-conditioning procedure at 1–2 months of age did not demonstrate impairment in the MWM until 6–8 months of age or later. Although these data must be interpreted with caution because many of these comparisons were made from different laboratories and with likely idiosyncrasies in the specific procedures employed, they do point out that the selection of particular strains of mice and the procedures to be employed must be done with great caution (see points later about the different strains carrying the *rd-1* allele and the effects this has on visual impairment that might account for some of the variability in the MWM). Although difficult, it would be ideal to have each AD strain evaluated in each of the procedures and to have these experiments conducted in the same laboratory.

Rats offer several advantages over mice as a rodent model of AD. They are physiologically, genetically, and morphologically closer to humans, possess a richer behavioral repertoire, and exhibit more complex social behavior (Jacob and Kwitek, 2002; DoCarmo and Cuello, 2013). Moreover, rats express all six isoforms of tau that are expressed in human neurons in contrast to mice that only express three (Hanes et al., 2009; McMillan et al., 2008). However, because of technical limitations such as the difficulty in producing viable rat embryonic stem cells (Tong et al., 2010) and practical limitations such as the length of gestation, the development of transgenic rat models of AD has lagged the development of mouse models. The first transgenic rat line was a double transgenic generated by Flood et al. (2003) that contained mutations in APP (K670N/M671L and V717F) and PS1 (M146V). Characterization of this line revealed the robust development of amyloid plaques in the hippocampus by 9 months, activated microglia, tau hyperphosphorylation, and deficits in spatial learning and memory (Liu et al., 2008); however, there was no neurofibrillary pathology or neuronal loss (Liu et al., 2008; Flood et al., 2009). Subsequently, the McGill-R-Thy1-APP rat was developed containing only human APP751 with the Swedish and Indiana mutations (Leon et al., 2010). This single transgene results in the accumulation of amyloid plaques, microglia, and spatial learning and memory deficits but no neurofibrillary pathology (Leon et al., 2010). More recently, the bigenic TgF344-AD rat expressing human APP695 with the Swedish mutation and PS1dE9 was developed (Cohen et al., 2013). This line develops age-related accumulation of Aβ, abundant oligomeric soluble Aβ, activated microglia, neurofibrillary tangles, neuronal loss, and cognitive impairment. Consequently, it appears to be the first rodent transgenic model that exhibits the full spectrum of age-dependent AD pathologies along with cognitive deficits (Cohen et al., 2013). It has been reported that a three-dimensional human neuronal cell culture model of AD produced by transfection with APP containing the Swedish and London mutations along with PS1dE9 exhibited Aβ accumulation and tauopathy that were both inhibited by treatment with a β or γ-secretase inhibitor (Choi et al., 2014). While much additional research needs to be done, this result provides additional support for the beta-amyloid hypothesis of AD and potential utility of the Tg344-AD rat as a model of AD in which to evaluate candidate therapeutics.

There have been additional efforts and suggestions to bring nontransgenic rat models more into the preclinical research area for pharmacological and behavioral assessments with the view that the rat has been relatively neglected as a tool for drug discovery in AD research (Lecanu and Papadopoulos, 2013). Exploration of different strains, together with the incorporation of aged rats, would appear to be of value because aged rats can provide a tractable model to examine the neurobiology and other pathological changes associated with age-related cognitive decline even though they do not develop AD pathology (Braidy et al., 2015; Rowe et al., 2007).

In attempting to make comparisons across the different transgenic strains as well as across the different behavioral procedures, it is clear that there are a number of key issues that should be acknowledged and addressed. Zeiss (2015) has provided a very insightful analysis of a large number of models that have been used to examine preclinical drug candidates for AD. In a number of cases, a precise definition of the rodent model, particularly those involving genetic manipulations in mice, was rarely provided. As one example, the widely used mouse APP/PS1 model, which has been used in over 24% of the studies using AD animal models, actually represents four different models. Although the model nomenclature defining the mutant allele was typically provided in the methods or reference sections, the background strain was rarely described. Zeiss noted that of the 16 strains that were analyzed, roughly comprising about 80% of those animals used in AD preclinical studies, eight of those strains carried the *rd-1* allele, an autosomal recessive allele that results in the degeneration of photoreceptors and causes blindness by 6–8 weeks of age. In light of the fact that many of the procedures used to assess cognitive impairment (eg, the MWM) rely on visually guided cues, these deficits could be quite independent of any specific AD-related pathology. These models are not the only ones known to harbor mutations that result in eye abnormalities with the general conclusion from this analysis being that 55% of the interventional studies using AD models in 2013 were conducted in populations potentially carrying mutations that impair vision and which, depending on the particular behavioral assay, could confound results. In summary, it is exceptionally difficult to compare the results of experiments using diverse transgenic models because of the variation in the strains and in the locus of AD pathology, and because some of the strains harbor background information potentially detrimental to or confounding the results.

It is certainly tempting to conclude on the basis of the limitations just described and the aforementioned failure rate in clinical trials that transgenic animal models of AD have little or no predictive utility. Before discarding these models, however, it is important to consider the complexity of clinical trials for AD and the challenge of designing a study that is truly definitive. For example, virtually all of the transgenic animal models are based on mutations found in autosomal dominant familial forms of AD that represent less than 1% of the AD patient population (Bekris et al., 2010). To date, only a very limited number of trials have been carried out exclusively in patients with the autosomal dominant form of AD, suggesting that the mismatch between the basis for the animal models and the treatment population may contribute to the lack of success. Another obvious discrepancy between the animal models and the human disorder is the time required for the pathology to produce behavioral symptoms. Animal models typically exhibit cognitive impairment between 1 and 6 months after the emergence of plaques and/or tangles, whereas clinical symptoms typically do not appear until 10–15 years after initial increases in Aβ (Selkoe and Hardy, 2016). Moreover, even after initial appearance, the cognitive decline is typically gradual and develops over multiple years leading to considerable uncertainty about how long to treat, when to initiate treatment, and when to anticipate measurable changes. What to measure is another confounding issue because it is well known that behavioral endpoints are notoriously variable and difficult to quantify but no surrogate biomarkers have been validated. Recent progress has been made in the development of imaging agents to measure some pathological hallmarks of AD that hold promise for use as diagnostic and pharmacodynamic measures (DeClercq et al., 2016). Moreover, a noncompetitive consortium of public and private organizations is pooling resources to address this issue (Carrillo et al., 2013). On the basis of these observations, it seems reasonable to conclude that the predictive validity of transgenic animal models has not been adequately tested and it would seem advisable to withhold final judgment on their utility in AD drug discovery and development until more definitive clinical trials are carried out.

INTEGRATION OF ALZHEIMER'S DISEASE MODELS AND BEHAVIORAL ANALYSES IN DRUG DISCOVERY

A wide variety of behavioral procedures have been used in conjunction with various transgenic models to evaluate potential new therapeutics for the treatment of AD. We will not provide an extensive review of this research, some of which has been mentioned in the preceding sections of this chapter, because there are multiple sources available for this information (Puzzo et al., 2014, 2015; Webster et al., 2014). Instead, we will highlight some of the more frequently used procedures, with a focus on their translational value. In addition to the use of behavioral assays in evaluating transgenic models as well as new therapeutics, it is also important to acknowledge the utility of other procedures, such as electrophysiological measures to analyze synaptic transmission and long-term potentiation (Sant'Angelo et al., 2003), as well as the use of in vivo two-photon imaging (Busche et al., 2015) and optogenetic techniques (Roy et al., 2016). These procedures, in conjunction with appropriate behavioral analyses, can provide additional insight into the evaluation of AD pathology as well as on the potential utility of targeted pharmacological interventions.

The primary behavioral procedures used to assess pathological impairment and to evaluate new compounds to treat AD are summarized in Table 12.2. As pointed out in earlier sections of this chapter, not all transgenic mouse models have been examined in each of these procedures, nor have all compounds that have been put forth into clinical development. In addition, the time at which these assays are conducted plays an important role in assessing the effects on cognition, particularly as the models each develop plaque pathology and other CNS effects at different time points. An important question about the measures of cognitive performance and Aβ levels is whether there is a relationship between these two critical parameters. Foley et al. (2015) performed a systematic review of 40 different transgenic AD mouse articles on the relationship between Aβ levels and measures of cognitive deficit in five different transgenic mouse lines [Tg2756, APP, PS1, 3xTg, and APP(OSK)-Tg], and also included analyses of gender and age. The behavioral assays consisted of escape latency times in the MWM or exploration of novel objects in the novel object recognition task (Table 12.2). Generally, although there was somewhat of a trend in the outcome of these studies, Foley et al. found that there was no statistically significant correlation between quantified Aβ levels and outcome measures of cognitive function.

TABLE 12.2 Behavioral Procedures to Assess Cognitive Function and Pharmacological Effects

Behavioral Procedure	Brief Description
Contextual fear conditioning	An environmental context or stimulus is associated initially with an electric shock and subsequent exposure to that context or stimulus is evaluated using freezing as the measure of prior learning.
Morris water maze	A small platform is placed below the surface of a circular pool of water that cannot be detected because of a substance added to the water. Location of the platform is typically provided by cues located outside the maze and finding the platform permits escape from the need to swim. Measures of time taken to find the platform are typically conducted over a number of days.
Novel object recognition	Rodents are exposed to and permitted to explore two objects that are identical and then, following a delay that can range from minutes to hours, are reexposed to one of the identical objects plus a novel object. Because rodents tend to explore novel objects, the time exploring the two objects provides a measure of retention over time.
Radial arm maze	This maze typically has a number of arms (6–8) radiating out from a central portion. Usually one of the arms contains a food reward and the task is to demonstrate learning to locate that reward. This maze is occasionally submerged under water and food is replaced by a platform that provides escape.

CONCLUSIONS

The urgency to discover effective therapeutics to prevent the onset of AD as well as to treat its occurrence is considerable. However, as imperfect as the rodent models of AD may be, at the present time it is inconceivable that the discovery of new drugs to treat this devastating disorder will not incorporate animal models into their preclinical assessment. The judicious use of transgenic rodent models that recapitulate the pathological CNS hallmarks of the disease together with the use of appropriate behavioral as well as other procedures is essential. The use of these approaches has, unquestionably, provided valuable information about the role of Aβ and tau in neuronal pathology and cognitive impairment, and about the impact of these neurodegenerative conditions on cognition and other measures associated with AD. Without the extensive analysis of these models and their incorporation into the drug discovery and development process, we would not be in a position to address many of the questions that have arisen from these studies. Based on the presently available information, a single transgenic model and a unitary behavioral phenotype is likely to be insufficient to provide the level of comfort needed to translate those findings into clinical development. The variability in both the pathology and behavior noted in the different transgenic mouse models is strongly influenced by the specific mutation, the promoter, and the expression levels in addition to the genetic background of the mouse. The role of gender on these models is notably absent, particularly in light of the fact that the incidence of AD is higher in females than in males. It has been demonstrated using transgenic Tg2576 mice that the amount of Aβ pathology is markedly influenced by mouse gender (Callahan et al., 2001). In this study, plaque load at 15 and 19 months was significantly greater in female than in male mice. This observation points to the importance of gender in amyloid production/deposition and highlights the need to take this variable into account in the design of studies carried out to examine both behavioral and pharmacological effects.

References

Alzheimer's Association, 2015. Alzheimer's disease facts and figures. Alzheimers Dement. 11, 332–384.

Bales, K.R., 2012. The value and limitations of transgenic mouse models used in drug discovery for Alzheimer's disease: an update. Expert Opin. Drug Discov. 7, 281–297.

Bartus, R.T., Dean, R.L., Beer, B., Lippa, A.S., 1982. The cholinergic hypothesis of geriatric memory dysfunction. Science 217, 408–414.

Becker, R.E., Greig, N.H., 2012. Increasing the success rate for Alzheimer's disease drug discovery and development. Expert Opin. Drug Discov. 7, 367–370.

Bekris, L., Yu, C.-E., Bird, T.D., Tsuang, D.W., 2010. Genetics of Alzheimer's disease. J. Geriatr. Psychiatry 23, 213–227.

Braidy, N., Poljak, A., Jayasena, T., Mansour, H., Inestrosa, N.C., Sachdev, P.S., 2015. Accelerating Alzheimer's research through 'natural' animal models. Curr. Opin. Psychiatry 28, 155–164.

Busche, M.A., Grienberger, C., Keskin, A.D., Song, B., Neumann, U., Staufenbiel, M., et al., 2015. Decreased amyloid-β and increased neuronal hyperactivity by immunotherapy in Alzheimer's models. Nat. Neurosci. 18, 1725–1727.

Callahan, M.J., Lipinski, W.J., Bian, F., Durham, R.A., Pack, A., Walker, L.C., 2001. Augmented senile plaque load in aged female beta-amyloid precursor protein-transgenic mice. Am. J. Pathol. 158, 1173–1177.

Carrillo, M.C., Blennow, K., Soares, H., Lewczuk, P., Mattsson, N., Oberoi, P., Umek, R., Vandijck, M., Salamone, S., Bittner, T., Shaw, L.M., Stephenson, D., Bain, L., Zetterberg, H., 2013. Global standardization measurement of cerebral spinal fluid for Alzheimer's disease: an update from the Alzheimer's Association Global Biomarkers Consortium. Alzheimers Dement. 9, 137–140.

Cavanaugh, S.E., Pippin, J.J., Barnard, N.D., 2014. Animal models of Alzheimer disease: historical pitfalls and a path forward. ALTEX 31, 279–302.

Choi, S.H., Kim, Y.H., Hebisch, M., Sliwinski, C., Lee, S., D'Avanzi, C., Chen, H., Hooli, B., Asselin, C., Muffat, J., Klee, J.B., Zhang, C., Wainger, B.J., Peitz, M., Kovacs, D.M., Woolf, C.J., Wagner, S.L., Tanzi, R.E., Kim, D.Y., 2014. A three-dimensional human neural cell culture model of Alzheimer's disease. Nature 515, 274–278.

Cohen, R.M., Rezai-Zadeh, K., Weitz, T.M., Rentsendorj, A., Gate, D., Spivak, I., Bholat, Y., Vasilevko, V., Glabe, C.G., Breunig, J.J., Rakic, P., Davtyan, H., Agadjanyan, M.G., Kepe, V., Bario, J.R., Bannykh, S., Szekely, C.A., Pechnick, R.N., Town, T., 2013. A transgenic Alzheimer rat with plaques, tau pathology, behavioral impairment, Oligomeric Aβ, and frank neuronal loss. J. Neurosci. 33, 6245–6256.

Craig, L.A., Hong, N.S., McDonald, R.J., 2011. Revisiting the cholinergic hypothesis in the development of Alzheimer's disease. Neurosci. Biobehav. Rev. 35, 1397–1409.

Cummings, J.L., Morstorf, T., Zhong, K., 2014. Alzheimer's disease drug-development pipeline: few candidates, frequent failures. Alzheimers Res. Ther. 6 (4), 37.

Davies, P., Maloney, A.J., 1976. Selective loss of central cholinergic neurons in Alzheimer's disease. Lancet 308, 1403.

DeClercq, L.D., Vandenberghe, R., Van Laere, K., Verbruggen, A., Bormans, G., 2016. Drug development in Alzheimer's disease: the contribution of PET and SPECT. Front. Pharmacol. http://dx.doi.org/10.3389/fphar.2016.00088.

DoCarmo, S., Cuello, A.C., 2013. Modelling Alzheimer's disease in transgenic rats. Mol. Neurodegener. 8, 37–48.

Flood, D.G., et al., 2003. Abeta Deposition in a Transgenic Rat Model of Alzheimer's Disease. Society for Neuroscience, Washington, DC.

Flood, D.G., Lin, Y.G., Lang, D.M., Trusko, S.P., Hirsch, J.D., Savage, M.J., Scott, R.W., Howland, D.S., 2009. A transgenic rat model of Alzheimer's disease with extracellular Abeta deposition. Neurobiol. Aging 30, 1078–1090.

Foley, A.M., Zmmar, Z.M., Lee, R.H., Mitchell, C., 2015. Systematic review of the relationship between amyloid-β levels and measures of transgenic mouse cognitive deficit in Alzheimer's disease. J. Alzheimer's Dis. 44, 787–795.

Games, D., Adams, D., Alessandrini, R., Barbour, R., Berthelette, P., Blackwell, C., et al., 1995. Alzheimer-type neuropathology in transgenic mice overexpressing V717F β-amyloid precursor protein. Nature 373, 523–527.

Gidyk, D.C., Deibel, S.H., Hong, N.S., McDonald, R.J., 2015. Barriers to developing a valid rodent model of Alzheimer's disease: from behavioral analysis to etiological mechanisms. Front. Neurosci. 9, 245.

Hackam, D.G., 2007. Translating animal research into clinical benefit. BMJ 334, 163–164.

Hackam, D.G., Redelmeier, D.A., 2006. Translation of research evidence from animals to humans. JAMA 296, 1731–1732.

Hanes, J., Zilka, N., Bartkova, M., Caletkova, M., Dobrota, D., Novak, M., 2009. Rat tau proteome consists of six tau isoforms: implication for animal models of human tauopathies. J. Neurochem. 108, 1167–1176.

Hsiao, K., Chapman, P., Nilsen, S., Eckman, C., Harigaya, Y., Younkin, S., et al., 1996. Correlative memory deficits, Abeta elevation and amyloid plaques in transgenic mice. Science 274, 99–103.
Holcomb, L., Gordon, M.N., McGowan, E., Yu, X., Benkovic, S., Jantzen, P., Wright, K., Saad, I., Mueller, R., Morgan, D., Sanders, S., Zehr, C., O'Campo, K., Hardy, J., Prada, C.M., Eckman, C., Younkin, S., Hsiao, K., Duff, K., 1998. Accelerated Alzheimer-type phenotype in transgenic mice carrying both mutant amyloid precursor protein and presenilin 1 transgenes. Nat. Med. 4, 97–100.
Ising, C., Stanley, M., Holtzman, D.M., 2015. Current thinking on the mechanistic basis of Alzheimer's and implications for drug development. Clin. Pharmacol. Ther. 98, 469–471.
Jacob, H.J., Kwitek, A.E., 2002. Rat genetics: attaching physiology and pharmacology to the genome. Nat. Rev. Genet. 3, 33–42.
Jankowsky, J.L., Fadale, D.J., Anderson, J., Xu, G.M., Gonzales, V., Jenkins, N.A., Copeland, N.G., Lee, M.K., Younkin, L.H., Wagner, S.L., Younkin, S.G., Borchelt, D.R., 2004. Mutant presenilins specifically elevate the levels of the 42 residue beta-amyloid peptide in vivo: evidence for augmentation of a 42-specific gamma secretase. Hum. Mol. Genet. 13, 159–170.
Justice, M.J., Dhillon, P., 2016. Using the mouse to model human disease: increasing validity and reproducibility. Dis. Model Mech. 9, 101–103.
Laursen, B., Mork, A., Plath, N., Kristiansen, U., Bastlund, J.F., 2013. Cholinergic degeneration is associated with increased plaque deposition and cognitive impairment in APPswe/PS1dE9 mice. Behav. Brain Res. 240, 146–152.
Lecanu, L., Papadopoulos, V., 2013. Modeling Alzheimer's disease with non-transgenic rat models. Alzheimer's Res. Ther. 5, 17.
Leon, W.C., Canneva, F., Partridge, V., Allard, S., Ferretti, M.T., DeWilde, A., Vercauteren, F., Atifeh, R., Ducatenzeiler, A., Klein, W., Szyf, M., Alhonen, L., Cuello, A.C., 2010. A novel transgenic rat model with a full Alzheimer's-like amyloid pathology displays pre-plaque intracellular amyloid-beta-associated cognitive impairment. J. Alzheimer's Dis. 20, 113–126.
Liu, L., Orozco, I.J., Planel, E., Wen, Y., Bretteville, A., Krishnamurthy, P., Wang, L., Herman, M., Figueroa, H., Yu, W.H., Arancio, O., Duff, K., 2008. A transgenic rat that develops Alzheimer's disease-like amyloid pathology, deficits in synaptic plasticity and cognitive impairment. Neurobiol. Dis. 31, 46–57.
Masters, C.L., Bateman, R., Blennow, K., Rowe, C.C., Sperling, R.A., Cummings, J.L., 2015. Alzheimer's disease. Nat. Rev. Dis. Primers Article No. 15056.
McGonigle, P., Ruggeri, B., 2014. Animal models of human disease: challenges in enabling translation. Biochem. Pharmacol. 87, 162–171.
McGowan, E., Eriksen, J., Hutton, M., 2006. A decade of modeling Alzheimer's disease in transgenic mice. Trends Genet. 22, 281–289.
McMillan, P., Korvatska, E., Poorkaj, P., Evstafjeva, Z., Robinson, L., Greenup, L., Leverenz, J., Schellenberg, G.D., D'Souza, I., 2008. Tau isoform regulation is region- and cell-specific in mouse brain. J. Comp. Neurol. 511, 788–803.
Morgan, P., Van der Graaf, P.H., Arrowsmith, J., Feltner, D.E., Drummond, K.S., Wegner, C.D., et al., 2012. Can the flow of medicines be improved? Fundamental pharmacokinetic and pharmacological principles toward improving Phase II survival. Drug Discov. Today 17, 419–424.
Oakley, H., Cole, S.L., Logan, S., Maus, E., Shao, P., Craft, J., et al., 2006. Intraneuronal beta-amyloid aggregates, neurodegeneration, and neuron loss in transgenic mice with five familial Alzheimer's disease mutations: potential factors in amyloid plaque formation. J. Neurosci. 26, 10129–10140.
Oddo, S., Caccamo, A., Shepherd, J.D., Murphy, M.P., Golde, T.E., Kayed, R., et al., 2003. Triple-transgenic model of Alzheimer's disease with plaques and tangles: intracellular Aβ and synaptic dysfunction. Neuron 39, 409–421.
Onos, K.D., Rizzo, S.J., Howell, G.R., Sasner, M., 2016. Toward more predictive genetic mouse models of Alzheimer's disease. Brain Res. Bull. 122, 1–11.
Pound, P., Bracken, M.G., 2014. Is animal research sufficiently evidence based to be a cornerstone of biomedical research? BMJ 348, g3387.
Puzzo, D., Gulisano, W., Palmeri, A., Arancio, O., 2015. Rodent models for Alzheimer's disease drug discovery. Expert Opin. Drug Discov. 10, 703–711.
Puzzo, D., Lee, L., Palmeri, A., Calabrese, G., Arancio, O., 2014. Behavioral assays with mouse models of Alzheimer's disease: practical considerations and guidelines. Biochem. Pharmacol. 88, 450–467.
Qian, X., Hamad, B., Dias-Lalcaca, G., 2015. The Alzheimer's disease market. Nat. Rev. Drug Discov. 14, 675–676.

Ramos-Rodriguez, J.J., Pacheco-Herrero, M., Thyssen, D., Murillo-Carretero, M.I., Berrocoso, E., Spires-Jones, T.L., Bacskai, B.J., Garcia-Alloza, M., 2013. Rapid [beta]-amyloid deposition and cognitive impairment after cholinergic denervation in APP/PS1 mice. J. Neuropathol. Exp. Neurol. 72, 272–285.

Rowe, W., Blalock, E., Chen, K., Kadish, I., Wang, D., Barrett, J.E., Porter, N., Rose, G., Landfield, P., 2007. Hippocampal expression analyses reveal selective association of immediate-early, neuroenergetic, and myelinogenic pathways with cognitive impairment in aged rats. J. Neurosci. 27, 3098–3110.

Roy, D.S., Arons, A., Mitchell, T.I., Pignatelli, M., Ryan, T.J., Tonegawa, S., 2016. Memory retrieval by activating engram cells in mouse models of early Alzheimer's disease. Nature 531, 508–512.

Sant'Angelo, A., Trinchese, F., Arancio, O., 2003. Usefulness of behavioral and electrophysiological studies in transgenic models of Alzheimer's disease. Neurochem. Res. 28, 1009–1015.

Selkoe, D.J., Hardy, J., 2016. The amyloid hypothesis of Alzheimer's disease at 25 years. EMBO. http://dx.doi.org/10.15252/emmm.201606210.

Stürchler-Pierrat, C., Abramowski, D., Duke, M., Wiederhold, K.H., Mistl, C., Rothacher, S., et al., 1997. Two amyloid precursor protein transgenic mouse models with Alzheimer disease-like pathology. Proc. Natl. Acad. Sci. U.S.A. 94, 13287–13292.

Tong, C., Li, P., Wu, N.L., Yan, Y., Ying, Q.L., 2010. Production of p53 gene knockout rats by homologous recombination in embryonic stem cells. Nature 467, 211–213.

Tsukamoto, T., 2016. Animal disease models for drug screening: the elephant in the room? Drug Discov. Today 21, 529–530.

Van Dam, D., De Deyn, P.P., 2006. Drug discovery in dementia: the role of rodent models. Nat. Rev. Drug Discov. 5, 956–970.

Van Dam, D., De Deyn, P.P., 2011. Animal models in the drug discovery pipeline for Alzheimer's disease. Brit. J. Pharmacol. 164, 1285–1300.

Van der Worp, H.B., Howells, D.W., Sena, E.S., Porritt, M.J., Rewell, S., O'Collins, V., et al., 2010. Can animal models of disease reliably inform human studies? PLoS Med. 7, e1000245.

Webster, S.J., Bachstetter, A.D., Nelson, P.T., Schmitt, F.A., Van Eldik, L.J., 2014. Using mice to model Alzheimer's dementia: an overview of the clinical disease and the preclinical behavioral changes in 10 mouse models. Front. Genet. 5, 88.

Zeiss, C., 2015. Improving the predictive value of interventional animal models data. Drug Discov. Today 20, 475–482.

Further Reading

Ribé, E.M., Perez, M., Puig, B., Gich, I., Lim, F., Cuadrado, T.S., et al., 2005. Accelerated amyloid deposition, neurofibrillary degeneration and neuronal loss in double mutant APP/tau transgenic mice. Neurobiol. Dis. 20, 814–822.

CHAPTER

13

Alzheimer's Disease Drugs in Clinical Trials

M. Sheerin, A. Adejare

OUTLINE

INTRODUCTION

Based on successfully meeting many milestones including scalability, in vitro and in vivo efficacy, and acceptable toxicity profile, a compound can be nominated to progress to first time in human studies. The Food and Drug Administration recommends assessments of the maximum tolerated dose and maximum feasible dose of the drug prior to the start of clinical trials (Fig. 13.1). The agency has provided a guidance document that recommends nonclinical studies on the basis of drug dosage.

Drug candidate and clinical information was obtained via Alzforum and/or clinicaltrials.gov. Search on clinicaltrials.gov indicated over 1300 studies at various stages from completed to terminated to recruiting. Structures of small molecule candidates were drawn using ChemDraw Pro Version 14. Structures of biomolecule candidates were accessed using the Protein Data Bank.

According to Alzforum, an internet-based resource for Alzheimer's disease (AD) researchers, there are currently over 90 potential treatments at various clinical trial points. These potential treatments demonstrate various targets, therapies, types, structures, and mechanisms of action. Lists of drugs currently in the various phases of clinical trials are provided in Tables 13.1–13.4. Provided are the names, synonyms, structures, and manufacturing or sponsoring company. The target type refers to the clinical feature in AD that the therapy is directed to modulate.

Drug Discovery Approaches for the Treatment of Neurodegenerative Disorders
http://dx.doi.org/10.1016/B978-0-12-802810-0.00013-1

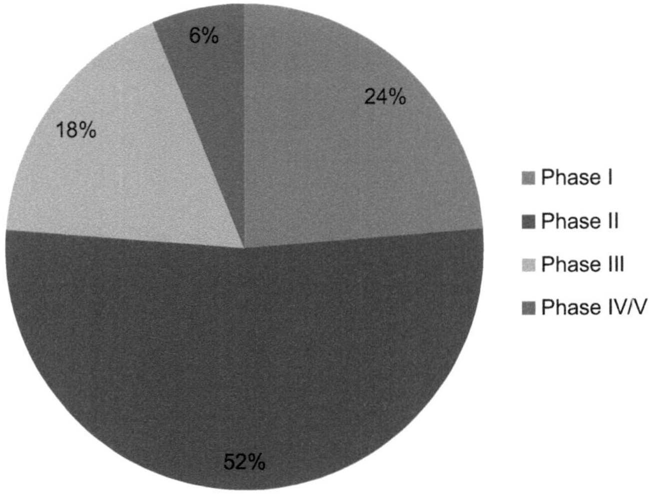

FIGURE 13.1 Percentages of Alzheimer's disease drugs in each stage of the clinical trials process.

Despite the seemingly flooded potential for new treatments, drug approval in the Alzheimer's market has proven to be a laborious effort with very low success rate (Fig. 13.2). The last approval for a new Alzheimer's treatment was that of memantine or Namenda in 2003. A new longer-acting version of Namenda, Namenda XR, was approved in 2014 (Lahiri et al., 2014). However, it is just an extended formulation of the same drug and not a new molecular entity (NME), which may bring advanced benefits to Alzheimer's and dementia patients.

A critical and initial step to the path of NME approval is validation of the drug's target (Fig. 13.3). This process begins with the identification of a certain enzyme, protein, gene, or other biomolecule, which is suspect in the propagation of a disease. This target is extensively studied in an effort to attain its biological functions, both beneficial and deleterious. The "target" for AD is unfortunately not clearly understood and there may be multiple players at every stage of the disease. Researchers have identified several potential targets for future therapies. A caveat to identifying a target and developing treatments is toxicity, which may result from manipulating the target and any physiological functions relying on that target.

Failure to effectively validate AD targets has contributed to billions in losses for clinical study sponsors. The "amyloid hypothesis" (Sommer, 2002) is an excellent example of misappropriation of potential therapy targets, the postulate of which places the driver of AD pathogenesis on the accumulation of amyloid beta (Aβ). Several drugs were developed to suppress the formation of Aβ using the amyloid precursor protein (APP) as a target. It was only when these therapies failed to show significant efficacy that the proposed target was called into question and complicating factors such as when to start treatment became appreciated. It also illustrated how a target in the APP processing cascade, for instance, γ-secretase, can be involved in both beneficial and deleterious effects.

TABLE 13.1 Alzheimer's Disease Drug Candidates in Phase I Clinical Trials

Name	Synonyms	Structure	Company	Target Type	Therapy Type	Mechanism of Action
AAB-003 (Nazem et al., 2015)	PF-05236812	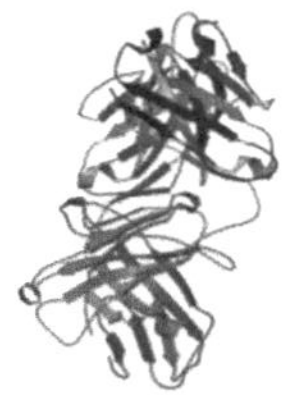 (Crespi et al., 2014)	Janssen, Pfizer	Amyloid related	Immunotherapy (passive)[a]	Binding and clearance of excess amyloid beta (Aβ)
AADvac-1 (Anand and Sabbagh, 2015)	Axon peptide 108 conjugated to keyhole limpet hemocyanin	Antibody	Axon Neuroscience SE	Tau	Immunotherapy (active)[b]	Binding and clearance of neurofibrillary tangles
ABT-957 (Pomytkin et al., 2015)		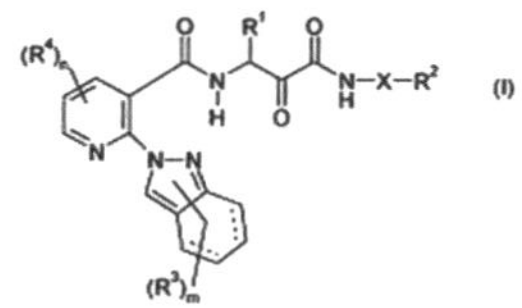	AbbVie	Other	Small molecule	Calpain inhibition
ACI-24 (Hickman et al., 2011)	Pal1-15 acetate salt	Antibody	AC Immune SA	Amyloid related	Immunotherapy (active)	Target, binding, and clearance of Aβ
ACI-35 (Hickman et al., 2011)		Antibody	AC Immune SA, Janssen	Tau	Immunotherapy (active)	Target, binding, and clearance of tau
Allopregnanolone (Turkmen et al., 2011)	3α,5α-Tetrahydro-progesterone	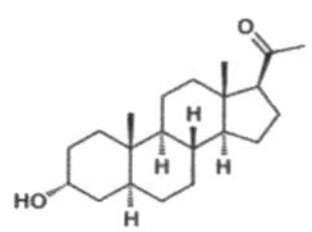	National Institutes of Health-funded study	Other neurotrans-mitters, other	Small molecule	Allosteric modulation of inhibitory γ-aminobutyric acid ($GABA_A$) receptors
GC 021109 (GC021109)		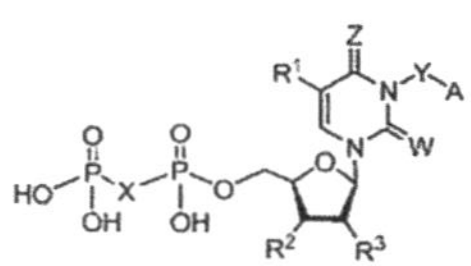	GliaCure	Inflammation	Small molecule	Reduction of inflammatory cytokines (2013)
GLN-1062 (Van Kampen et al., 2012)	Memogain	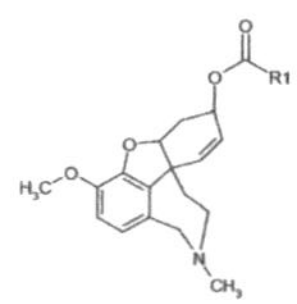	Galantos Pharma, Neurodyn	Cholinergic system	Small molecule	Inhibition of cholinesterase

(Continued)

TABLE 13.1 Alzheimer's Disease Drug Candidates in Phase I Clinical Trials—cont'd

Name	Synonyms	Structure	Company	Target Type	Therapy Type	Mechanism of Action
GSK2647544 (Chen et al., 2015)	GSK-2647544	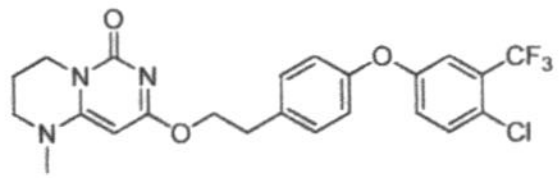	GlaxoSmithKline (GSK)	Cholesterol	Small molecule	Modulation of cholesterol metabolism
LY3002813 (LY3002813)	N3pG-Aβ monoclonal antibody	Antibody	Eli Lilly & Co.	Amyloid related	Immunotherapy (passive)	Binding and clearance of excess Aβ
MEDI1814 (Froestl et al., 2014)		Antibody	AstraZeneca	Amyloid related	Immunotherapy (passive)	Recognition of nonmonomeric Aβ. Modulation of synaptotoxic activity of such species
SAR228810 (SAR228810)		Antibody	Sanofi	Amyloid related	Immunotherapy (passive)	Binding and clearance of protofibrillar and fibrillar species of Aβ
S-Equol (Setchell et al., 2005)	Aus-131	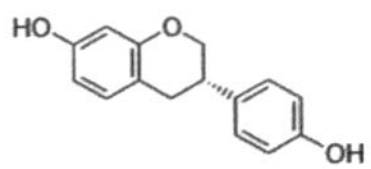	Ausio Pharmaceuticals, LLC	Other	Small molecule	Potentiation of neuronal mitochondrial function
SUVN-G3031 (Babu et al., 2014)		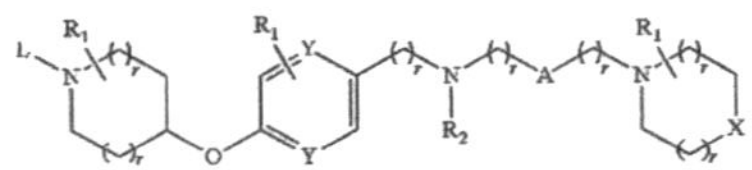	Suven Life Sciences Ltd	Cholinergic system, other neurotransmitters	Small molecule	Receptor antagonist of histamine H_3
TPI 287 (Adam, Corticobasal)	Abeotaxane	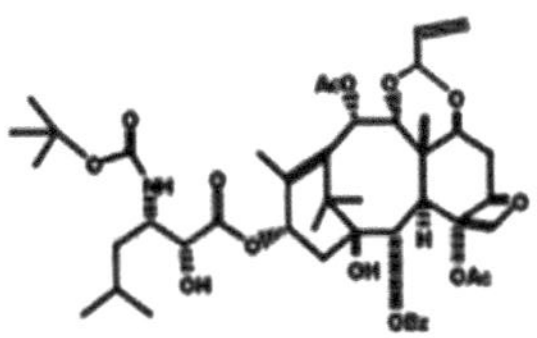 TPI-287	Cortice Biosciences	Tau	Small molecule	Binding of tubulin for stabilization of cytoskeleton

[a] *Passive immunotherapy—antibodies administrated to patient to combat disease.*
[b] *Active immunotherapy—treatment administered in an effort to stimulate patient's own immune response.*
Alzforum, (n.d.). Retrieved 19 Jan 2016, from http://www.alzforum.org/research-models/5xfad.

TABLE 13.2 Alzheimer's Disease Drug Candidates in Phase II Clinical Trials

Name	Synonyms	Structure	Company	Target Type	Therapy Type	Mechanism of Action
Acitretin (Endres et al., 2014)	Soriatane	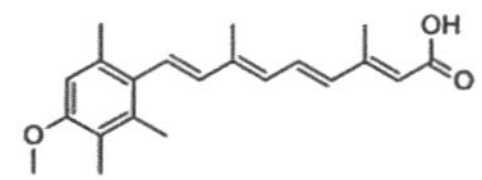	Actavis, Allergan plc	Amyloid related	Small molecule	Promotion of non-amyloidogenic processing of amyloid precursor protein (APP)
Affitope AD02 (Mattson et al., 1998)		Antibody	AFFiRiS AG	Amyloid related	Immunotherapy (active)	Recognition of amyloid beta (Aβ) Aβ without reacting with APP
Anavex 2-73 (McDonald, Potential)	Tetrahydro-*N*,*N*-dimethyl-2,2-diphenyl-3-furanmethanamine hydrochloride	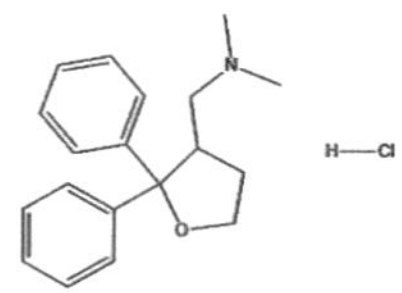	Anavex Life Science Corp.	Other	Small molecule	Antagonism of the intracellular sigma-1 chaperone protein
BAN2401 (Lannfelt et al., 2014)		Antibody	Biogen, Eisai Co., Ltd.	Amyloid related	Immunotherapy (passive)	Selective binding of large, soluble Aβ protofibrils
Bexarotene (Tousi, 2015)	Targretin	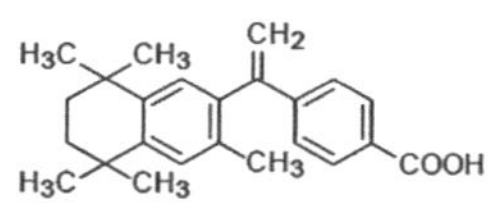	Ligand Pharmaceuticals, Inc., ReXceptor Inc.	Amyloid related, unknown	Small molecule	Increases ApoE concentration Reduction in Aβ levels and amyloid deposition
BI 409306 (BI 409306)	SUB 166499	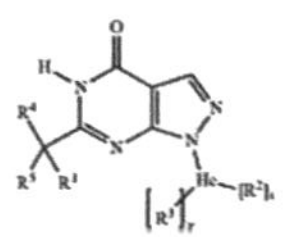	Boehringer Ingelheim	Other neurotransmitters, other	Small molecule	Inhibition of phosphodiesterase 9A
Cerebrolysin (Masliah and Díez-Tejedor, 2012)		Protein mixture	Ebewe Pharmaceutical	Other	Other	Regulation of glycogen synthase kinase-3β and cyclin-dependent kinase 5 activities

(Continued)

TABLE 13.2 Alzheimer's Disease Drug Candidates in Phase II Clinical Trials—cont'd

Name	Synonyms	Structure	Company	Target Type	Therapy Type	Mechanism of Action
Circadin (NPS)	Melatonin	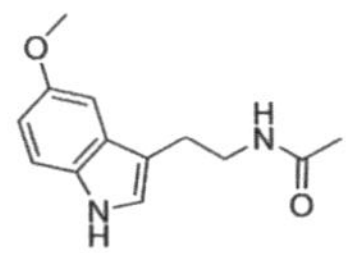	Neurim Pharmaceuticals Ltd.	Other	Small molecule	Sleep aid
Crenezumab (Genentech, Inc.,)	MABT5102A	Antibody	Genentech	Amyloid related	Immunotherapy (passive)	Recognition of oligomeric and fibrillar species
Curcumin (Huang et al., 2012)	Diferuloylmethane	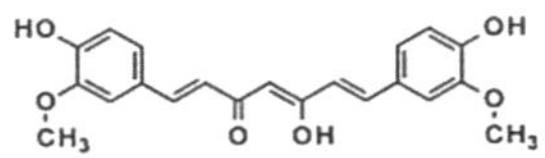	Verdure Sciences	Other, unknown	Dietary supplement	Inhibition of Aβ aggregation
E2609 (Bernier et al., 2013)	BACE inhibitor	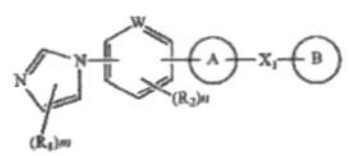	Biogen, Eisai Co., Ltd.	Amyloid related	Small molecule	Inhibition of BACE
EHT 0202 (Désiré et al., 2013)	Etazolate	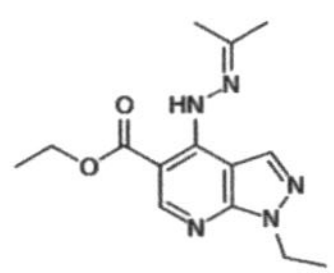	ExonHit Therapeutics	Other	Small molecule	Positive allosteric modulation of the γ-aminobutyric acid ($GABA_A$) receptor at barbiturate site
ELND005 (Abushakra et al., 2014)	AZD-103	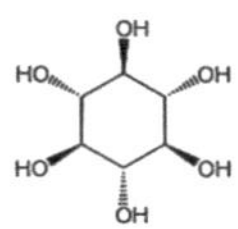	Elan Corporation, Speranza Therapeutics, Transition Therapeutics, Inc.	Amyloid related	Small molecule	Prevention of development of Aβ plaques
Etanercept (Spencer-Green, 2000)	Enbrel	Antibody	Amgen, Inc., Pfizer	Inflammation	Immunotherapy (passive)	Neuroinflammatory protectant
EVP-0962 (Apter, 2010; Rogers et al., 2012)	EVP 0015962	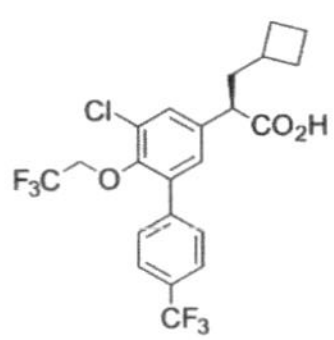	FORUM Pharmaceuticals Inc.	Amyloid related	Small molecule	Modulation of APP secretase

Exendin-4 (Kim et al., 2009)	Exenatide	H-His-Gly-Glu-Gly-Thr-Phe-Thr-Ser-Asp-Leu-Ser-Lys-Gln-Met-Glu-Glu-Glu-Ala-Val-Arg-Leu-Phe-Ile-Glu-Trp-Leu-Lys-Asn-Gly-Gly-Pro-Ser-Ser-Gly-Ala-Pro-Pro-Pro-Ser-NH_2 (Runge et al., 2008)	Amylin Pharmaceuticals	Other	Peptide	Regulation of glucose metabolism
G-CSF (Boyd et al., 2010)	Filgrastim	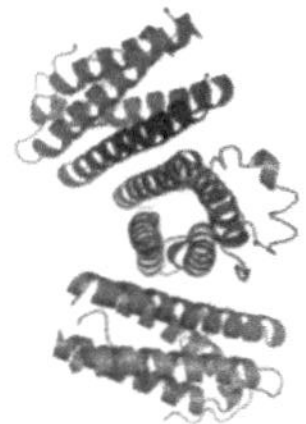 (Aritomi et al., 1999)	Amgen	Other	Small molecule	Regulation of glucose metabolism
Liraglutide (Talbot, 2014)	Victoza	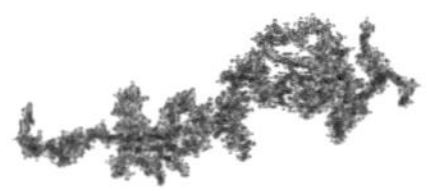 (Steensgaard et al., 2013)	Novo Nordisk A/S	Other	Small molecule	Regulation of glucose metabolism
Minocycline (Zhang and Zhao, 2014)	Solodyn	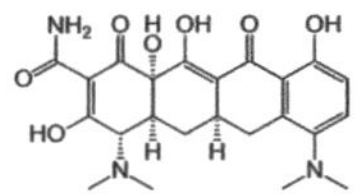	King's College London	Inflammation	Small molecule	Inhibition of microglia
MK-7622 (Blot et al., 2015)	Donepezil	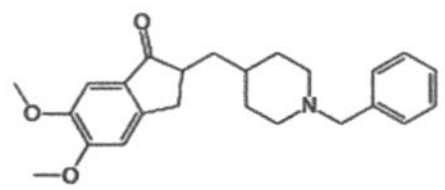	Merck	Unknown	Small molecule	Inhibition of cholinesterase
MSDC-0160 (Shah et al., 2014)	Mitoglitazone	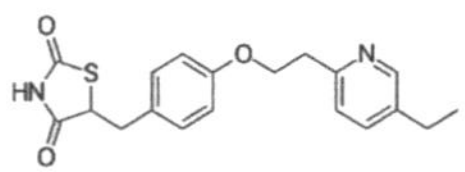	Metabolic Solutions Development Company	Other	Small molecule	Modulation of mitochondrial target of thiazolidinediones
Nasal insulin (Bryant et al., 2013)	Detemir	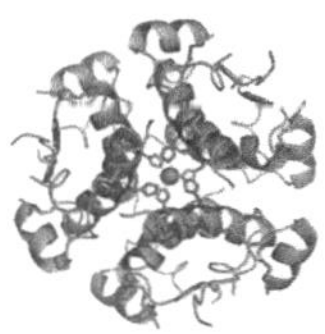	Novo Nordisk	Amyloid related, other	Small molecule, other	Regulation of glucose metabolism
NIC5-15 (Hampel et al., 2009)	Pinitol	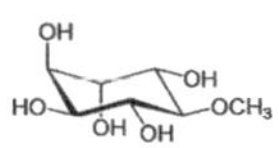	Humanetics Pharmaceuticals Corporation	Amyloid related, other	Small molecule, dietary supplement	Modulation of γ-secretase

(Continued)

TABLE 13.2 Alzheimer's Disease Drug Candidates in Phase II Clinical Trials—cont'd

Name	Synonyms	Structure	Company	Target Type	Therapy Type	Mechanism of Action
Nicotinamide (Mai et al., 2009)	Enduramide	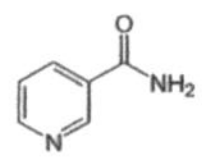	Endur	Other	Small molecule	Restoration of cognition
ORM-12741 (Gleichmann and Mattson, 2010)		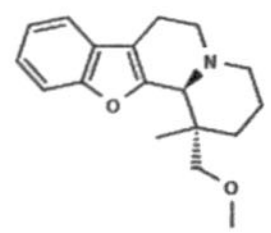	Orion Pharma	Other neurotransmitters	Small molecule	Antagonism of alpha-2c adrenoceptor
PBT2 (Faux et al., 2010)	PBT-2	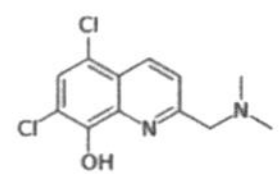	Prana Biotechnology Limited	Amyloid related, metals	Small molecule	Analog of 8-hydroxyquinoline
PF-05212377 (Bruin and Kruse, 2015)	PF-5212377, WYE-103760, SAM-760	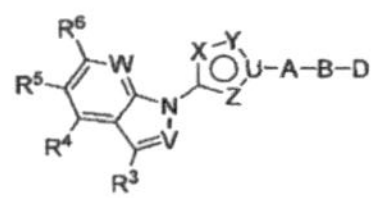	Pfizer	Other neurotransmitters	Small molecule	Antagonist of the serotonin 6 receptor ($5\text{-}HT_6$)
PQ912 (Bouter et al., 2015)		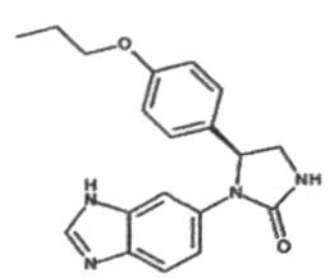	Probiodrug AG	Amyloid related, inflammation	Small molecule	Inhibitor of glutaminyl cyclase
Repetitive transcranial magnetic stimulation (Bentwich et al., 2011)	rTMS		Neuronix Ltd	Other	Procedural intervention	Direct neural stimulation
Rilapladib (Frishman and Pallerla, 2012; Maher-Edwards et al., 2014)	SB-659032	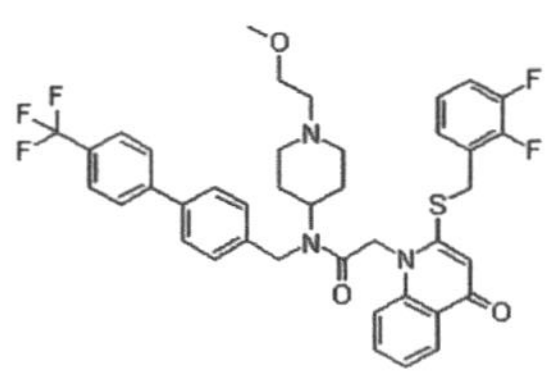	GlaxoSmithKline (GSK)	Other	Small molecule	Inhibition of lipoprotein-associated phospholipase A2
Riluzole (Coric et al., 2005)	Rilutek	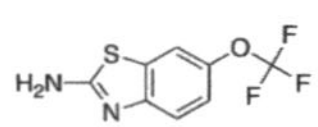	Sanofi	Other neurotransmitters, other	Small molecule	Inhibition of glutamate release and signaling

R-pramipexole (Truong et al., 2003)	RPPX	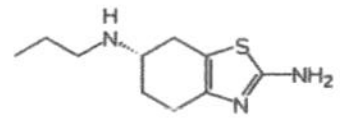	Biogen, Knopp Biosciences LLC, Virginia Commonwealth University	Other neurotransmitters, other	Small molecule	Agonist of dopamine
RVT-101 (Maher-Edwards et al., 2015)	SB-742457	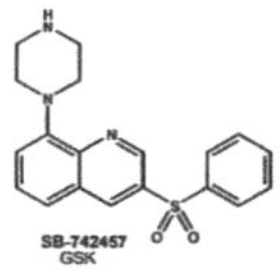	Axovant Sciences Ltd.	Other neurotransmitters	Small molecule	Selective antagonism of 5-HT_6 receptor
SAR110894D (Griebel et al., 2012)	Difumarate monohydrate	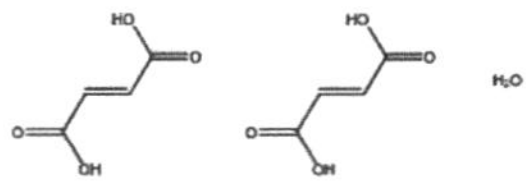	Sanofi	Other	Small molecule	Attenuation of neurotransmitter release
Saracatinib (Nygaard et al., 2015)	AZD0530	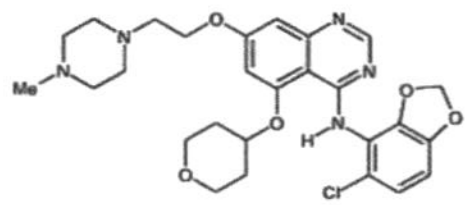	AstraZeneca	Other	Small molecule	Inhibition of Src and Abl kinases1
Sargramostim (Gleichmann and Mattson, 2010)	Leukine	Polypeptide	Genzyme, Sanofi	Inflammation, other, unknown	Other	Immunostimulation
SUVN-502 (Filip and Bader, 2009; Nirogi et al., 2009)		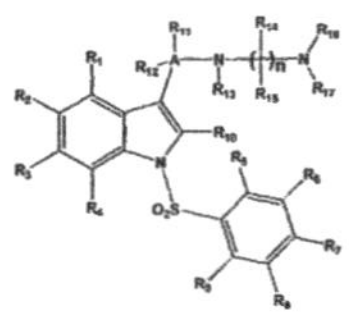	Suven Life Sciences Ltd.	Other neurotransmitters	Small molecule	Selective antagonism of the 5-HT_6 serotonin receptor
T-817MA (Takamura et al., 2014)	T817MA	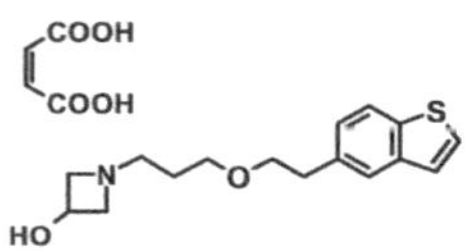	Toyama Chemical Co., Ltd.	Other, unknown	Small molecule	Neuroprotection
VX-745 (Duffy et al., 2011)		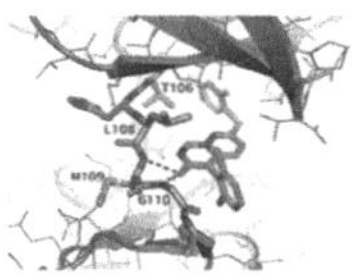	EIP Pharma, LLC	Inflammation	Small molecule	Selective inhibition of p38α kinase inhibitor

TABLE 13.3 Alzheimer's Treatment Candidates in Phase III Clinical Trials

Name	Synonyms	Structure	Company	Target Type	Therapy Type	Mechanism of Action
AC-1204 (Appleby et al., 2013; Doody et al., 2012)	Caprylic triglyceride	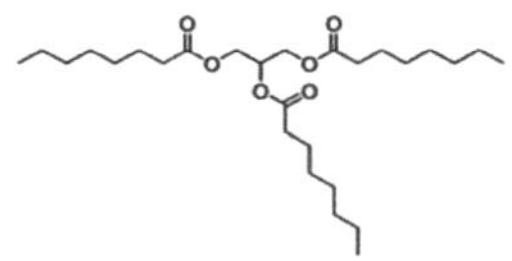	Accera, Inc.	Other	Dietary supplement	Regulation of brain glucose levels
AZD3293 (AZD 3293)	LY3314814	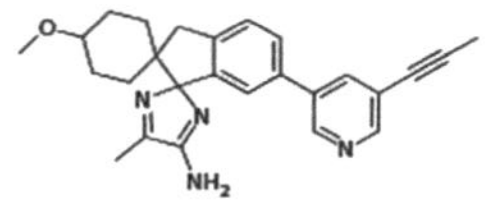	AstraZeneca	Amyloid related	Small molecule	Inhibition of beta-site amyloid precursor protein cleaving enzyme (BACE)
CAD106 (Winblad et al., 2012)	B-cell epitope (Aβ1–6)	Polypeptide	Novartis Pharmaceuticals Corporation	Amyloid related	Immunotherapy (active)	Vaccine against amyloid beta (Aβ) peptides
CNP520 (Norvatis, Inc.)	BACE inhibitor	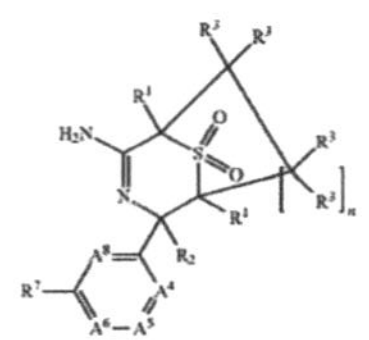	Amgen, Inc., Novartis Pharmaceuticals Corporation	Amyloid related	Small molecule	Inhibition of BACE
Encenicline (Barbier et al., 2015)	EVP-6124	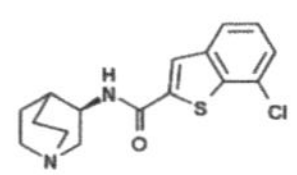	FORUM Pharmaceuticals Inc., Mitsubishi Tanabe Pharma	Cholinergic system	Small molecule	Partial agonist of the α7 nicotinic receptor
Epigallocatechin gallate (EGCG) (Kaviarasan et al., 2011)	Sunphenon EGCg	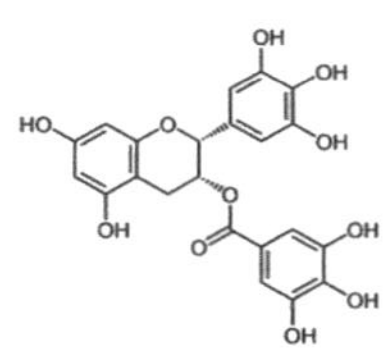	Taiyo International	Amyloid related, inflammation, other	Dietary supplement	Candidate neuroprotective
Gamunex (Smith et al., 2013)	Intravenous immunoglobulin	Antibody	Grifols Biologicals Inc.	Amyloid related, inflammation	Immunotherapy (passive)	Intravenous immunotherapy

Idalopirdine (Wilkinson et al., 2014)	Lu AE58054	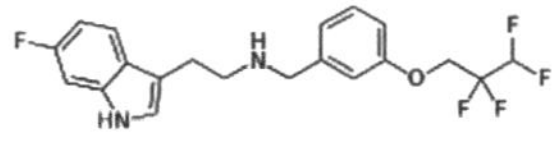	Eli Lilly & Co., H. Lundbeck, Otsuka Pharmaceutical Co., Ltd.	Other neurotrans-mitters	Small molecule	Selective antagonism $5\text{-}HT_6$ receptor
JNJ-54861911 (Khachaturian and Khachaturian, 2015)	BACE inhibitor	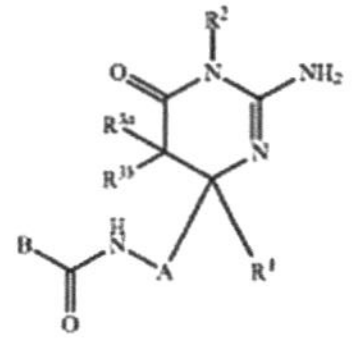	Janssen, Shionogi Pharma	Amyloid related	Small molecule	Inhibition of amyloid precursor protein (APP) cleavage by BACE
Masitinib (Folch et al., 2015)	Masivet	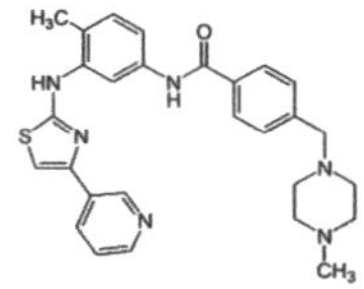	AB Science	Other	Small molecule	Inhibition of tyrosine kinase
Resveratrol (Harikumar and Aggarwal, 2008)	*trans*-3,4′,5-Trihydroxystilbene	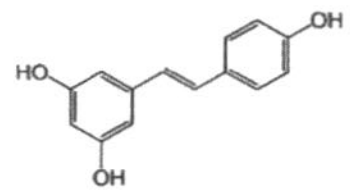	Other	Other	Small molecule, dietary supplement	Potential neuroprotective
Thalidomide (He et al., 2013)	Thalomid	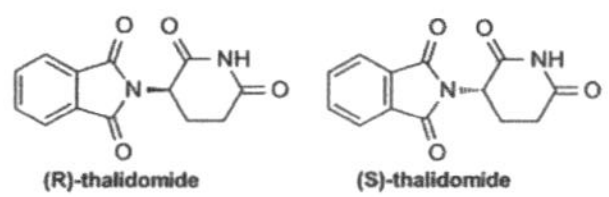	Celgene Corporation	Amyloid related, inflammation	Small molecule	Inhibition of beta-site APP cleaving enzyme 1 (BACE1) expression
TRx0237 (Berk and Sabbagh, 2013)	LMT-X, methylene blue	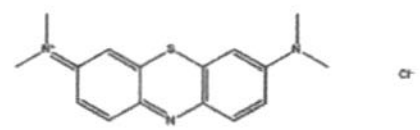	TauRx Therapeutics Ltd.	Tau	Small molecule	Inhibition of protein aggregation

TABLE 13.4 Alzheimer's Treatment Candidates in Phase IV Clinical Trials (https://clinicaltrials.gov)

Name	Synonyms	Structure	Company	Target Type	Therapy Type
AVP-923	Nuedexta	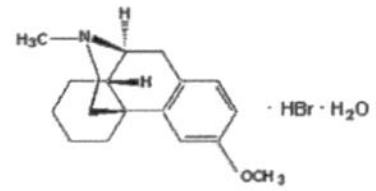	Avanir Pharmaceuticals	Other neurotransmitters	Small molecule
Donepezil	Aricept	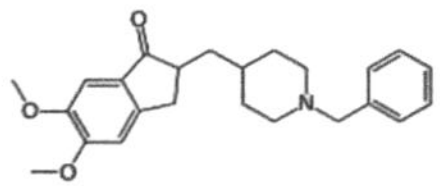	Eisai Co., Ltd., Pfizer	Cholinergic system	Small molecule
Galantamine	Razadyne	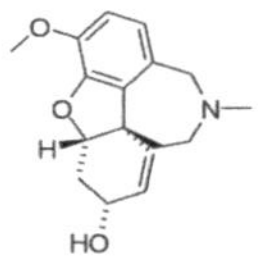	Multiple	Cholinergic system	Small molecule
Memantine	Ebixa	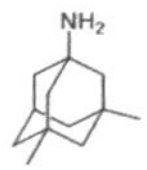	Forest Laboratories, Inc., H. Lundbeck, Merz Pharma	Other neurotransmitters	Small molecule
Rivastigmine	Exelon	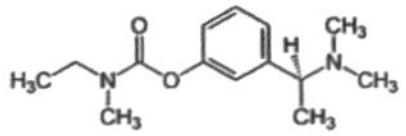	Novartis Pharmaceuticals Corporation	Cholinergic system	Small molecule
Tacrine	Cognex	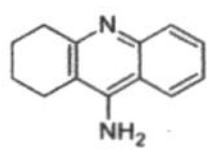	Pfizer, Shionogi Pharma	Cholinergic system	Small molecule

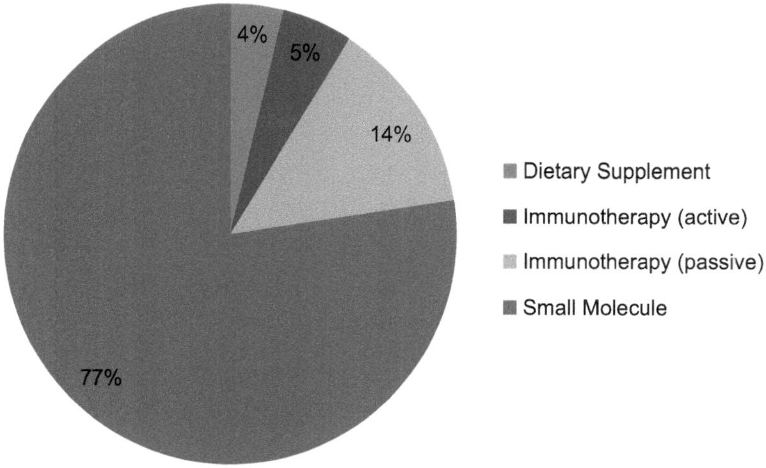

FIGURE 13.2 Percentages of Alzheimer's disease treatments by therapy type.

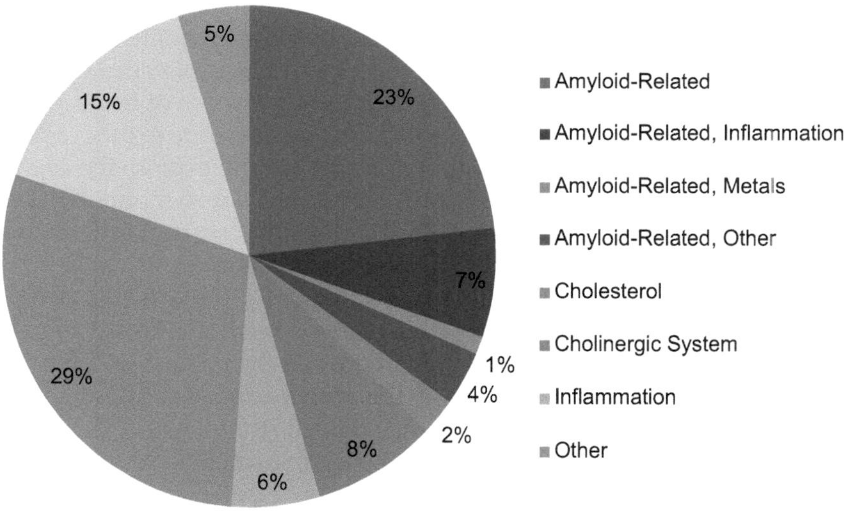

FIGURE 13.3 Percentages of Alzheimer's disease treatments by target type.

Still, lackluster target validation, failure to be effective, and toxicity are not the only causes for such high clinical failure rates. AD is a devastating disease with unpredictable prognosis depending on each victim. For double-blind studies, there must be a placebo group that is affected by the disease yet receives no candidate treatment. The rates of decline for AD patients vary greatly. There have been scenarios where the cognitive decline of the placebo population cohort plateaus at the same time as the treated cohort, and it cannot be argued that the candidate demonstrated efficacy versus the untreated population, even if the drug demonstrated efficacy in the dosed cohort. In addition, many clinical trials fail in proving bioequivalence or noninferiority against current marketed treatments.

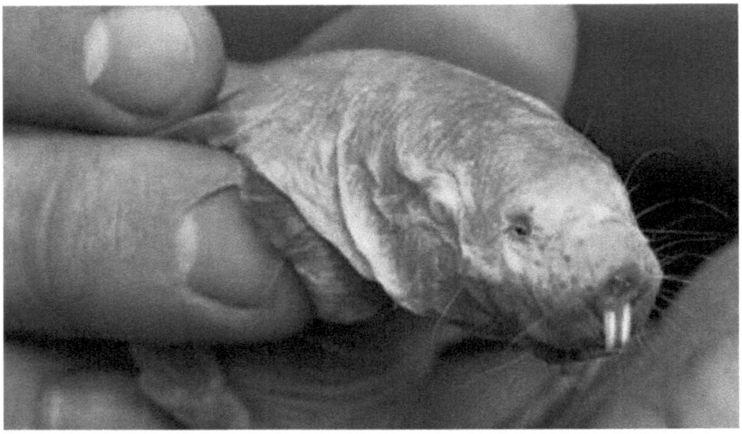

FIGURE 13.4 Naked mole rat as depicted with handler from *National Geographic*.

Animal models serve as a means of bolstering the validation of a drug candidate. Efficacy of an AD drug candidate on memory and behavior can be directly observed and evaluated by using rat and/or mice models. Behaviors studied by animal scientists include those that are impaired and decline during the progression of the disease: reference memory, working memory, and executive function. These can be tested using a series of reward-driven mazes. Quite often, mice, rats, or other rodents are genetically engineered to express a higher level of a biomarker such as APP and therefore begin to phenotypically express the cognitive effects of the disease. However, there are concerns about how relevant such models are to the disease and use of aged rats is being advocated. Two earlier chapters in this book fully examine animal models from the simple *Caenorhabditis elegans* to rodents.

Animal models can be particularly useful in anticipating the performance of a candidate as they mimic in vivo human behavior and drug effects. One key limitation to any animal study is the lack of capability of vocal communication between the cohorts and the investigators during trials. Nevertheless, much useful information can be deduced by studying the behavior patterns and disruptions in a well-documented animal study.

Recent developments in AD animal models have begun to include unconventional species. The naked mole rat (*Heterocephalus glaber*), which has an anticipated and unrivaled rodent lifespan of approximately 30 years, has the potential to displace the well-established rodent models (Fig. 13.4). Preliminary nuclear magnetic resonance proteomic studies have demonstrated that the naked mole rats express greater genotypic homology with human Aβ. Mice express three fewer amino acids in their Aβ sequence than that of humans while the mole rat Aβ is only one amino acid away from the full human sequence. The lifespan of the naked mole rat is significantly greater than other members of the rodent family, making it a worthwhile in vivo model for the cognitive decline seen in AD. The mole rats have also demonstrated a greater innate propensity to develop amyloid plaques similar to that of humans (Shanks et al., 2009).

In conclusion, this chapter has described proposed and current treatments for AD in the various stages of the clinical trial process. This information can be overwhelming, and this chapter is intended to summarize this information to assist AD sufferers, caregivers, and researchers in identifying the options available.

References

Abushakra, S.R., Kesslak, P., Kurth, M., Fan, F., Bairu, M., Miller, D.S., Lyketsos, C., 2014. Drug development for agitation and aggression in Alzheimer's disease (AD): study design and outcome measures in phase 2 study of scyllo-inositol (ELND005 studyag201). Alzheimer's and Dementia. http://ovidsp.ovid.com/ovidweb.cgi?T=JS&PAGE=reference&D=emed12&NEWS=N&AN=71627925.

Adam, B., Corticobasal Syndrome or Progressive Supranuclear Palsy Phase 1 Trial of TPI-287 | UCSF Memory and Aging Center. http://memory.ucsf.edu/research/clinical-trials/tpi-287-4r.

Anand, K., Sabbagh, M., August 1, 2015. Early investigational drugs targeting tau protein for the treatment of Alzheimer's disease. Expert Opin. Investig. Drugs Informa Healthcare 24 (10), 1355–1360.

Appleby, B., Nacopoulos, D., Milano, N., Zhong, K., Cummings, J., 2013. A review: treatment of Alzheimer's disease discovered in repurposed agents. Dementia Geriatr Cog Disorder 35, 1–22.

Apter, J.T., 2010. Abstract# 1: EVP-6124 elicits pro-cognitive effects in Alzheimer's patients. Neurotherapeutics 7 (3), 328.

Aritomi, M., Kunishima, N., Okamoto, T., Kuroki, R., Ota, Y., Morikawa, K., 1999. Nature 401, 713–717.

AZD 3293-AdisInsight. http://adisinsight.springer.com/drugs/800037439.

Babu, M.R., Muddana, N., Mekala, V.R., Jayarajan, P., Kanamarlapudi, V.B., Faheem, M.A., Shinde, A., Irappanavar, S., Goyal, V.K., Pandey, S.K., Gangadasari, P.N., Ponnamaneni, R., Nirogi, R., 2014. Alzheimer's Dement. 10 (4), P459–P460.

Barbier, A.J., Hilhorst, M., Van Vliet, A., Snyder, P., Palfreyman, M.G., Gawryl, M., Dgetluck, N., Massaro, M., Tiessen, R., Timmerman, W., Hilt, D.C., 2015. Clin. Ther. 37 (2), 311–324.

Bentwich, J., Dobronevsky, E., Aichenbaum, S., Shorer, R., Peretz, R., Khaigrekht, M., Marton, R.G., Rabey, J.M., 2011. Beneficial effect of repetitive transcranial magnetic stimulation combined with cognitive training for the treatment of Alzheimer's disease: a proof of concept study. Journal of Neural Transmission 118 (3), 463–471.

Berk, C., Sabbagh, M.N., 2013. Drugs Aging 30 (10), 783–792.

Bernier, F., Sato, Y., Matijevic, M., Desmond, H., McGrath, S., Burns, L., Kaplow, J.M., Albala, B., 2013. Alzheimer's Dement. 9 (4), P886.

BI 409306 for Cognitive Impairment Due to Alzheimer's Disease | National Institute on Aging. https://www.nia.nih.gov/alzheimers/clinical-trials/bi-409306-cognitive-impairment-due-alzheimers-disease.

Blot, K., Kimura, S.I., Bai, J., Kemp, A., Manahan-Vaughan, D., Giros, B., Tzavara, E., Otani, S., 2015. Cereb. Cortex 25 (5), 1348–1361.

Bouter, Y., Noguerola, J.S.L., Tucholla, P., Crespi, G.A.N., Parker, M.W., Wiltfang, J., Miles, L.A., Bayer, T.A., 2015. Acta Neuropathol. 130 (5), 713–729.

Boyd, T.D., Bennett, S.P., Mori, T., Governatori, N., Runfeldt, M., Norden, M., Padmanabhan, J., Neame, P., Wefes, I., Sanchez-Ramos, J., Arendash, G.W., Potter, H., 2010. J. Alzheimer's Dis. 21 (2), 507–518.

Bruin, N.M.W.J. de, Kruse, C.G., 2015. Curr. Pharm. Des. 21 (26), 3739–3759.

Bryant, G.A., McDanel, D.L., Horner, K.E., Farris, K.B., Newkirk, E.N., 2013. Pharmacotherapy 33 (1), 56–62.

Chen, X., Xu, W., Wang, K., Mo, M., Zhang, W., Du, L., Yuan, X., Xu, Y., Wang, Y., Shen, J., 2015. J. Med. Chem. 58 (21), 8529–8541.

Coric, V., Taskiran, S., Pittenger, C., Wasylink, S., Mathalon, D.H., Valentine, G., Saksa, J., Wu, Y.T., Gueorguieva, R., Sanacora, G., Malison, R.T., Krystal, J.H., 2005. Biol. Psychiatry 58 (5), 424–428.

Crespi, G.A.N., Ascher, D.B., Parker, M.W., Miles, L.A., 2014. Acta Crystallogr. Sect. F, Struct. Biol. Commun. 70 (Pt 3), 374–377.

Désiré, L., Blondiaux, E., Carrière, J., Haddad, R., Sol, O., Fehlbaum-Beurdeley, P., Einstein, R., Zhou, W., Pando, M.P., 2013. J. Alzheimer's Dis. 34 (2), 469–483.

Doody, R., Galvin, J., Farlow, M., Shah, R., Doraiswamy, P.M., Ferris, S., Zetlaoui, J., Henderson, S., Isaacson, R.S., 2012. J. Nutr. Health Aging 868.

Duffy, J.P., Harrington, E.M., Salituro, F.G., Cochran, J.E., Green, J., Gao, H., Bemis, G.W., Evindar, G., Galullo, V.P., Ford, P.J., Germann, U.A., Wilson, K.P., Bellon, S.F., Chen, G., Taslimi, P., Jones, P., Huang, C., Pazhanisamy, S., Wang, Y.M., Murcko, M.A., Su, M.S.S., 2011. ACS Med. Chem. Lett. 2 (10), 758–763.

Endres, K., Fahrenholz, F., Lotz, J., Hiemke, C., Teipel, S., Lieb, K., Tüscher, O., Fellgiebel, A., 2014. Neurology 83 (21), 1930–1935.

Filip, M., Bader, M., 2009. Overview on 5-HT receptors and their role in physiology and pathology of the central nervous system. Pharmacological Reports 61 (5), 761–777.

Faux, N.G., Ritchie, C.W., Gunn, A., Rembach, A., Tsatsanis, A., Bedo, J., Harrison, J., Lannfelt, L., Blennow, K., Zetterberg, H., Ingelsson, M., Masters, C.L., Tanzi, R.E., Cummings, J.L., Herd, C.M., Bush, A.I., 2010. J. Alzheimer's Dis. 20 (2), 509–516.

Folch, J., Petrov, D., Ettecho, M., Pedrós, I., Abad, S., Beas-Zarate, C., Lazarowski, A., Marin, M., Olloquequi, J., Auladell, C., Camins, A., 2015. Expert Rev. Neurother. 10, 1–10.

Frishman, W.H., Pallerla, K., 2012. Cardiol. Rev. 102–110.

Froestl, W., Pfeifer, A., Muhs, A., 2014. J. Alzheimer's Dis. 42 (4), 1079–1149.

GC021109 for Mild to Moderate Alzheimer's Disease | National Institute on Aging. https://www.nia.nih.gov/alzheimers/clinical-trials/gc021109-mild-moderate-alzheimers-disease.

Genentech, Inc., Crenezumab for Mild to Moderate Alzheimer Disease | National Institute on Aging. https://www.nia.nih.gov/alzheimers/clinical-trials/crenezumab-mild-moderate-alzheimer-disease.

Gleichmann, M., Mattson, M.P., 2010. Neuromolecular Med. 12 (1), 44–47.

Griebel, G., Pichat, P., Pruniaux, M.P., Beeské, S., Lopez-Grancha, M., Genet, E., Terranova, J.P., Castro, A., Sánchez, J.A., Black, M., Varty, G.B., Weiner, I., Arad, M., Barak, S., De Levie, A., Guillot, E., 2012. Pharmacol. Biochem. Behav. 102 (2), 203–214.

Hampel, H., Broich, K., Hoessler, Y., Pantel, J., 2009. Dialogues Clin. Neurosci. 11 (2), 141–157.

Harikumar, K.B., Aggarwal, B.B., 2008. Cell Cycle 1020–1037.

He, P., Cheng, X., Staufenbiel, M., Li, R., Shen, Y., 2013. PLoS One 8 (2), e55091.

Hickman, D.T., López-Deber, M.P., Ndao, D.M., Silva, A.B., Nand, D., Pihlgren, M., Giriens, V., Madani, R., St-Pierre, A., Karastaneva, H., Nagel-Steger, L., Willbold, D., Riesner, D., Nicolau, C., Baldus, M., Pfeifer, A., Muhs, A., 2011. J. Biol. Chem. 286 (16), 13966–13976.

Huang, H.-C., Chang, P., Dai, X.-L., Jiang, Z.-F., 2012. Neurochem. Res. 37 (7), 1584–1597.

Kaviarasan, S., Sivakumar, A.S., Barik, A., Kunwar, A., Naik, G.H., Priyadarsini, K.I., 2011. J. Food Biochem. 35 (2), 596–612.

Khachaturian, Z.S., Khachaturian, A.S., 2015. Mol. Aspects Med. 43–44, 3–15.

Kim, S., Moon, M., Park, S., 2009. J. Endocrinol. 202 (3), 431–439.

Lahiri, D.K., Ray, B., Balaraman, Y., Bailey, J.A., Erickson, C.E., Nurnberger, J.I., 2014. Biol. Psychiatry 1, 389S.

Lannfelt, L., Möller, C., Basun, H., Osswald, G., Sehlin, D., Satlin, A., Logovinsky, V., Gellerfors, P., 2014. Alzheimer's Res. Ther. 6 (2), 16.

LY3002813 for Mild Cognitive Impairment and Alzheimer's Disease | National Institute on Aging. https://www.nia.nih.gov/alzheimers/clinical-trials/ly3002813-mild-cognitive-impairment-and-alzheimers-disease.

Maher-Edwards, G., De'Ath, J., Barnett, C., Lavrov, A., Lockhart, A., 2014. A 24-week study to evaluate the effect of Rilapladib on cognition and CSF markers of Alzheimer's disease. Alzheimer's & Dementia: The Journal of the Alzheimer's Association 10 (4), P301–P302.

Maher-Edwards, G., Watson, C., Ascher, J., Barnett, C., Boswell, D., Davies, J., Fernandez, M., Kurz, A., Zanetti, O., Safirstein, B., Schronen, J.P., Zvartau-Hind, M., Gold, M., 2015. Alzheimer's Dement. Transl. Res. Clin. Interv. 1 (1), 23–36.

Mai, A., Rotili, D., Valente, S., Kazantsev, A.G., 2009. Curr. Pharm. Des. 15 (34), 3940–3957.

Masliah, E., Díez-Tejedor, E., 2012. Drugs Today (Barc). 48 (Suppl. A), 3–24.

Mattson, M.P., Partin, J., Begley, J.G., 1998. Brain Res. 807 (1–2), 167–176.

McDonald, I., Potential Alzheimer's disease treatment "ANAVEX 2–73" shows promising results in mouse studies | Alzheimer's Australia Dementia Research Foundation (AADRF). http://dementiaresearchfoundation.org.au/blog/potential-alzheimer%E2%80%99s-disease-treatment-%E2%80%98anavex-2-73%E2%80%99-shows-promising-results-mouse-studies.

Nazem, A., Sankowski, R., Bacher, M., Al-Abed, Y., 2015. J. Neuroinflammation 12 (1), 74.

Nirogi, R., Kandikere, V., Mudigonda, K., Bhyrapuneni, G., Jasti, V., 2009. Alzheimer's Dement 5 (4), 250–251.

Norvatis, Inc., CAD106 and CNP520 to Prevent or Delay Symptoms of Alzheimer's Disease (Generation). https://www.nia.nih.gov/alzheimers/clinical-trials/cad106-and-cnp520-prevent-or-delay-symptoms-alzheimers-disease-generation.

NPS. Better choices, Better health. Melatonin prolonged-release tablets (Circadin) for primary insomnia in older people. http://www.nps.org.au/publications/health-professional/nps-radar/2010/may-2010/melatonin.

Nygaard, H.B., Wagner, A.F., Bowen, G.S., Good, S.P., MacAvoy, M.G., Strittmatter, K.A., Kaufman, A.C., Rosenberg, B.J., Sekine-Konno, T., Varma, P., Chen, K., Koleske, A.J., Reiman, E.M., Strittmatter, S.M., van Dyck, C.H., 2015. Alzheimers Res. Ther. 7 (1), 35.

Pomytkin, I.A., Chernopiatko, A., Andreeva, L., 2015. Nutrients Solutions for Enhancement of Cognitive Function. http://www.freepatentsonline.com/y2015/0374745.html.

Rogers, K., Felsenstein, K.M., Hrdlicka, L., Tu, Z., Albayya, F., Lee, W., Hopp, S., Miller, M.J., Spaulding, D., Yang, Z., Hodgdon, H., Nolan, S., Wen, M., Costa, D., Blain, J.F., Freeman, E., De Strooper, B., Vulsteke, V., Scrocchi, L., Zetterberg, H., Portelius, E., Hutter-Paier, B., Havas, D., Ahlijanian, M., Flood, D., Leventhal, L., Shapiro, G., Patzke, H., Chesworth, R., Koenig, G., 2012. Modulation of γ-secretase by EVP-0015962 reduces amyloid deposition and behavioral deficits in Tg2576 mice. Mol. Neurodegener. 7, 61.

Runge, S., Thogersen, H., Madsen, K., Lau, J., Rudolph, R., 2008. J. Biol. Chem. 283, 11340–11347.

SAR228810-Product Profile – BioCentury. http://www.biocentury.com/products/sar228810.

Setchell, K.D., Clerici, C., Lephart, E.D., Cole, S.J., Heenan, C., Castellani, D., Wolfe, B.E., Nechemias-Zimmer, L., Brown, N.M., Lund, T.D., Handa, R.J., Heubi, J.E., 2005. Am. J. Clin. Nutr. 81 (5), 1072–1079.

Shah, R.C., Matthews, D.C., Andrews, R.D., Capuano, A.W., Fleischman, D.A., VanderLugt, J.T., Colca, J.R., 2014. Curr. Alzheimer Res. 11 (6), 564–573.

Shanks, N., Greek, R., Greek, J., 2009. Philos. Ethics Humanit. Med. 4 (1), 2.

Smith, L.M., Coffey, M.P., Klaver, A.C., Loeffler, D.A., 2013. Int. Immunopharmacol. 16 (4), 424–428.

Sommer, B., 2002. Curr. Opin. Pharmacol. 2 (1), 87–92.

Spencer-Green, G., 2000. Ann. Rheum. Dis. 59 (Suppl. 1), i46–i49.

Steensgaard, D.B., Schluckebier, G., Strauss, H.M., Norrman, M., Thomsen, J.K., Friderichsen, A.V., Havelund, S., et al., 2013. Ligand-controlled assembly of hexamers, dihexamers, and linear multihexamer structures by the engineered acylated insulin degludec. Biochemistry 52 (2), 295–309.

Takamura, Y., Ono, K., Matsumoto, J., Yamada, M., Nishijo, H., 2014. Neurobiol. Aging 35 (3), 532–536.

Talbot, K., 2014. Neurodegener. Dis. Manag. 4 (1), 31–40.

Tousi, B., 2015. Neuropsychiatr. Dis. Treat. 11, 311–315.

Truong, J.G., Rau, K.S., Hanson, G.R., Fleckenstein, A.E., 2003. Eur. J. Pharmacol. 474 (2–3), 223–226.

Turkmen, S., Backstrom, T., Wahlstrom, G., Andreen, L., Johansson, I.-M., 2011. Br. J. Pharmacol. 162 (2), 311–327.

Van Kampen, J., Kay, D., Baranowski, D., Maelicke, A., Kopke, A., 2012. Alzheimer's Dement. 8 (4), P392–P393.

Wilkinson, D., Windfeld, K., Colding-Jørgensen, E., 2014. Lancet Neurol. 13 (11), 1092–1099.

Winblad, B., Andreasen, N., Minthon, L., Floesser, A., Imbert, G., Dumortier, T., Maguire, R.P., Blennow, K., Lundmark, J., Staufenbiel, M., Orgogozo, J.M., Graf, A., 2012. Lancet Neurol. 11 (7), 597–604.

Zhang, L., Zhao, J., 2014. Neuropsychiatr. Dis. Treat. 10, 1103–1111.

CHAPTER

14

Nonpharmacological Treatment Approaches

D.Y. Hu, C.Y. Hu, E.C. Corum

OUTLINE

INTRODUCTION

Hallmark features of dementia include a progressive loss of memory, language, problem solving, communication, and other cognitive functions. At its peak, these cognitive impairments can negatively impact a person's ability to perform activities of daily living. This loss of function significantly alters a patient's interaction with the environment and other individuals around them, ultimately leading to a decline in quality of life. Alzheimer's disease (AD), a degenerative neurologic disease, is the leading cause of dementia. According to 2015 statistics,

Drug Discovery Approaches for the Treatment of Neurodegenerative Disorders
http://dx.doi.org/10.1016/B978-0-12-802810-0.00014-3

an estimated 5.3 million Americans have AD. As can be expected, the prevalence of the disease increases proportionately with age. Approximately 11% of people older than 65 years of age suffer from the disease while 32% of people aged greater than 85 years of age are affected. More descriptively, 81% of individuals that are affected by AD are greater than 75 years of age (Alzheimer's Association, 2015).

As the American population increases in age, so does the incidence of AD. It is estimated that there will be 473,000 newly diagnosed AD patients in 2015. More specifically, these estimates translate into two new cases per 100,000 people age 65–74, 13 new cases per 100,000 people age 75–84, and 39 cases per 100,000 people age greater than 85 years. These estimates equate to a new diagnosis of AD every 64 s. This rapid increase in incidence is expected to continue over the next 10 years. By 2025, it is projected that every state within the country will experience an increase of at least 14% in the number of people with the disease. With the advancement of medical therapies, the number of people surviving into their 80s and 90s will increase. By 2030, people aged greater than 65 will constitute 20% of the population—an increase of 17% from 2010 (Alzheimer's Association, 2015).

AD is associated with a high degree of morbidity and mortality. Among people aged 70 years or older with AD, 61% are expected to die before the age of 80; whereas, of the patients aged greater than 70 years without AD, 30% are expected to die before the age of 80. It is estimated that 700,000 patients in the United States will die with AD in 2015. Although deaths because of other causes, such as cardiovascular disease, have declined over time, deaths caused by AD have increased. Between 2000 and 2013, deaths caused by AD increased by 71%. From a morbidity standpoint, patients with AD have three times more hospital stays per year than those patients without AD (Alzheimer's Association, 2015).

The large disease burden of AD on society requires a substantial amount of attention and caregiving. According to the Alzheimer's Association, there are over $217 billion of unpaid caregiving hours related to AD. This equates to over 17 billion hours of caregiving time dedicated to the management of the disease (Alzheimer's Association, 2015). Long-term care or hospice care for those with AD is also quite costly. Costs per person for assisted living facilities average $42,000 a year and nursing homes average $77,380 a year. The overall health care costs associated with AD are staggering as well. Health care for those with AD was predicted to be over $220 billion by 2015. Medicaid payments per AD patient averaged $11,021 as compared to $574 for similar Medicaid patients without AD (Alzheimer's Association, 2015).

Overall, the manifestations of AD can be classified into two hallmark categories: clinical cognitive decline and the neuropsychiatric symptoms (NPS). Typically, both manifestations are treated with pharmacological interventions.

Medications such as donepezil and memantine are intended to slow cognitive degeneration through the potentiation of acetylcholine; however, individual responses to therapy are highly variable. Additionally, there is some evidence that there is some degree of tachyphylaxis with these medications (Schletrens and Feldman, 2003). Although the clinical effectiveness of these Food and Drug Administration (FDA)-approved agents have been illustrated in clinical trials, tolerability and side effects still pose a barrier to compliance. For example, the rate of discontinuation for dose-titrated donepezil is 13% (Aricept package insert, 2013). Currently, no medication has been approved for the reversal or prevention of AD (Alzheimer's Association, 2015; California Workgroup, 2008).

Those with AD exhibit NPS in several forms: agitation, aggression, hallucinations, and verbal and physical outbursts (Lyketsos et al., 2006). Currently, there are no FDA-approved agents for the management of NPS associated with AD, and, because of this, caregivers and clinicians resort to using atypical antipsychotics such as olanzapine and haloperidol (Schletrens and Feldman, 2003; California Workgroup, 2008). Not only are these agents not FDA approved for these indications, they are associated with significant adverse events. Some of these adverse events are minor, such as somnolence, but there are many that are severe, such as neuroleptic malignant syndrome or torsades de pointes (Zyprexa package insert, 2014). A large randomized controlled trial published in 2006 concluded that the adverse effects associated with the use of atypical antipsychotics in AD patients offset any therapeutic benefit. The authors concluded that the use of these agents in this patient population should be limited (Schneider et al., 2006). In 2008, the FDA issued an alert that the use of both typical and atypical antipsychotics in the elderly with dementia or AD was associated with an increased risk of mortality (Food and Drug Administration Alert, 2008). As a result of these findings, the off-label use of these agents to manage behavioral symptoms in the AD patient population was added to the boxed warnings (Zyprexa package insert, 2014).

AD is associated with an enormous economic and social burden. The catastrophic effects of this disease include decreased quality of life for patients and caregivers, large financial implications, and a drain on health care resources. Because of these reasons, there is an overwhelming degree of research being conducted in search of therapies that can either decrease cognitive decline or slow pathological progression. It is well recognized that the causes of AD are multifactorial; therefore the approach to the patient with AD should be multifaceted. The mainstay of research has been in the realm of pharmacological agents. While current pharmacological therapies are widely utilized in the management of disease, costs, lack of efficacy, and side effects can be limiting factors. There is an abundant amount of research that reviews the effectiveness of nonpharmacological interventions (NPIs) in the setting of AD. The advantages of NPIs include low cost, ease of reproducibility, and little to no side effects. Moreover, the employment of NPIs as an adjunctive approach to pharmacological therapy supports a multifaceted approach to the disease.

In this chapter, we will describe the current evidence and rationale behind the use of NPIs in the management of AD. The interventions are grouped into those that aid in delaying cognitive decline through the enhancement of cognitive reserve and those interventions that can be used to address neuropsychiatric behaviors associated with AD.

NONPHARMACOLOGICAL INTERVENTIONS AND COGNITIVE RESERVE

Mild cognitive impairment (MCI) is defined as the noticeable, cognitive decline that does not impair activities of daily living (Alzheimer's Association, 2015). Although there is much controversy regarding whether MCI is synonymous with mild AD, there is much consensus that MCI is a definite risk factor for the development of AD (Duara et al., 2009). At the 2008 Sixth Annual Mild Cognitive Impairment Symposium, the keynote speaker, Denis Evans, MD, suggested that the search for disease modification should center around three main concepts. First, AD does not arise from a single cause but rather a cumulative result of many risk factors, and therapy must include a multifaceted approach. Second, the border between normality and disease is not abrupt but continuous because the onset of the disease is gradual over a long period of time. Lastly, as the population continues to age, the disease burden from

AD will continue to increase. Based upon these three concepts, Evans emphasized that the management of AD should largely focus on prevention rather than treatment (Duara et al., 2009). Because of the focus on preventive strategies, the early identification and management of MCI is imperative to the long-term treatment of AD. To date, there have been numerous studies that link NPIs and the delayed onset of AD-associated cognitive decline. Understanding the underlying pathogenic mechanisms behind MCI and AD creates a strong foundation to the nonpharmacological approach to cognitive decline in the AD patient.

Pathogenic Mechanisms of Cognitive Impairment in Alzheimer's Disease

Hallmark findings in AD include beta amyloid (Aβ) plaques, neurofibrillary tangles composed of hyperphosphorylated tau, and neuronal and synaptic loss. Although there has been extensive research in all of these pathological features, little has been established on the relative importance of each.

Three types of amyloid-related plaques in the brain have been identified as usual findings in the AD patient. Diffuse plaques contain no amyloid core, but contain stable amyloid immunoreactive proteins. These plaques are thought to represent the early stages of plaque formation. Diffuse plaques are typically found in areas of the brain that are unrelated to symptoms identified throughout the course of AD such as the cerebellum and cerebral hemisphere. The second type of plaque found in AD is the spherical classical neuritic plaques. These plaques, unlike diffuse plaques, are composed of an amyloid core surrounded by dystrophic neurites. The classical neuritic plaques also contain tau proteins, antichymotrypsin, apolipoprotein E (APOE), and other components. Although diffuse plaques contain amyloid similar to that of the classical neuritic plaque, they are smaller in size, do not contain neurites, and do not have evidence of adjacent neuronal injury. The last type of plaque related to the pathogenesis of AD is the "burnt out" plaque, which is composed of an isolated dense amyloid core. Evidence of inflammation is often found within or immediately surrounding the neuritic plaque. Additionally, acute phase reactants such as α_1-antichymotrypsin and immune mediators such as interleukin-1 are present within the neuritic plaques (Cummings et al., 1998).

Neurofibrillary tangles are a second key feature to the pathogenesis of AD. The tangles are composed of paired helical filaments that occupy the cell body and may extend into the dendrites. The paired helical filaments consist of protofilaments arranged to form a tubule, which contain abnormal amounts of phosphorylated tau protein. The distribution of neurofibrillary tangles occurs in a systematic order beginning in the transentorhinal cortex, progressing into the limbic cortical regions, and finally extending into the neocortical areas. The pattern of neurofibrillary tangle distribution matches that of symptomatic progression from early memory abnormalities to the development of aphasia and apraxia. Furthermore, early and extensive involvement of the limbic cortex is associated with a variety of NPS. Because neurofibrillary tangles are present in many other neurodegenerative diseases such as postencephalitic Parkinson's disease, neurofibrillary tangles are less specific to AD than the neuritic plaques. The histopathological criteria for AD have evolved over time. Recently, through a joint work group between the National Institute on Aging and the Reagan Institute of the Alzheimer's Association, clearer criteria for the diagnosis of AD have been established. These criteria emphasize that the diagnosis must include the presence of both neuritic plaques and neurofibrillary tangles in the neuronal cortex (Cummings et al., 1998).

Nerve cell loss, particularly in the larger neurons of the superficial cortex, is another feature of AD. Synaptic alterations are also characteristic of AD. Presynaptic terminal density has been found to be reduced up to 45% after autopsy in AD patients. As stated earlier, the neuronal injury and loss seen in AD does not occur around the diffuse plaques but around the classical neuritic plaques. There is a strong direct correlation between the degree of synaptic loss and cognitive alterations in AD (Cummings et al., 1998).

Cognitive Reserve Hypothesis

The cognitive reserve hypothesis posits that patients manifest different thresholds for symptom occurrence based upon the degree of brain dysfunction (Cummings et al., 1998; Liberati et al., 2012). Individuals with greater cognitive reserve, according to the hypothesis, can sustain more pathogenic mechanisms of AD prior to the clinical manifestation of cognitive impairment symptoms. Both genetic and environmental factors contribute to the amount of cognitive reserve. Genetic factors may influence synaptic density relating to native intellectual ability. Environmental factors include education, age, culture, and history of head trauma. Fig. 14.1 illustrates the relationship between Aβ, cognitive reserve, and symptom threshold (Cummings et al., 1998). The rightmost curve of the figure represents normal aging with a very gradual production of Aβ at a rate that would prohibit cognitive impairment manifestations within the normal human lifespan. Conversely, the leftmost curve represents down syndrome in which patients have both reduced cognitive reserve and overproduction of Aβ, leading to dementia syndromes early in life. Consistent with the cognitive reserve hypothesis, those patients with higher educational levels, or that did well in early education, are less likely to present with AD (Cummings et al., 1998; Liberati et al., 2012).

Although no therapies to date have illustrated reversal of AD pathogenesis, there is overwhelming consensus that prevention or disease slowing is the most important approach to the AD patient (Duara et al., 2009; California Workgroup, 2008; Alzheimer's Association, 2015; Segal-Gidan, 2011). The hypothesis of cognitive reserve postulates that the further enhancement of this reserve may increase the threshold at which clinical symptoms are manifested. Essentially, larger cognitive reserve corresponds to a higher degree of brain dysfunction that

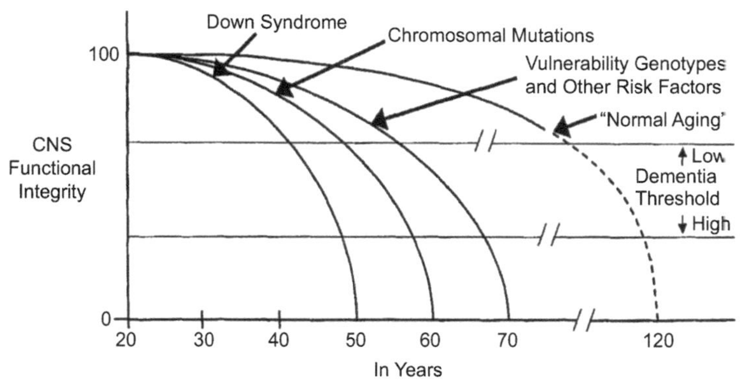

FIGURE 14.1 Interaction of Aβ, cognitive reserve, and symptom threshold (Cummings et al., 1998).

can be experienced before clinical symptoms appear, thus delaying the onset of disease. AD is associated with a large human, social, and economic burden. However, the postponement of AD onset by 5 years may halve the projected AD prevalence in the future (Brookmeyer et al., 1998; Jorn et al., 2005; Kivipelto et al., 2013).

Cognitive Training

Based upon the theory of cognitive reserve, there is a great deal of focus around cognitive training and continuous mental stimulation. This hypothesis is based on the concept that cognitive reserve is not fixed and at any time throughout life it can be affected by a combination of experiences and exposures. Increasing cognitive reserve in AD patients can allow the maintenance of everyday functioning for longer periods of time later in life and thus delay the manifestations of progressive neuronal injury. In a study of lifestyle practices in adults, positron emission tomography imaging indicated that participation in cognitive stimulation across an individual's lifespan was associated with reduced Aβ deposition (Davey, 2014; Landau et al., 2012). There are a variety of cognitive interventions that have been shown to enhance memory and function in the AD patient.

The spaced retrieval technique (SRT) involves the incorporation of progressive increases in the intervals between the presentation of information to be remembered and the recall of that information. The SRT was first described by Landauer and Bjork in 1978 and has been recognized as an effective technique to enhance memory recollection (Acevedo and Loewenstein, 2007; Bird and Kinsella, 1996; Camp, 1989; Camp et al., 2000; Camp and Stevens, 1990; Clare et al., 2002; Davis et al., 2001). SRT efficacy has been shown in memory of common household objects, personal names, face–name associations, and object–location associations. In the SRT, information is learned and retained by making active recall attempts over progressively longer time intervals. A patient is taught a piece of information that is then tested at retention intervals that systematically lengthen over successful recall periods (5, 10, 20, 40, 60 s). If a recall trial is failed, feedback is provided, and the trial is repeated at the recall interval of the last successful trial. Cherry et al. (2010) were able to successfully illustrate the benefits of SRT in four older adults with AD through recollection of name–face and occupation association. In their analysis, there was modest evidence of transfer of the name–face–occupation association to the actual person.

Another technique that has been effectively employed in AD patients is the activation of procedural motor memory. Motor memory tends to be well preserved in mild-to-moderately impaired AD patients. AD patients may demonstrate severe impairment in episodic memory but are able to achieve normal motor learning and skill retention in procedural motor tasks. Procedural motor learning includes tasks such as mirror tracing and learning to dance. These procedural motor tasks have been retained in patients with AD as compared to age-matched controls (Acevedo and Loewenstein, 2007; Hirono et al., 1997). The resiliency of procedural motor memory in AD patients is attributed to the relative preservation of the basal ganglia circuitry and sensory motor cortex in the early stages of the disease. Techniques of procedural motor memory have been expanded to include cognitive procedural learning training. This technique is similar to that of procedural motor learning except that it accounts for the three qualitatively different phases (cognitive, associative, and autonomous). An example of a cognitive procedural learning protocol is the Tower of Hanoi (TH). In this cognitive procedural task, patients are given a variety of blocks, pegs, and discs along with two cognitive rules. A group of French investigators studied the results of the TH protocol and cognitive procedural learning in 18 AD patients. The study concluded that cognitive procedural learning was retained and enhanced in this group of AD patients (Beaunieux et al., 2012).

Dual cognitive support is another cognitive intervention technique in AD patients. Dual cognitive support involves the extensive use of support at the encoding and retrieval stages of learning and memory processes. Support at encoding can be achieved by using stimuli that facilitate a high degree of organization, activation of prior knowledge, or by anchoring the recall of events. Support at retrieval includes the provision of recall cues that incorporate techniques at encoding. Dual cognitive support has been shown to facilitate memory in patients with AD (Acevedo and Loewenstein, 2007; Bachman and Small, 1998).

Aside from the aforementioned single, targeted approaches to cognitive training, there are many multimodal rehabilitation paradigms that utilize a multifaceted approach to cognitive training. Quayhagen and colleagues evaluated the effect of a cognitive stimulation program that consisted of memory, problem solving, and conversational exercises that were delivered as 1-h sessions 6 days a week. The study duration was 12 weeks. At the 9-month follow-up, the control group had declined in two of four outcome measurements while the experimental group had returned to baseline after initial improvement after the intervention (Quayhagen and Quayhagen, 1989). Zanetti and colleagues compared the performance of 10 healthy older adults to that of 10 older adults with AD after participation in a cognitive training program. The program focused on activities of daily living and included 1-h sessions 5 days a week over 3 weeks. At the end of the analysis, those patients with AD were able to complete trained and untrained tasks at a faster speed. These results suggest that the cognitive training program utilized by the investigators can be generalized to those untrained tasks (Zanetti et al., 1997).

Lifestyle Influences on Alzheimer's Disease

There are a handful of lifestyle factors that have been shown to reduce the risk and/or delay the onset of cognitive impairment associated with AD. The augmentation of many of these factors in those patients with AD or MCI has been shown to increase cognitive reserve.

Exercise

Within the last two decades, the benefits of exercise on cognitive function have been well accepted. Studies have shown that exercise has the capacity to enhance learning and memory (Vaynman and Gomez-Pillani, 2006; Suominen-Troyer et al., 1986; Rogers et al., 1990; van Praag et al., 1999). A systematic review of neurodegenerative disorders has indicated that physical activity decreased the risk of AD. The authors concluded that physical activity should be a key component in the preventive approach to AD (Colcombe and Kramer, 2003). There are many proposed mechanisms to this relationship. First, physical activity has been shown to have a direct correlation to mood and depression (Ardern and Rotondi, 2013; Penedo and Dahn, 2005; Potter et al., 2011; Heyn et al., 2004), and untreated depression worsens the severity of cognitive decline (Bennett and Thomas, 2014; Chung et al., 2015). Second, experimental research suggests that physical activity may promote the maintenance of gray matter brain volume and thus delay the onset of cognitive decline (Ardern and Rotondi, 2013; Heyn et al., 2004). Third, physical activity is known to decrease vascular disease risk (cerebrovascular and cardiovascular), the most significant risk factors of AD (Yancy et al., 2013; Sacco et al., 2006). Lastly, the antioxidant effects of aerobic activity may preserve neuronal integrity in adults (Hayes et al., 2014; Swain et al., 2003).

It is also noteworthy that different types of exercise can have positive effects on brain function. In a Swedish analysis, investigators used structural and functional magnetic resonance imaging (MRI) diagnostics to evaluate the relationship between aerobic and nonaerobic fitness training on brain function and cognition. The investigators also performed functional connectivity seeding analysis to examine age-related differences in connectivity. Older adults were randomized to an aerobic program (walking) or a nonaerobic program (flexibility, toning, and balance) three times per week. Participants underwent both structural and functional MRI to evaluate coherence of cognitively relevant and sensory brain networks. Functional connectivity was reviewed through seeding analysis based on anatomical hubs known to be altered with age. The study found that the walking group had increased connectivity after 12 months in the regional connections supported by the default mode network and the frontal executive network, two brain networks that are central to brain dysfunction in aging. More interesting was that both the aerobic and nonaerobic groups illustrated increased connectivity in those areas of the brain that are sensitive to age-related disruption. Based upon these results, the authors concluded that exercise can indeed induce functional plasticity of the brain in the aging adult. The authors further extrapolate these findings to patients with AD (Voss et al., 2010). There is also evidence that resistance training positively impacts brain function in seniors. In a single-blinded randomized study, patients were assigned to twice weekly resistance training, aerobic training, or balance and tone training. Functional MRI was used to evaluate functional brain plasticity and the Stroop test was used to measure the primary outcome of attention and conflict resolution. At the end of 6 months, the resistance training group had a larger change in Stroop test scores (9.13) as compared to the balance and tone group (1.37) and the aerobic group (8.83). The study included elderly women aged 70–80 years diagnosed with MCI (Lindsey et al., 2012). Although this study may be hard to generalize as it only included women, these results still illustrate the profound relationship between physical activity and brain plasticity.

Diet

Diet, which is often studied with exercise and is a strong influencer on vascular disease and diabetes, is a lifestyle factor that influences MCI and AD. Dietary patterns have been linked to AD. Diets characterized by a high intake of meat, butter, high-fat dairy products, eggs, and refined sugars have been found in AD patients. The Western diet is characterized by a high intake of red and processed meats, refined grains, sweets, and desserts. Conversely, a Japanese diet is characterized by increased intake of fish and plant foods (soybean products, seaweeds, vegetables, and fruits) and decreased intake of refined carbohydrates and animal fats. In an analysis of over 1000 Japanese persons followed for 15 years, a diet consisting of a high intake of soybeans and soybean products, vegetables, algae, milk, and dairy products with low intake of rice was associated with a reduced risk of AD (Hu et al., 2013; Ozawa et al., 2013). In addition to geographically based diets, specific diet plans have also been shown to decrease the risk of AD. The Dietary Approaches to Stop Hypertension (DASH) diet contains a high intake of plant foods, fruits, vegetables, fish, poultry, whole grains, low-fat dairy products, and nuts while minimizing intake of red meat, sodium, sweets, and sugar. In a study of over 100 patients with hypertension, those patients on the DASH diet exhibited greater neurocognitive improvements (Hu et al., 2013; Smith et al., 2010). Because hypertension is a risk factor for AD, it is plausible that the reduction of blood pressure, secondary to the DASH diet, is the mechanism behind this cognitive finding. Lastly, although it is hypothesized that calorie restriction may decrease risks associated with AD, this finding has only been evaluated in mouse models and should not be extrapolated to the AD patient population (Pasinetti et al., 2011). Because of this, it is recommended that patients engage in a healthy lifestyle (as previously described) to decrease AD risk rather than employing techniques of fasting or severe calorie restriction.

Vascular Risk

Though highly related to exercise and diet, reduction in vascular risk has also been shown to delay the onset of AD. Vascular risk includes that of cardiovascular and cerebrovascular disorders. Most consensus guidelines on the management of vascular risk support an initial nonpharmacological approach to treatment. Nonpharmacological approaches to vascular risk reduction include weight control, low fat and sodium diets, and limiting toxins such as smoking and alcohol. The successful management of metabolic and vascular risk factors not only delays the onset of AD, but also decreases the morbidity and mortality risk in the AD population (Yancy et al., 2013; Sacco et al., 2006).

Diabetes

Multiple epidemiological studies have indicated that the risk of developing AD is 50–150% higher in type II diabetics than in the general population (Li et al., 2015; Biessels et al., 2006; Cukierman et al., 2005; Strachman et al., 1997). The trifecta of diabetic risk factors—obesity, hyperinsulinemia, and metabolic syndromes—has been linked to risk of developing AD. A metaanalysis concluded that the incidence of AD increased in men who gained weight between the ages of 30 and 45 years of age and in women with a body mass index greater than 30 (Li et al., 2015; Beydoun et al., 2008). There is currently much research into the relationship between insulin resistance and cognitive decline. It is hypothesized that impaired cerebral glucose uptake and utilization may contribute to the cognitive impairment seen in AD (Li et al., 2015; Peila et al., 2002; Luchsinger, 2012; Okereke et al., 2012). The exact pathophysiological link between type II diabetes and AD is unclear; however, there are multiple proposed mechanisms. These include insulin resistance and deficiency, impaired insulin growth factor signaling, glucose toxicity, abnormal protein glycation, cerebrovascular injury, and vascular inflammation. Despite the uncertainty surrounding the mechanistic link between type II diabetes and AD, diabetes is well accepted as a major risk factor for the development of AD. In this regard, the focus of lifestyle modifications that improve risk associated with diabetes can be utilized to also decrease the risk associated with AD. Such lifestyle modifications include exercise, weight control, smoking cessation, and abstinence from alcohol.

Sleep

It is well established that sleep has a major effect on memory. Studies further show a relationship between AD and too little, too much, and poor sleep. In a study that used the Finnish Twin Cohort as a sample base, Virta et al. (2013) showed that persons who had less than 7h of sleep a day or more than 8h of sleep per day in their midlife had lower cognitive scores later in life than participants sleeping 7–8h per day. Likewise, in a Nurses' Health Study, women aged greater than 70years who got either less than 5h or more than 9h of sleep a night were at increased risk of cognitive decline compared to women who slept 7h per night (Brauser, 2012). Both of these studies are consistent with other research that has shown that long sleep duration is associated with an increased risk of dementia (Benito-Leon et al., 2009; Loerbroks et al., 2010). Poorer sleep consolidation (ie, interrupted sleep) has also been associated with worsening cognition (Lim et al., 2013; Blackwell et al., 2006; Blackwell et al., 2011). As an extension of research regarding the relationship between the APOE genotype and AD, the investigators sought to evaluate the effect of consolidated sleep and cognition. The work included data from the Rush Memory and Aging Project, and concluded that the APOE genotype is associated with cognitive decline and AD. Over the 3.5-year study, 98 patients developed AD. In the sleep subgroup analysis, it was determined that every standard deviation increase in sleep consolidation attenuated the impact of the APOE genotype on AD risk by nearly 50% (Lim et al., 2013).

NONPHARMACOLOGICAL INTERVENTIONS AND NEUROPSYCHIATRIC SYMPTOMS

Noncognitive NPS associated with AD are among the most challenging issues that caregivers and clinicians face (Teri et al., 1988; Mohamad et al., 2010; Lyketsos et al., 2006). NPS, often also referred to as behavioral symptoms, can be broken down into two categories of symptoms: psychotic (positive) and negative symptoms. Psychotic behavioral symptoms include agitation, aggression, hallucinations, and anxiety. Negative behavioral symptoms include passive resistance, depression, apathy, wandering, and vocalization (Yusupov and Galvin, 2014). The most severe NPS typically occur during the later stages of AD, but other more mild forms of NPS are pervasive at virtually all stages of the disease. Over a 2-year cohort study of nursing home residents with moderately severe-to-severe dementia, 97% were shown to display NPS (Wetzels et al., 2010a). Further confounding the difficulties associated with AD, these NPS become more frequent and worse over time (Steinberg et al., 2008). Because of the negative impact behavioral symptoms have on caregivers and patients, these symptoms are the most frequent trigger to utilization of pharmacological agents (Wetzels et al., 2010b). However, as described in the introduction to this chapter, these pharmacological interventions are associated with high costs, potentially low efficacy, and adverse effects.

There is a high cost associated with managing NPS both financially on the facility (Murman et al., 2002; Livingston et al., 2014) and emotionally on the well-being of the caregiver (Mohamed et al., 2010; Donaldson et al., 1997; Ballard et al., 1996). There is a direct relationship with cost of care and agitation level (Livingston et al., 2014). The progressive worsening of NPS typically leads to the eventual admission to a nursing home (Steele et al., 1990; Morris et al., 1988).

The growing spotlight on AD has sparked a focus on the quality of personal care delivered in a long-term care environment (nursing homes and specialized assisted living facilities). Specifically, the culture change movement within long-term care facilities is intended to promote a higher level of individualized and effective care for institutionalized persons thereby increasing their quality of life (Kolanowski et al., 2010). At the forefront of the culture change movement is the effective use of NPIs to help increase quality of life through the reduction of NPS that can be common among those who suffer from AD (Alzheimer's Association, 2015; California Workgroup, 2008).

Current guidelines stress using NPIs as the initial approach to the management of agitation after an appropriate assessment. The initial assessment should work to identify any potential medical problems that may cause the behavioral symptom (Alzheimer's Association, 2015; California Workgroup, 2008; Lyketsos et al., 2006). However, to follow these guidelines, it is important to find effective, evidence-based techniques for reducing NPS.

There are several different types of NPIs that can be used to treat the NPS of those with AD. Broadly, NPIs for the management of NPS can be separated into those that target environmental modification, communicative strategies, sensory training, and activity-based therapies.

Environmental Modifications

One of the main causes of NPS in AD is the loss of the patient's internal mapping abilities. Environmental modification strategies are based on the concept of relying on an environment to dictate its appropriate use rather than the knowledge in a patient's head. By structuring an environment that innately directs its correct care, the positive behavioral symptoms associated with patient-centered frustrations can be avoided. In a *New England Journal of Medicine* article, Dr. Edward Campion identifies the physical environment of AD patients as a major therapeutic focus in the management of disease (Campion, 1996). Environmental design works to reduce the demands on the patient's already challenged perceptions thereby reducing frustration and behavioral symptom manifestations. Moreover, an environment that promotes security, sense of belonging, and mastery allows AD patients to feel comfortable within their environment and improves quality of life (Zeisel et al., 2003).

Environmental modifications include modifications to lighting, color, noise, and furniture placement. Examples of these include:

- Low levels of lighting during meals (improves eating habits).
- Simply furnished spaces with minimal distractions.
- Consistent background noise (musical or nature sounds).
- Placing objects that cue memories in clear view (photographs, mementoes).
- Ensuring privacy and personalized space.

Aside from these general environmental changes, there is an abundance of literature that evaluates the environmental structure in Alzheimer's Special Care Units. A few environmental modifications in an Alzheimer's Specialty Care Unit that have been shown to decrease NPS (Zeisel et al., 2003) are:

- Camouflaging exits reduce the risk of elopement and wandering (Dickinson and Mclain-Kark, 1998).
- Privacy reduces aggression and agitation and improves sleep (Morgan and Stewart, 1998).
- Common spaces with a unique noninstitutional character are associated with reduced social withdrawal (Gotestam and Melin, 1987).
- Sensory comprehension reduces verbal agitation (Cohen-Mansfield and Werner, 1998).
- Walking paths with multisensory activity nodes decrease exit seeking, improve mood, and engage family members (Cohen-Mansfield and Werner, 1998).
- Therapeutic garden access reduces elopement attempts and improves sleep (Stewart, 1995).
- Increased safety leads to improved independence and fewer falls (Capezuti et al., 1998).

Communicative Strategies and Person-Centered Care

Many of the NPS are a result of AD patient frustration with the inability to perform tasks, communicate with others, or understand their environment. To ease these sources of frustration, caregivers can implement proactive communication and caregiving strategies.

One technique in communication with the AD patient is the use of validation therapy. Validation therapy is based on the concept of communicating and accepting an AD patient's reality rather than attempting to correct it. The theory is that this validation and respect of a person's identity will help to reduce both physically and verbally aggressive behaviors (Cohen-Mansfield et al., 2015; Toseland et al., 1997). There is wide diversity in the implementation of validation therapy; however, most interventions involve group activities and can incorporate communication, music, and reminiscence (Ballard et al., 2009). The ease of use in an institutionalized setting is one of the benefits of validation therapy. Though a randomized trial demonstrated validation therapy to have improvements in reducing NPS as compared to socialization, the improvements were only modest, thereby creating a need for more conclusive studies (Livingston et al., 2005).

Another technique is the use of redirection. Redirection involves the distraction of the patient away from an activity or thought process. It is imperative for the caregiver to remain sensitive to the patient's sense of reality and independence while performing this technique. The use of redirection has been shown to decrease the negative NPS of vocalization (Yusopov and Galvin, 2014). Additionally, memory cueing is an effective communication strategy that is recognized by the Alzheimer's Association. Memory cueing incorporates the use of words and visuals that cue old or recent memories. It has been shown that a familiar residential character, which aids in memory cueing, is associated with reduced social withdrawal, greater independence, improved sleep, and more family visits (Zeisel et al., 2003).

There are several approaches to caregiver training that have been shown to ease stress for both caregivers and patients associated with NPS. The first, the Antecedent-Behavior-Consequence (ABC) approach, is a well-established method that provides caregivers a better understanding of the NPS to allow appropriate modifications to the context in which the behavioral symptom(s) occurs. The ABC behavioral analysis approach seeks to identify the precipitants (Antecedents) of a specific behavior (Behavior) and its effects on the patient, caregivers, and others (Consequence) (California Workgroup, 2008; Teri, 1990; Teri et al., 2002). A second approach to the AD patient with behavioral symptoms is the 3Rs approach (Repeat, Reassure, and Redirect). In this strategy, the caregiver repeats an instruction or an answer to a question, validates the patient's reaction, and then redirects the patient to another activity to divert attention from a problematic situation (Sadowsky and Galvin, 2012).

Person-centered care is a holistic approach designed to address all of the needs of a person with AD while maintaining the notion of their personhood. Practical delivery of person-centered care typically involves developing individual care plans and techniques for the person with AD (Edvardsson et al., 2008). This can include training for caregivers (both professional and family) on skills such as communication techniques and how to tailor approaches when performing routine caregiving tasks. A person-centered approach to personal bathing and grooming, one of the most challenging issues for caregivers, demonstrated a reduction in the agitation and aggressive behavior associated with these tasks (Sloane et al., 2004). The authors of one study compared person-centered care to dementia-care mapping and usual care by training staff members in nursing homes on subjects that included understanding NPS manifestation as a form of communication, focusing on individual expression of feelings, and how to modify care according to the patient's particular needs. This approach demonstrated a significant reduction in NPS, particularly agitation, as compared to the usual care group (Chenoweth et al., 2009). Another study compared the efficacy of a systematic algorithm designed to identify the underlying cause of NPS then provide NPI solutions for individual patients in nursing homes. This person-centered method demonstrated a greater decrease in agitation as compared to a placebo group (Cohen-Mansfield et al., 2007).

Sensory-Related Strategies

Sensory interventions target the theoretical understimulation of the AD patient's five senses, and have been shown to improve both burgeoning as well as severe NPS. Therapy that involves touch is an intervention that targets a single sense through the therapeutic touching or massaging of an individual with AD. Such therapies have been shown to effectively reduce agitation events even while the individual with AD is demonstrating these symptoms. A method known as the acupressure-presence-Montessori method uses acupressure, a variant of acupuncture meant to stimulate particular points on one's body, and was shown to be effective at reducing NPS when delivered daily for a 4-week period of time (Lin et al., 2009). However, longer-term and residual effects of touch therapy are unknown.

The typical example of multisense stimulatory NPI involves the usage of so-called *Snoezelen* rooms (*Snoezelen* is the registered trademark of Rompa in the United Kingdom). *Snoezelen* rooms were pioneered in the Netherlands in the 1970s and are specially created multisensory rooms outfitted with special equipment meant to stimulate four senses: touch, sight, auditory, and smell. The stimulation of these four senses will theoretically replace the effects of negative stimuli, thus helping to relax the user. A study that utilized a control group within a nursing home setting determined daily *Snoezelen* room therapy over the course of 18 months was highly effective in reducing NPS during morning care, as assessed by staff (van Weert et al., 2005). Another study did not show a statistically relevant improvement using *Snoezelen* therapy as compared to reminiscence therapy, another activity-based NPI, though no control group was used (Ballion et al., 2004).

There have been a few randomized control studies that have demonstrated the positive effect of aromatherapy as a treatment for NPS, specifically on agitation, though there could be some experimental limitations because of rating bias (Livingston et al., 2014). Lavender oil and lemon balm (*Melissa officinalis*) were either applied topically in oil form or used in aroma-stream form and showed significant improvement in agitation when compared to a placebo group (Akhondzadeh et al., 2003; Ballard et al., 2002; Lin et al., 2007). The benefit of such therapies is in the ease of translating the same methods used in the research study to the daily routine of care providers.

Activity-Based Strategies

Music therapy, when carried out twice a week by a trained therapist, has been shown to be effective at decreasing agitation levels in care homes (Lin et al., 2010; Ledger and Baker, 2007;

Sung et al., 2012). Typical music therapy interventions involve playing a familiar song to the participant followed by a period where the participant is encouraged to sing along. This therapy was determined to be particularly effective in decreasing burgeoning agitation, but remains inconclusive for participants with more severe agitations.

One theory regarding the cause of NPS in AD patients is based on the thought that these symptoms are caused by the inability to communicate when a basic need (both internal and external) is not being met (Algase et al., 1996; Cohen-Mansfield et al., 2015). These needs can include the inability to express physical discomfort, notification of hunger/thirst, improper room temperature, overstimulation, or inadequate stimulation. Therefore several NPIs are focused on fulfilling the basic need requirements of people with AD, thereby removing the stimulus that may cause an NPS. One area of significant unmet needs is in proper stimulatory activity. Studies have shown that a variety of activities (such as gardening, cooking, word games, painting, dance), when delivered consistently, can be effective in reducing agitation and passivity among residents in facilities (Kolanowski et al., 2011). Activity-based interventions are most successful when tailored to the individual's interests and cognitive ability.

Physical activity, which has been established as a mechanism to delay the onset of AD, has also been shown as an effective NPI treatment for those with AD. Winchester and colleagues evaluated cognitive function through use of the mini-mental status exam (MMSE) in sedentary AD patients as compared to those who walked 1 h, or 2 or more hours per week over a 1-year time period. The results of the study indicated that the sedentary study group had a dramatic decline in cognitive function, while the group who walked an hour a week experienced less of a decline in function. Most importantly, the study illustrated an improvement in MMSE scoring in the group that walked 2 or more hours per week (Winchester et al., 2013). As described previously, there is a direct relationship between decreased cognitive function and the advent of NPS. The progressive decline in cognition results in AD patient frustrations, which, in turn, manifests as uncontrolled NPS. Physical activity aids in mood stabilization, and to some degree, attenuated cognitive decline. These results cumulatively aid in managing the occurrence of NPS. Thus physical activity for persons with AD can have a positive impact on reducing the caregiver burden through the reduction of NPS manifestations in the AD patient.

CONCLUSION

There are two main components to the management of AD: cognitive decline and NPS manifestations. Although unique in themselves, these components are closely related to one another. Progressive cognitive decline yields to patient frustrations that manifest as behavioral symptoms.

No therapy to date, whether it is pharmacological or nonpharmacological, actively reverses the pathogenic results of AD. Because of this, there is an overwhelming consensus surrounding the prevention of disease. The theory of cognitive reserve supports the concept that continued and constant cognitive stimulation can delay the onset of cognitive impairment in the AD patient population. Although these efforts do not reverse the physical disease, NPI aimed at increasing cognitive reserve can attenuate the adversity associated with cognitive decline. Furthermore, extensive literature has indicated that adherence to a healthy lifestyle focused on decreased comorbid risk can also delay the onset of cognitive decline symptoms.

The results of persistent cognitive decline and progression of AD then lead to the most visible aspect of AD, behavioral symptoms. There are several strategies that both caregivers and family members can utilize to reduce the severity and frequency of NPS. NPIs should include multiple strategies that focus on a combination of environmental, communication, sensory, and activity-based techniques. One of the benefits of NPIs used to manage NPS is the avoidance of adverse effects of pharmacological agents. The use of NPIs as first line to prevent or treat NPS is supported within the guidelines. The success of NPIs in the management of NPS benefits both caregivers and the patient.

Although NPIs result in positive effects related to cognitive decline and NPS, the implementation of these approaches prove to be quite challenging. Some of the difficulties surrounding NPIs in the AD patient are in the actual delivery of care in an institutionalized setting. Studies have identified barriers that staff members face when attempting some of these interventions. These barriers include lack of time, budgetary constraints, and proper staff education (Kolanowski et al., 2010; Cohen-Mansfield et al., 2012). Lastly, there are great challenges in translating controlled study design methods into an institutionalized setting (Ballard et al., 2009).

The key to the treatment of most disease states, whether it is heart disease, diabetes, or cerebrovascular disease, is rooted in a multifaceted approach. AD is no exception. NPIs employed in the management of AD should involve a multipronged approach that includes interventions that address both cognitive decline and behavioral symptoms. Moreover, the overarching approach to the AD patient should include a combination of nonpharmacological and pharmacological therapies. The crux behind this multifaceted approach is that these two techniques are both cumulative and complementary. Both pharmacological and nonpharmacological interventions should largely target the prevention of disease.

References

Acevedo, A., Loewenstein, D.A., 2007. Nonpharmacological cognitive interventions in aging and dementia. J. Geriatr. Psychiatry Neurol. 20 (4), 239–248.

Akhondzadeh, S., et al., 2003. Melissa officinalis extract in the treatment of patients with mild to moderate Alzheimer's disease: a double blind, randomized, placebo controlled trial. J. Neurol. Neurosurg. Psychiatry 74 (7), 863–866.

Algase, D.L., et al., 1996. Need-driven dementia-compromised behavior: an alternative view of disruptive behavior. Am. J. Alzheimers Dis. Other Demen. 11, 10–19.

Alzheimer's Association, 2015. 2015 Alzheimer's disease facts and figures. Alzheimer's Demen. 11 (3), 332.

Ardern, C.I., Rotondi, M., February, 2013. The Role of Physical Activity in the Prevention and Management of Alzheimer's Disease – Implications for Ontario. Ontario Brain Institute.

Aricept® [package insert], 2013. Pfizer Inc, New York City, NY.

Bachman, L., Small, B.J., 1998. Influences of cognitive support on episodic remembering: tracing the process of loss from normal aging to Alzheimer's disease. Psychol. Aging 13 (2), 267–276.

Ballard, C.G., et al., 1996. A follow up study of depression in the carers of dementia sufferers. BMJ 312 (7036), 947.

Ballard, C.G., et al., 2002. Aromatherapy as a safe and effective treatment for the management of agitation in severe dementia: the results of a double-blind, placebo-controlled trial with Melissa. J. Clin. Psychiatry 63 (7), 553–558.

Ballard, C.G., et al., 2009. Management of agitation and aggression associated with Alzheimer disease. Nat. Rev. Neurol. 5 (5), 245–255.

Ballion, S., et al., 2004. A comparison of the effects of Snoezelen and reminiscence therapy on the agitated behaviour of patients with dementia. Int. J. Geriatr. Psychiatry 19 (11), 1047–1052.

Beaunieux, H., et al., 2012. Cognitive procedural learning in early Alzheimer's disease: impaired processes and compensatory mechanisms. J. Neuropsychol. 6, 31–42.

Benito-Leon, J., et al., 2009. Total daily sleep duration and the risk of dementia: a prospective population-based study. Eur. J. Neurol. 16, 990–997.
Bennett, S., Thomas, A., 2014. Depression and dementia: cause, consequence or coincidence? Maturitas 79, 184–190.
Beydoun, M.A., et al., 2008. Association of adiposity status and changes in early to mid-adulthood with incidence of Alzheimer's disease. Am. J. Epidemiol. 168 (10), 1179–1189.
Biessels, G.J., et al., 2006. Risk of dementia in diabetes mellitus: a systematic review. Lancet Neurol. 5 (1), 64–74.
Bird, M., Kinsella, G., 1996. Long-term cued recall of tasks in senile dementia. Psychol. Aging 11, 45–56.
Blackwell, T., et al., 2006. Poor sleep is associated with impaired cognitive function in older women: the study of osteoporotic fractures. J. Gerontol. A Biol. Sci. Med. Sci. 61 (4), 405–410.
Blackwell, T., et al., 2011. Association of sleep characteristics and cognition in older community-dwelling men: the MrOS sleep study. Sleep 34 (10), 1347–1356.
Brauser, D., July 2012. Sleep quality now may affect cognition later. In: Presented at Alzheimer's Association International Conference Vancouver, BC, Canada.
Brookmeyer, R., et al., 1998. Projections of Alzheimer's disease in the United States and the public health impact of delaying disease onset. Am. J. Public Health 88, 1337–1342.
position statement. California Workgroup on Guidelines for Alzheimer's Disease Management Guidelines for the Alzheimer's Disease Management, 2008. Retrieved from: http://www.cdph.ca.gov/programs/alzheimers/Documents/professional_GuidelineFullReport.pdf.
Camp, C.J., Stevens, A.B., 1990. Spaced-retrieval: a memory intervention for dementia of the Alzheimer's type (DAT). Clin. Gerontol. 10, 58–60.
Camp, C.J., Bird, M.J., Cherry, K.E., 2000. Retrieval strategies as a rehabilitation aid for cognitive loss in pathological aging. In: Hill, R.D., Backman, A., Stigsdotter, N. (Eds.), Cognitive Rehabilitation in Old Age. Oxford University Press, New York, NY, pp. 224–248.
Camp, C.J., 1989. Facilitation of new learning in Alzheimer's disease. In: Gilmore, G., Whitehouse, P., Wykle, M. (Eds.), Memory and Aging: Theory, Research and Practice. Springer, New York, NY, pp. 212–225.
Campion, E.W., 1996. When a mind dies. NEJM 334 (12), 791–792.
Capazeti, E., et al., 1998. The relationship between physical restraint removal and falls and injuries among nursing home residents. J. Gerontol. A Biol. Sci. Med. Sci. 53A, M47–M52.
Chenoweth, L., et al., 2009. Caring for Aged Dementia Care Resident Study (CADRES) of person-centred care, dementia-care mapping, and usual care in dementia: a cluster-randomised trial. Lancet Neurol. 8 (4), 317–325.
Cherry, K.E., et al., 2010. Spaced retrieval enhances memory for a name-face-occupation association in older adults with probable Alzheimer's disease. J. Genet. Psychol. 171 (2), 168–181.
Chung, J.K., et al., 2015. Lifetime history of depression predicts increased amyloid-β accumulation in patients with mild cognitive impairment. J. Alzheimers Dis. 45 (3), 907–919.
Clare, L., et al., 2002. Relearning face-name associations in early Alzheimer's disease. Neuropsychocology 16, 538–547.
Cohen-Mansfield, J., Werner, P., 1998. The effects of an enhanced environment on nursing home residents who pace. Gerontologist 28, 199–208.
Cohen-Mansfield, J., et al., 2007. Nonpharmacological treatment of agitation: a controlled trial of systematic individualized intervention. J. Gerontol. A Biol. Sci. Med. Sci. 62 (8), 908–916.
Cohen-Mansfield, J., et al., 2012. What are the barriers to performing nonpharmacological interventions for behavioral symptoms in the nursing home? J. Am. Med. Dir. Assoc. 13 (4), 400–405.
Cohen-Mansfield, J., et al., 2015. The use of nonpharmacological interventions for behavioral symptoms in dementia: an exploratory study. Am. J. Geriatr. Psychiatry 23 (2), 160–170.
Colcombe, S.J., Kramer, A.F., 2003. Fitness effects on the cognitive function of older adults: a meta-analysis study. Psychol. Sci. 14, 125–130.
Cukierman, T., et al., 2005. Cognitive decline and dementia in diabetes – systematic overview of prospective observational studies. Diabetologia 48 (12), 2460–2469.
Cummings, J.L., et al., 1998. Etiologies, pathophysiology, cognitive reserve, and treatment opportunities. Neurology 51 (Suppl. 1), S2–S17.
Davey, D., 2014. Alzheimer's disease and vascular dementia: one potentially preventable and modifiable disease? Part II: management, prevention and future perspective. Neurodegener. Dis. Manag. 4 (3), 261–270.
Davis, R.N., et al., 2001. Cognitive intervention in Alzheimer's disease: a randomized placebo-controlled study. Alzheimer Dis. Assoc. Disord. 15, 1–9.

Dickinson, J.L., McLain-Kark, J., 1998. Wandering behavior and attempted exits among residents diagnosed with dementia-related illnesses: a qualitative approach. J. Women Aging 10, 23–45.

Donaldson, C., et al., 1997. The impact of the symptoms of dementia on caregivers. Br. J. Psychiatry 170, 62–68.

Duara, R., et al., 2009. The basis for disease-modifying treatments for Alzheimer's disease: the Sixth Annual Mild Cognitive Impairment Symposium. Alzheimer's Demen. 5, 66–74.

Edvaardson, D., et al., 2008. Person-centred care of people with severe Alzheimer's disease: current status and ways forward. Lancet Neurol. 7 (4), 362–367.

Gotestam, K.G., Melin, L., 1987. Improving well-being for patients with senile dementia by minor changes in the ward environment. In: Levi, L. (Ed.), Society, Stress and Disease. Oxford University Press, Oxford, England, pp. 295–297.

Hayes, S.M., et al., 2014. The effects of aerobic exercise on cognitive and neural decline in aging and cardiovascular disease. Curr. Geriatr. Rep. 3 (4), 282–290.

Heyn, P., et al., 2004. The effects of exercise training on elderly persons with cognitive impairment and dementia: a meta-analysis. Arch. Int. Med. 85 (10), 1694–1704.

Hirono, M., et al., 1997. Procedural memory in patients with mild Alzheimer's disease. Dement. Geriatr. Cogn. Disord. 8, 210–216.

Hu, N., et al., 2013. Nutrition and the risk of Alzheimer's disease. BioMed. Res. Int. 1–12, 2013.

Jorn, A.F., et al., 2005. Projections of future numbers of dementia cases in Australia with and without prevention. Aust. N.Z. J. Psychiatry 39 (959), 963.

Kivipelto, M., et al., 2013. The Finnish Geriatric Intervention Study to Prevent Cognitive Impairment and Disability (FINGER): study design and progress. Alzheimer's Demen. 9, 657–685.

Kolanowski, A., et al., 2010. It's about time: use of nonpharmacological interventions in the nursing home. J. Nurs. Scholarsh. 42 (2), 214–222.

Kolanowski, A., et al., 2011. A randomized clinical trial of theory-based activities for behavioral symptoms of dementia in nursing home residents. J. Am. Geriatr. Soc. 59 (6), 1032–1041.

Landau, S.M., et al., 2012. Association of lifetime cognitive engagement and low β-amyloid deposition. Arch. Neurol. 69, 623–629.

Landauer, T.K., Bjork, R.A., 1978. Optimal rehearsal patterns and name learning. In: Gruneberg, M.M., Harris, P.E., Sykes, R.N. (Eds.), Practical Aspects of Memory. Academic Press, New York, NY, pp. 625–632.

Ledger, A.J., Baker, F.A., 2007. An investigation of long-term effects of group music therapy on agitation levels of people with Alzheimer's disease. Aging Ment. Heath 11, 330–338.

Li, X., et al., 2015. Link between type 2 diabetes and Alzheimer's disease: from epidemiology to mechanism and treatment. Clin. Interv. Aging 10, 549–560.

Liberati, G., et al., 2012. Cognitive reserve and its implications for rehabilitation and Alzheimer's disease. Cogn. Process. 13, 1–12.

Lim, A.S., et al., 2013. Sleep modifies the relation of APOE to the risk of Alzheimer disease and neurofibrillary tangle pathology. JAMA Neurol. 70 (12), 1–15.

Lin, P.W., et al., 2007. Efficacy of aromatherapy (*Lavandula angustifolia*) as an intervention for agitated behaviours in Chinese older persons with dementia: a cross-over randomized trial. Int. J. Geriatr. Psychiatry 22 (5), 405–410.

Lin, L.C., et al., 2009. Using acupressure and Montessori-based activities to decrease agitation for residents with dementia: a cross-over trial. J. Am. Geriatr. Soc. 57 (6), 1022–1029.

Lin, Y., et al., 2010. Effectiveness of group music intervention against agitated behavior in elderly persons with dementia. Int. J. Geriatr. Psychiatry 26 (7), 670–678.

Lindsey, S., et al., 2012. Resistance training promotes cognitive and functional brain plasticity in seniors with probable mild cognitive impairment: a 6-month randomized controlled trial. Arch. Int. Med. 172 (8), 666–668.

Livingston, G., et al., 2005. Systematic review of psychological approaches to the management of neuropsychiatric symptoms of dementia. Am. J. Psychiatry 162 (11), 1996–2021.

Livingston, G., et al., 2014. A systematic review of the clinical effectiveness and cost-effectiveness of sensory, psychological and behavioural interventions for managing agitation in older adults with dementia. Health Technol. Assess. 18 (39), 1–256.

Loerbroks, A., et al., 2010. Nocturnal sleep duration and cognitive impairment in a population-based study of older adults. Int. J. Geratr. Psychiatry 25, 100–109.

Luchsinger, J.A., 2012. Type 2 diabetes and cognitive impairment: linking mechanisms. J. Alzheimer's Dis. 30 (Suppl. 2), S185–S198.

Lyketsos, C.G., et al., 2006. Position statement of the American Association for Geriatric Psychiatry regarding principles of care for patients with dementia resulting from Alzheimer disease. Am. J. Geriatr. Psychiatry 14 (7), 561–573.

Mohamed, S., et al., 2010. Caregiver burden in Alzheimer's disease: cross sectional and longitudinal patient correlates. Am. J. Geriatr. Psychiatry 18 (10), 917–927.

Morgan, D.J., Stewart, M.J., 1998. Multiple occupancy versus private rooms on dementia care units. Environ. Behav. 30, 487–504.

Morris, L.W., et al., 1988. The relationship between marital intimacy, perceived strain and depression in spouse caregivers of dementia sufferers. Br. J. Med. Psychol. 61, 231–236.

Murman, D.L., et al., 2002. The incremental direct costs associated with behavioral symptoms in AD. Neurology 59 (11), 1721–1729.

Okereke, O.I., et al., 2012. Fasting plasma insulin, C-peptide and cognitive change in older men without diabetes: results from the Physicians' Health Study II. Neuroepidemiology 34 (4), 200–207.

Osawa, M., et al., 2013. Dietary patterns and risk of dementia in an elderly Japanese population: the Hisayama study. Am. J. Clin. Nutr. 97 (5), 1076–1082.

Pasinetti, G.M., et al., 2011. Calorie intake, dietary lifestyles, macronutrient composition, and Alzheimer's disease dementia. Int. J. Alzheimer's Dis. 1–12, 2011.

Peila, R., et al., 2002. Fasting insulin and incident dementia in an elderly population of Japanese–American men. Neurology 63 (2), 228–233.

Penedo, F.J., Dahn, J.R., 2005. Exercise and well-being: a review of mental and physical health benefits associated with physical activity. Curr. Opin. Psychiatry 18 (2), 189–193.

Potter, R., et al., 2011. A systematic review of the effects of physical activity on physical functioning, quality of life and depression in older people with dementia. Int. J. Geriatr. Psychiatry 26 (10), 1000–1011.

Quayhagen, M.P., Quayhagen, M., 1989. Differential effects of family based strategies on Alzheimer's disease. Gerontologist 29, 150–155.

Rogers, R.L., et al., 1990. After reaching retirement age physical activity sustains cerebral perfusion and cognition. J Am. Geriatr. Soc. 38, 123–128.

Sacco, R.L., et al., 2006. Guidelines for prevention of stroke in patients with ischemic stroke or transient ischemic attack. Stroke 37, 577–617.

Sadowsky, C.H., Galvin, J., 2012. Guidelines for the management of cognitive and behavioral problems in dementia. J. Am. Board Fam. Med. 25 (3), 350–366.

Schelterns, P., Feldman, H., 2003. Treatment of Alzheimer's disease; current state and new perspectives. Lancet Neurol. 2 (9), 539–547.

Schneider, L.S., et al., 2006. Effectiveness of atypical antipsychotic drugs in patients with Alzheimer's disease. NEJM 355 (15), 1525–1538.

Segal-Gidan, F., et al., 2011. Alzheimer's disease management guideline: update 2008. Alzheimer's Demen. 7, e51–e59.

Sloane, P.D., et al., 2004. Effect of person-centered showering and the towel bath on bathing-associated aggression, agitation, and discomfort in nursing home residents with dementia: a randomized, controlled trial. J. Am. Geriatr. Soc. 52 (11), 1795–1804.

Smith, P.J., et al., 2010. Effects the dietary approaches to stop hypertension diet, exercise and calorie restriction on neurocognition in overweight adults with high blood pressure. Hypertension 55 (6), 1331–1338.

Steele, C., et al., 1990. Psychiatric symptoms and nursing home placement of patients with Alzheimer's disease. Am. J. Psychiatry 147 (8), 1049–1051.

Steinberg, M., et al., 2008. Neuropsychiatric Symptoms in Dementia: The Cache County Study Int. J. Geriatr. Psychiatry 23 (2), 170–177.

Stewart, J.T., 1995. Management of behavior problems in the demented patient. Am. Fam. Physician 52, 2311–2320.

Strachan, M.W., et al., 1997. Is type II diabetes associated with an increased risk of cognitive dysfunction? A critical review of published studies. Diabetes Care 20 (3), 438–445.

Sung, H., et al., 2012. A group music intervention using percussion instruments with familiar music to reduce anxiety and agitation of institutionalized older adults with dementia. Int. J. Geriatr. Psychiatry 27 (6), 621–627.

Suominem-Troyer, S., et al., 1986. Impact of physical fitness on strategy development in decision-making tasks. Percept. Mot. Skills 62, 71–77.

Swain, R.A., et al., 2003. Prolonged exercise induces angiogenesis and increases cerebral blood flow volume in primary motor cortex the rat. Neuroscience 117 (4), 1037–1046.

Teri, et al., 1988. Behavioral disturbance in dementia of Alzheimer's type. J. Am. Geriatr. Soc. 36, 1–6.

Teri, et al., 2002. Nonpharmacologic treatment of behavior disturbances in dementia. Med. Clin. North Am. 86, 641–656.
Teri, L., 1990. Managing and Understanding Behavior Problems in Alzheimer's Disease and Related Disorders. Video tape training program. University of Washington, Seattle.
Toseland, R.W., et al., 1997. The impact of validation group therapy on nursing home residents with dementia. J. Appl. Gerontol. 16, 31–50.
U.S. Food and Drug Administration, 2008. Information for Healthcare Professionals: Conventional Antipsychotics. FDA alert Retrieved from: http://www.fda.gov/Drugs/DrugSafety/PostmarketDrugSafetyInformationforPatientsandProviders/ucm124830.htm.
van Praag, H., et al., 1999. Running enhances neurogenesis, learning and long term potentiation in mice. PNAS 96 (1), 13427–13434.
van Weert, J.C.M., et al., 2005. Behavioral and mood effects of snoezelen integrated into 25-hour dementia care. J. Am. Geriatr. Soc. 53 (1), 24–33.
Vaynman, S., Gomez-Pinilla, F., 2006. Revenge of the "sit": how lifestyle impacts neuronal and cognitive health through molecular systems that interface energy metabolism with neuronal plasticity. J. NeuroSci. Res. 84, 699–715.
Virta, J.J., et al., 2013. Midlife sleep characteristics associated with late life cognitive function. Sleep 36 (10), 1533–1541A.
Voss, M.W., et al., 2010. Plasticity of brain networks in a randomized intervention trial of exercise training in older adults. Front. Aging Neurosci. 2 (32), 1–17.
Wetzels, R.B., et al., 2010a. Course of neuropsychiatric symptoms in residents with dementia in nursing homes over 2-year period. Am. J. Geriatr. Psychiatry 18 (12), 1054–1065.
Wetzels, R.B., et al., 2010b. Determinants of quality of life in nursing home residents with dementia. Dement Geriatr. Cogn. Disord. 29, 189–197.
Winchester, J., et al., 2013. Walking stabilizes cognitive functioning in Alzheimer's disease (AD) across one year. Arch. Gerontol. Geriatr. 56 (1), 96–103.
Yancy, C.W., et al., 2013. 2013 ACC/AHA guidelines for the management of heart failure. Circulation 128, e240–e327.
Yusupov, A., Galvin, J., 2014. Vocalization in dementia: a case report and review of the literature. Case Rep. Neurol. 6, 126–133.
Zanetti, O., et al., 1997. Procedural memory stimulation in Alzheimer's disease: impact of a training programme. Acta Neurol. Scand. 95, 152–157.
Zeisel, J., et al., 2003. Environmental correlates to behavioral health outcomes in Alzheimer's special care units. Gerontologist 43 (5), 697–771.
Zyprexa® [package insert], 2014. Eli Lilly and Company, Indianapolis, IN.

Further Reading

Alzheimer's Association, n.d. Alzheimer's and Dementia. Retrieved from: https://www.alz.org/.
Research Advances from 2014. Alzheimer's Association International Conference. Two-Year Clinical Trial of Multi-faceted Lifestyle-Based Intervention Provides Cognitive Benefits for Older Adults at Risk of Dementia [article, 2014]. Retrieved from: http://www.alz.org/aaic/releases_2014/mon-730pm-finger.asp.

Index

'*Note:* Page numbers followed by "f" indicate figures and "t" indicate tables.'

Kolibri 360 GmbH
Ferdinand-Jühlke-Straße 7
99095 Erfurt, Deutschland
produktsicherheit@kolibri360.de